Acute Stroke Management
in the First 24 Hours

T0177633

Acute Stroke Management in the First 24 Hours

A Practical Guide for Clinicians

EDITED BY

MAXIM MOKIN, MD, PHD

ASSISTANT PROFESSOR OF NEUROLOGY AND NEUROSURGERY
UNIVERSITY OF SOUTH FLORIDA
MEDICAL DIRECTOR OF NEUROINTERVENTIONAL SERVICES
TAMPA GENERAL HOSPITAL
TAMPA, FL

EDWARD C. JAUCH, MD, MS

PROFESSOR, CHAIR, DEPARTMENT OF EMERGENCY MEDICINE
PROFESSOR, DEPARTMENT OF NEUROLOGY
MEDICAL UNIVERSITY OF SOUTH CAROLINA
CHARLESTON, SC
ADJUNCT PROFESSOR, DEPARTMENT OF BIOENGINEERING
CLEMSON UNIVERSITY
CLEMSON, SC

ITALO LINFANTE, MD, FAHA

MEDICAL DIRECTOR OF INTERVENTIONAL NEURORADIOLOGY
AND ENDOVASCULAR NEUROSURGERY
MIAMI CARDIAC AND VASCULAR INSTITUTE
AND BAPTIST NEUROSCIENCE INSTITUTE
CLINICAL PROFESSOR OF RADIOLOGY AND NEUROSCIENCE
HERBERT WERTHEIM COLLEGE OF MEDICINE
FLORIDA INTERNATIONAL UNIVERSITY
MIAMI, FL

ADNAN SIDDIQUI, MD, PHD, FAHA

VICE-CHAIRMAN AND PROFESSOR OF NEUROSURGERY AND RADIOLOGY
DIRECTOR OF NEUROENDOVASCULAR FELLOWSHIP PROGRAM
JACOBS SCHOOL OF MEDICINE AND BIOMEDICAL SCIENCES
THE STATE UNIVERSITY OF NEW YORK AT BUFFALO
DIRECTOR OF THE NEUROSURGICAL STROKE SERVICE
KALEIDA HEALTH
BUFFALO, NY

ELAD LEVY, MD, MBA, FACS, FAHA

CHAIRMAN OF NEUROLOGICAL SURGERY
PROFESSOR OF NEUROSURGERY AND RADIOLOGY
JACOBS SCHOOL OF MEDICINE AND BIOMEDICAL SCIENCES
THE STATE UNIVERSITY OF NEW YORK AT BUFFALO
MEDICAL DIRECTOR OF NEUROENDOVASCULAR SERVICES
GATES VASCULAR INSTITUTE
BUFFALO, NY

OXFORD
UNIVERSITY PRESS

Oxford University Press is a department of the University of Oxford. It furthers
the University's objective of excellence in research, scholarship, and education
by publishing worldwide. Oxford is a registered trade mark of Oxford University
Press in the UK and certain other countries.

Published in the United States of America by Oxford University Press
198 Madison Avenue, New York, NY 10016, United States of America.

Library of Congress Cataloging-in-Publication Data
Names: Mokin, Maxim, editor. | Jauch, Edward C., editor. |
Linfante, Italo, editor. | Siddiqui, Adnan, editor. | Levy, Elad, editor.
Title: Acute stroke management in the first 24 hours: a practical guide for clinicians /
edited by Maxim Mokin, Edward C. Jauch, Italo Linfante, Adnan Siddiqui, Elad Levy.
Description: Oxford; New York: Oxford University Press, [2018] |
Includes bibliographical references.
Identifiers: LCCN 2017054218 | ISBN 9780190856519 (pbk.: alk. paper)
Subjects: | MESH: Stroke–diagnosis | Stroke–therapy | Critical Care–methods |
Emergency Treatment–methods
Classification: LCC RC388.5 | NLM WL 356 | DDC 616.8/1–dc23
LC record available at https://lccn.loc.gov/2017054218

9 8 7 6 5 4 3

Printed by Webcom Inc., Canada

CONTENTS

FOREWORD

TUDOR G. JOVIN ■

The dream of being able to reverse a stroke by opening the occluded cerebral artery from within started in the early days of neuroendovascular therapies pioneered by the neurologist Egaz Moniz and has become reality in the era of modern mechanical thrombectomy. After years of stagnation that followed publication of the landmark NINDS iv t-PA trial in 1995, which led to the implementation of intravenous t-PA as the standard and only proven treatment for acute ischemic stroke, the past years have witnessed disruptive changes in the delivery of acute stroke care. Remarkable technological advances, spearheaded by physicians and industry along with a maturation process on the part of stroke care providers with regards to patient selection, workflow, and peri- and intra-procedural care culminated in no less than eight completed and strongly positive randomized trials of thrombectomy for acute stroke due to large vessel occlusion. These studies, which together have enrolled over 2,000 patients, have not only demonstrated a treatment effect only a handful of other procedural based therapies can claim in medicine but have also widened the therapeutic time window to a previously unimaginable 24 hours. Highly effective as these interventions are, favorable outcomes are still observed in only about half of the patients treated. Furthermore, a substantial proportion of patients potentially eligible for this procedure remain untreated. Much work remains ahead to establish more effective approaches that will not only lead to more patients treated but also result in higher rates of favorable outcomes

Not unlike ischemic stroke prior to the recent developments, intracerebral hemorrhage has been plagued by decades of therapeutic nihilism. And while this area of vascular neuroscience has not yet achieved a breakthrough similar to that observed with ischemic stroke, there are exciting new minimally invasive approaches that hold great promise for the future.

Considering the exquisite time-sensitive benefit of thrombectomy, dramatic paradigm shift implementation required at both individual and system levels for the care of patients with acute stroke represents a formidable challenge. Among the many interventions necessary for an effective change in the delivery of acute stroke care, healthcare provider education is of paramount importance.

From that standpoint, *Acute Stroke Management in the First 24 Hours* is a much needed and timely contribution that fills a real void in knowledge as it represents a comprehensive overview of most aspects related to the care of the acute ischemic and hemorrhagic stroke patient. Furthermore, as a novel and refreshing approach, it follows the logical progression of care from evaluation and management in the pre-hospital setting to the in-hospital hyperacute intervention (when indicated) and through to the critical stage of early post-admission care. This practical yet well-grounded in science material represents the result of a collaborative work by a multispecialty group of widely acknowledged experts in the field of cerebrovascular diseases. Given the complexity of acute stroke care and the fact that knowledge included and easily accessible in this book can be life (or brain) saving, every physician and healthcare provider involved in the care of patients with acute stroke could benefit from adding a copy of *Acute Stroke Management in the First 24 Hours* to their library.

Tudor G. Jovin, MD
Professor of Neurology and Neurosurgery
Director, University of Pittsburgh Medical Center (UPMC) Stroke Institute
Director, UPMC Center for Neuroendovascular Therapy
Pittsburgh, PA

The last two decades have ushered a dramatic evolution in management of acute stroke patients through promising advances in medical, endovascular, and open surgical procedures. Physicians who are at the vanguard of treating the acute stroke patient are faced with ever increasing challenges and race against time to achieve the best possible clinical outcomes. Navigating the complexities of the stroke system of care starts with time-sensitive identification of the acute stroke patient in the prehospital setting, followed by appropriate hospital triage, and continues in hospital with selection of a suitable and individualized treatment.

The treatment of acute ischemic stroke has become considerably more complex now that endovascular thrombectomy has proved its high safety and efficacy as treatment option. While some patients are candidates for only one particular type of revascularization therapy (either intravenous thrombolysis or endovascular thrombectomy), others may benefit from both therapies combined; making proper patient selection and triage more challenging. Randomized trials focusing on medical and surgical management of intracerebral and subarachnoid hemorrhage have expanded our understanding of patients with cerebrovascular diseases. Although promising, these results have further confounded clinical decision making for hemorrhagic stroke patients. Furthermore, the evaluation and treatment protocols for acute stroke frequently exclude patients whose clinical presentation does not fall within the established guidelines.

Aware of these challenges, neurologists, neurosurgeons, interventionalists, and emergency medicine specialists who traditionally practice within a narrow scope now find themselves assuming new roles to achieve optimal patient outcomes. Clinician collaboration within a multidisciplinary team that includes first responders and hospital administration is vital to the establishment of stroke outreach programs and updated, progressive triage protocols. *Acute Stroke Management in the First 24 Hours* is a practical, collaborative road map for a broad audience of health-care providers involved in the initial evaluation and management of acute stroke patients. It benefits from the experience of its authors who expertly understand the burgeoning need of a cooperative approach to acute stroke treatment.

CONTRIBUTORS

Siviero Agazzi, MD, MBA, FCAS
Professor, College of Medicine
   Neurosurgery
Director, Division of Cranial Surgery
Department of Neurosurgery and
   Brain Repair
University of South Florida
Tampa, FL

Clara Barreira, MD
Clinical Research Fellow
Department of Neurology
Emory University School
   of Medicine
Atlanta, GA

Mandy J. Binning, MD
Assistant Professor
Stroke Director
Department of Neurosurgery
Drexel University
Philadelphia, PA

Laura Bishop, MD
Assistant Professor, Neurology
Department of Neurology
Wake Forest University
Winston-Salem, NC

Andrew Blake Buletko, MD
Vascular Neurology Fellow
Cerebrovascular Center,
   Neurological Institute
Cleveland Clinic
Cleveland, OH

Noella J. Cypress West, ARNP
Vascular Neurology Nurse Practitioner
Tampa General Hospital
Tampa, FL

Travis Dailey, MD
PGY-3 Resident
Department of Neurosurgery
   and Brain Repair
University of South Florida
Tampa, FL

Lucas Elijovich, MD, FAHA
Associate Professor
Departments of Neurology and
   Neurosurgery
Semmes-Murphey Neurologic
   Institute
University of Tennessee Health
   Sciences Center
Memphis, TN

Kyle M. Fargen, MD, MPH
Assistant Professor,
   Neurosurgery
Department of Neurological Surgery
Wake Forest University
Winston-Salem, NC

Daniel R. Felbaum, MD
Department of Neurosurgery
Drexel University
Philadelphia, PA

Casey Frey, MS
Department of Neurological
    Surgery
Wake Forest University
Winston-Salem, NC

Shreyas Gangadhara, MD
Department of Neurology
University of Mississippi
    Medical Center
Jackson, MS

Waldo R. Guerrero, MD
Neuroendovascular Surgery
    Fellow Associate
Department of Neurology,
    Stroke Division
University of Iowa Carver
    College of Medicine
Iowa City, IA

Diogo Hauseen, MD
Assistant Professor
Grady Memorial Hospital
Emory University School
    of Medicine
Atlanta, GA

M. Shazam Hussain, MD
Associate Professor, Cleveland Clinic
    Lerner College of Medicine
Director, Cerebrovascular Center
    Neurological Institute
Cleveland Clinic
Cleveland, OH

Violiza Inoa, MD
Assistant Professor
Departments of Neurology and
    Neurosurgery
Semmes-Murphey Neurologic
    Institute
University of Tennessee Health
    Sciences Center
Memphis, TN

Kaustubh Limaye, MD
Clinical Assistant Professor of
    Neurology, Cerebrovascular Diseases
Department of Neurology
University of Iowa Carver College of
    Medicine
Iowa City, IA

Vladimir Ljubimov, MD
PGY-2 Resident
Department of Neurosurgery and
    Brain Repair
University of South Florida
Tampa, FL

Jason Mathew, DO
Vascular Neurology Fellow
Cerebrovascular Center,
    Neurological Institute
Cleveland Clinic
Cleveland, OH

Raul G. Nogueira, MD
Director, Neuroendovascular
    Division
Marcus Stroke & Neuroscience
    Center
Grady Memorial Hospital
Emory University School
    of Medicine
Atlanta, GA

Santiago Ortega-Gutierrez, MD, MSC
Clinical Assistant Professor
Director of the Neurointerventional
    Surgery in Neurology
Associate Program Director of the
    Neuroendovascular Surgery
    Fellowship Program
Department of Neurology, Stroke
    Division
University of Iowa Carver
    College of Medicine
Iowa City, IA

Aparna Pendurthi, MD
Instructor
Department of Neurology
University of Kansas Medical
    Center
Kansas City, KS

Juan Ramos-Canseco, MD
Vascular Neurology
Palm Beach Neuroscience Institute
West Palm Beach, FL

Andrew Russman, DO
Head, Cleveland Clinic Stroke
    Program
Cerebrovascular Center
Neurological Institute
Cleveland Clinic
Cleveland, OH

Edgar A. Samaniego, MD
Clinical Assistant Professor
Department of Neurology
    Stroke Division
University of Iowa Carver
    College of Medicine
Iowa City, IA

Robert Sawyer, MD
Associate Professor
Department of Neurology
University at Buffalo, the State
    University of New York
New York, NY

Vera Sharashidze, MD
Resident
Department of Neurology
Emory University School
    of Medicine
Atlanta, GA

Lila Sheikhi, MD
Vascular Neurology Fellow
Cerebrovascular Center
Neurological Institute
Cleveland Clinic
Cleveland, OH

Shashank Shekhar, MD, MSc
Vascular Neurology Fellow
Department of Neurology
University of Mississippi
    Medical Center
Jackson, MS

Rebecca Sugg, MD, FAHA
Associate Professor, Vice Chair,
    and Director
Department of Neurology
University of Mississippi
    Medical Center
Jackson, MS

Tapan Thacker, MD
Vascular Neurology Fellow
Cerebrovascular Center
Neurological Institute
Cleveland Clinic
Cleveland, OH

Lawrence R. Wechsler, MD
Henry B. Higman Professor
    and Chair
Department of Neurology
Vice President of Telemedicine
    Services
Physician Services Division
University of Pittsburgh Schools of
    the Health Sciences
Pittsburgh, PA

Stacey Q. Wolfe, MD
Program Director and Associate
    Professor
Department of Neurological
    Surgery
Wake Forest University
Winston-Salem, NC

Acute Stroke Management in the First 24 Hours

Basic Clinical Syndromes and Definitions

APARNA PENDURTHI AND MAXIM MOKIN ■

CONTENTS

1 INTRODUCTION

Stroke remains the single leading cause of long-term care disability in the United States and the fifth leading cause of death, killing nearly 133,000 people a year.[1] The goal for neurological evaluation in the Emergency Department (ED) is to appropriately route potential acute ischemic or hemorrhagic stroke patients toward medical intervention in the most expedient manner possible. Emergency medical services are the primary access point for stroke evaluations, with providers performing the initial diagnostic workup and care. Patients aged 75 and over had the highest rate of emergency room visits from 2001 to 2011 for stroke and transient ischemic attacks (TIAs), with nearly a 10% increase in admissions/transfer from EDs in that time.[2]

Even before radiographic scans, quick and thorough neurological evaluations can establish the likelihood of acute stroke syndromes and mobilize providers toward appropriate therapies. This chapter focuses on familiarizing the reader with stroke subtypes and clinical manifestations associated with specific syndromes. This information can assist in rapid identification of common stroke presentations.

2 CLASSIFICATION

Acute neurologic episodes being evaluated in the emergent setting for stroke workup can be divided into broad categories based on duration of symptoms and findings from basic imaging. Box 1.1 and Figure 1.1 describe the common types of cerebral infrarctions that are freqeuntly encountered in an acute setting.

Question 1.1: How often does magnetic resonance imaging (MRI) detect acute stroke in patients with transient episodes of neurologic dysfunction?

Answer: It is critical that all patients with suspected TIAs receive a brain MRI. Research shows that between 9% and 67% of patients fitting the clinical definition of TIAs have evidence of acute stroke on MRI.

Box 1.1

Ischemic stroke
- Imaging or pathological evidence of cerebral, retinal, or spinal cord focal ischemic injury in a defined vascular distribution
- OR focal ischemic injury based on symptoms lasting ≥24 hours

Silent infarction
- Imaging (such as MRI or CT) or pathological evidence of CNS infarction without a corresponding clinical deficit

TIA
- Transient episode of neurological dysfunction
- AND no acute infarction on brain, retinal, or spinal cord imaging

ICH
- A focal collection of blood within the brain parenchyma

Intraventricular hemorrhage
- A type of intarcerebral hemorrhage with blood present in the ventricular system

Subarachnoid hemorrhage
- Focal or diffuse collection of blood within the subarachnoid space

Subdural and epidural hematomas
- Bleeding external to the brain and subarachnoid space. Mostly as a result of trauma but can be spontaneous.
- Are not considered strokes by the 2013 American Heart Association statement, given the differences in mechanisms and pathology

Cerebral venous thrombosis
- Ischemic infarction and/or hemorrhage caused by thrombosis of draining veins and venous sinuses

Adapted from the 2013 Statement for Healthcare Professionals from the American Heart Association[4]

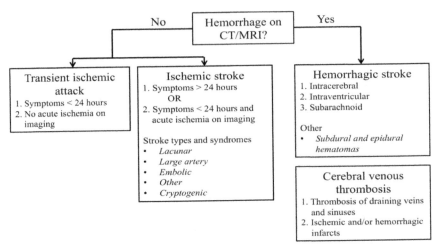

Figure 1.1 Types of cerebral infarctions based on clinical and radiographic characteristics.
SOURCE: Adapted from the 2013 Statement for Healthcare Professionals from the American Heart Association.

2.1 Transient ischemic attack

TIAs are episodes of focal neurologic dysfunction caused by disruption in cerebral blood flow without complete obstruction. TIAs present with the same symptoms associated with stroke, such as acute onset hemibody weakness or numbness, aphasia (inability to speak), dysarthria (slurred speech), and visual deficits that correspond to specific vascular regions. However, these events do not lead to permanent neuronal cell damage seen on radiographic imaging and typically last less than one hour.[3]

In the past, before the widespread use of MRI, TIAs used to be defined as neurologic events lasting less than 24 hours. The 24-hour mark was chosen arbitrarily, and studies subsequently proved that many of these patients would have evidence of acute ischemia detected with MRI imaging. The modern definition of a TIA therefore includes both clinical and radiographic criteria. A TIA is a **transient** episode of neurological dysfunction caused by focal brain, spinal cord, or retinal ischemia, **without acute infarction** (Case 1.1).[4,5]

TIAs secondary to periods of interrupted blood flow do not cause persistent clinical impairment but are considered to be events that increase long-term stroke risk and, as such, require thorough evaluation. These episodes contribute to between 200,000 and 500,000 neurologic evaluations in the United States yearly in the ED and outpatient setting.[6] There are various potential underlying causes for transient flow reductions, including atherosclerosis of intra- or extra-cranial arteries, cardioembolic sources, inflammation of the arteries, sympathomimetic drugs, or hypercoaguable conditions.

As TIA symptoms often resolve prior to physician evaluation, the goals of assessment are to uncover any subtle, persistent neurological deficits and risk stratify for future ischemic events. Adequate history and review of previous medical records is vital, as alternate diagnoses, including focal seizures, arrythmia, or migraine headaches, can often be mistaken for TIAs. Initial diagnostic evaluation can be achieved by obtaining basic vital signs, including blood pressure, heart rate and rhythm evaluation, laboratory workup, and imaging in the ED. Hypoglycemia, blood pressure abnormalities, electrolyte derangements, and cardiac and vestibular etiologies are all non-neurologic sources of transient mentation changes that can quickly be elucidated by providers.

Once the likelihood of transient ischemia has been determined, further assessment can assist with estimation of short-term stroke risk. The ABCD^2 score, first introduced in 2007, has aided medical providers with a numerical scale to assess benefits of hosptialization and further diagnostic workup. Originally developed for outpatient evaluation of TIA, it has since been shown that as the ABCD^2 score increases, the risk of subsequent stroke also increases across multiple settings.[7,8] The score is based on various stroke risk factors including age, blood pressure values, clinical featues, duration, and pre-existing diabetes. It is used to gauge the risk of stroke within 2, 7, 30, and 90 days after a TIA and has become a mainstay of ED evaluations (Box 1.2).[9]

Box 1.2

ABCD^2 SCORE TO PREDICT STROKE RISK AFTER A TRANSIENT ISCHEMIC ATTACK EPISODE AND ITS RECOMMENDED INTERPRETATION BY THE AMERICAN HEART ASSOCIATION

ABCD^2 score calculation (0–7 points)
- Age ≥ 60 years = 1 point
- Blood pressure ≥140/90 mm Hg on first evaluation = 1 point
- Symptoms of focal weakness or speech impairment lasting ≥ 60 minutes = 2 points OR
- Symptoms of focal weakness or speech impairment lasting 10–59 minutes = 1 point
- Diabetes mellitus = 1 point

The 2-day risk of stroke
- 0% for score of 0 or 1
- 1.3% for score 2 or 3,
- 4.1% for score 4 or 5
- 8.1% for score 6 or 7

Patients with a recent (within 72 hours of symptoms occurrence) TIA should be hospitalized when
- Total score ≥3
- OR total score is 0–2 but unable to compete diagnostic workup within 2 days

Adapted from the 2009 Statement for Healthcare Professionals from the American Heart Association on evaluation of TIAs[5]

For patients deemed low risk via the ABCD^2 criteria (score 0–3), an outpatient workup including further vascular imaging, antithrombotic therapy, cardiac event monitoring, and statin therapy may be most appropriate; the details of such further management are discussed in subsequent chapters. For patients considered high risk (ABCD^2 score >3), hospital admission may be advisable to expedite such interventions.

2.2 Stroke

Stroke, in comparison to TIAs, is an acute, persistent neurological deficit with associated central nervous system (CNS) injury from interrupted blood supply. Brain injury associated with vascular deficiencies is often focal and localizes to specific cerebral regions, producing characteristic clinical deficits. Similar to TIAs, acute stroke can present with acute weakness, numbness, and verbal or visual deficits; however, the impairment does not resolve and is usually present at the time of assessment by medical providers. Physiologically, neuronal tissue undergoes irreversible damage and death in the absence of oxygen, with the average patient losing approximately 120 million neurons each hour (equivalent to 3.6 years of normal aging).[10]

Nearly 800,000 people in the United States suffer strokes yearly, with three-fourths of these events being first-time occurrences. The majority of these represent ischemic strokes, which occur in the absence of blood flow to the cerebral tissue, and account for 85% of all strokes. Hemorrhagic strokes, caused by arterial leakage into brain parenchyma, comprise the remaining 15%.

Further clinical differentiation can be made into cortical versus subcortical infarcts, which broadly specify the location of the infarcted territory. As their name implies, cortical strokes affect regions of the cerebral cortex such as the frontal, parietal, temporal, and occipital lobes. Cortical strokes may disrupt higher cognitive functioning, producing symptoms like aphasia (the inability to produce or express language), alexia (inability to read), agraphia (inability to write), and hemibody neglect. Subcortical strokes, by comparison, affect regions below the cortex, such as the internal capsule, thalamus, basal ganglia, brainstem, and cerebellum. Subcortical strokes do not classically affect higher cognitive functioning. While all subtypes of acute stroke are associated with permanent neuronal damage, the etiology and management vary significantly with respect to thrombolytic use, supportive parameters, medication recommendations, and need for neurosurgical evaluations.

3 ISCHEMIC STROKE

Ischemic stroke results from obstruction within a blood vessel, prohibiting flow to a portion of the CNS. This originates from atherosclerotic plaque buildup within the arteries, blood clot (thrombus) formed at the site of occlusion, or an embolism that travels from another portion of the circulatory system to distally occlude cerebral vasculature. Small vessel, or **lacunar strokes**, are the most common type of ischemic stroke; they can occur from closing off small arteries that supply deep brain structures including the internal capsule, basal ganglia, thalamus, and paramedian regions of the brain.[11] These are often considered the end-organ effects of systemic hypertension and atheromatous disease. **Artery-to-artery embolism** refers to infarcts that arise from atherosclerotic lesions in proximal arteries that fragment and travel to distal vessels, occluding them. **Large artery thrombosis** often occurs as atherosclerotic plaque builds up to create progressive stenosis, with final artery occlusion resulting from thrombosis of the narrowed lumen. Embolic material can originate from a variety of sources, including mural thrombi/platelet aggregates from extracranial vasculature, cardiac thrombus, or less frequently, calcific plaques and fat embolism.[12,13] Determining the source of embolic material often requires multiple vascular imaging modalities; however, despite extensive evaluation and the use of various techniques (discussed in future chapters), the sources of 17% of all presumed embolic strokes have not been identified.[14]

Question 1.2: Are lacunar strokes common?

Answer: Lacunar infarcts are common, accounting for 25–40% of all ischemic strokes. Some studies indicate that lacunar stroke is the most common type of ischemic stroke in general population.

3.1 Lacunar stroke syndromes

Lacunar strokes are considered small (≤15 mm in diameter) subcortical strokes associated with the occlusion of a penetrating branch of one artery.[11] These strokes are thought to occur from small vessel disease, likely related to end-organ effects of systemic hypertension, lipohylanosis, or microatheromas.[15] Uncontrolled stroke-associated risk factors, such as aging, hypertension, diabetes, hyperlipidemia, and smoking, are considered the most significant factors for the development of lacunar infarcts. They are estimated to represent 15–25% of all ischemic strokes in the United States. Ischemic stroke outcomes are variable depending on size, comorbidities, and interventions available. Lacunar stroke outcomes are better than for other stroke subtypes, with 96% having a 30-day survival rate and 70–80% of patients having functional independence at one year.[16] Over 20 lacunar syndromes have been described, including the classic 5 lacunar syndromes first established by Dr. Charles Miller Fisher in the 1960s, which continue to be used today. Detailed in the following discussion, they have been validated for predictive value between physical examination findings and radiographic stroke correlation.[17]

3.1.1 PURE MOTOR HEMIPARESIS

Pure motor stroke is the most common lacunar syndrome, comprising 45–57% of lacunar syndromes.[18] This syndrome primarily affects the posterior limb of the internal capsule, which carries descending corticospinal and corticobulbar tracts, thus interrupting descending motor relay signals. Lesions can also be seen in the pons. Clinically, the patient presents with hemiparesis (weakness) or hemiplegia (paralysis) of the face, arm, and leg contralateral to the infarcted region; it is not typically associated with sensory, vocal, or visual deficits.

3.1.2 PURE SENSORY STROKE

Pure sensory stroke is estimated to encompass 7–18% of lacunar strokes[19] and most consistently localizes to the ventral posterolateral nucleus of the thalamus. This stroke presents as a contralateral numbness of the face, arm, and leg and in the absence of motor, verbal, or visual deficits. The sensory loss associated with this syndrome is usually noted to cease at the midline, which is characteristic of lesions to the thalamus.

3.1.3 SENSORIMOTOR STROKE

This lacunar syndrome is an infarct that affects both thalamus and the adjacent portion of the internal capsule's posterior limb, effectively causing both sensory and motor symptoms. Patients with this pattern describe contralateral hemibody weakness and sensory impairment of the face, arm, and leg.

3.1.4 ATAXIC HEMIPARESIS

Ataxic hemiparesis, the second most frequent lacunar stroke, has been shown to have a 95% positive predictive value for corresponding radiologic lesions.[16] This syndrome results from damage to the corticospinal and cerebellar pathways by infarction of the pons or internal capsule. Ataxic hemiparesis features both cerebellar and motor symptoms, including weakness and clumsiness on the ipsilateral side of the body, with the lower extremities typically more involved than the upper extremities. A combination of pyramidal signs (hemiparesis, hyperreflexia, Babinski sign) and cerebellar ataxia may be present on the affected side.

3.1.5 DYSARTHRIA-CLUMSY HAND SYNDROME

Dysarthria-clumsy hand syndrome is the least common of all lacunar syndromes, accounting for 2–6% of lacunar strokes in a case series review.[17] It is sometimes considered a variant of ataxic hemiparesis, as it also involves infarction of the pons or internal capsule. However, this syndrome differs in its characteristic dysarthria and contralateral hand weakness, which is often best provoked by testing the patient's handwriting. With a pontine lesion, facial, and tongue weakness may also be seen.

> **Question 1.3:** What is the most common occlusion site in large vessel occlusion strokes?
> **Answer:** Proximal (M1 segment) middle cerebral artery (MCA).

3.2 Large vessel stroke syndromes

In contrast to small lacunar infarctions, thrombosis of higher diameter vessels can produce infarct in large arteries supplying significant neuronal tissue. As previously described, thrombotic ischemic events are associated with elevated blood pressure, hyperlipidemia, diabetes, tobacco use, and age. Progressive atherosclerosis acts to impede blood flow to cerebral vascular territories, with thrombosis ultimately terminating blood supply to distal cerebral structures. Large vessel thrombotic disease can encompass extracranial (common carotid and internal carotid arteries), posterior cerebral circulation (vertebral arteries), and intracranial artery (Circle of Willis and its more proximal divisions) territories. Figures 1.2 and 1.3 illustrate the normal cranial and cervical anatomy of major arteries supplying the brain. As stenosis impedes blood flow, fragments from these obstructed arteries can break off as emboli to travel distally; like embolic strokes from elsewhere in the circulatory system, stroke occurs as the emboli reach arteries too small to transverse. While atherosclerosis is the most common cause of thrombotic ischemic strokes, other pathologies affecting these vessels, including dissection, arteritis, fibromuscular dysplasia, and vasculopathies, can similarly produce infarction.[19]

Acute ischemic strokes affecting large arteries produce characteristic neurologic deficits based on the area of neuronal tissue impacted. Once familiarized with the clinical characteristics of large vessel occlusion syndromes, a clinical provider can easily and reliably localize the likely area of at risk neuronal tissue prior to radiographic findings. In scenarios when imaging availability is limited or delayed, such knowledge can assist in rapidly mobilizing medical and surgical interventions.

3.2.1 ANTERIOR CIRCULATION STROKES

The blood supply comprising the anterior portion of the cerebral hemispheres is derived from the common carotid arteries, which further divides into internal and external division at the level of the fourth cervical vertebra. The internal carotid divisions travel into the cranium to supply the brain, while the external carotid branches travel superficially to supply the neck and face. Within the skull, the left and right internal carotid arteries further divide into corresponding cerebral branches, comprised of

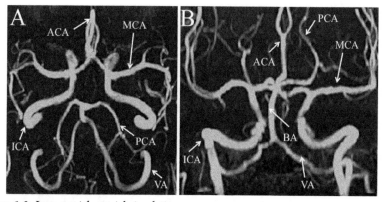

Figure 1.2 Intracranial arterial circulation.
(A) Axial and (B) coronal views of the MR angiography of the head showing normal vascular anatomy.
ABBREVIATIONS: ACA, anterior cerebral artery; BA, basilar artery, ICA, internal carotid artery; MCA, middle cerebral artery; PCA, posterior cerebral artery; VA, vertebral artery.

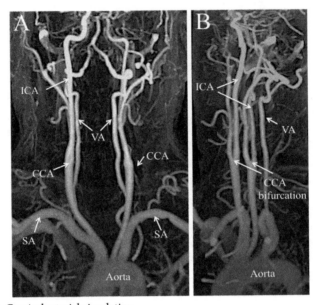

Figure 1.3 Cervical arterial circulation.
(A) Coronal and (B) oblique lateral views of the magnetic resonance angiography of the neck showing normal vascular anatomy.
ABBREVIATIONS: CCA, common carotid artery; ICA, internal carotid artery; SA, subclavian artery; VA, vertebral artery.

left and right anterior cerebral and middle cerebral arteries. These arteries supply large areas of eloquent tissue over the frontal, parietal, and temporal lobes.

3.2.1.1 Middle cerebral artery stroke

Acute occlusion of the internal carotid and left MCA produces characteristic clinical deficits, with the MCA being the artery most often occluded in stroke.[20] The MCAs are the primary blood supply for the motor and sensory cortices involving the head, neck, trunk, and arm; the basal ganglia; and the anterior portion of the internal capsule. In over 90% of the population, the left cerebral hemisphere is also the dominant hemisphere conferring language comprehension and fluency.[21]

The MCA then further bifurcates into two main branches: the superior and inferior divisions. Often, the MCA is classified into four segments based on nearby anatomic landmarks.[22] The sphenoidal segment (M1) is the origin of the MCA to the bifurcation. The second M2 segment, also known as the insular segment, encompasses the bifurcation to the insula. The more distal M3 segment (opercular branches) lay within the Sylvian fissure, and the M4 region describes the branches over the outer convexity of the brain. Infarction to any branch of the MCA can produce clinically evident stroke syndromes.

A large stroke affecting the main trunk of the MCA prior to its bifurcation will produce contralateral hemiplegia, deviation of the head and eyes toward the side of the infarct, contralateral sensory loss, and hemianopia (partial visual loss secondary to visual radiation tract involvement) (Case 1.2).[23] In addition, if the stroke is located in the dominant hemisphere, global aphasia will also occur as speech and language centers become impaired. In the non-dominant hemisphere, neglect and impaired awareness of the stroke is expected. When the infarct is large with significant brain tissue involvement, there is risk for decline and herniation secondary to development of cytotoxic edema in the region, known as malignant infarction.[24] Malignant infarctions usually require an escalation in acute management, either with medical or neurosurgical management.

MCA strokes distal to the superior/inferior branch bifurcation will produce symptoms similar to those of a complete artery occlusion, though likely less severe. A superior division MCA occlusion in the dominant hemisphere will produce weakness and sensory deficits to the contralateral hemibody and is likely to produce **expressive (Broca's) aphasia.**[25,26] This type of aphasia, which occurs with damage to the inferior frontal gyrus, affects the ability to speak fluently but spares comprehension. In a non-dominant stroke to the superior division, weakness and sensory loss may be present with some degree of visual/spatial neglect; language is not usually impaired.[27]

An inferior division MCA stroke often spares the motor and sensory regions but does involve verbal and visual areas. In a left dominant hemisphere stroke of the inferior MCA, the primary examination findings may be contralateral **homonymous hemianopia** (visual field loss on the right side of the vertical midline) and **receptive (Wernicke's) aphasia.**[23,24]

3.2.1.2 Anterior cerebral artery stroke

The anterior cerebral artery (ACA) occlusion represents between 0.6% and 3% of all ischemic strokes.[28,29] The ACA extends upwards from the internal carotid artery and supplies the frontal lobes, the parts of the brain that control personality, logical thought, and lower extremity movement. Stroke within the ACA territory produces ischemia within the paracentral lobule, usually resulting in sensory loss and weakness in the contralateral leg. Weakness is usually greater in the distal lower extremity than proximally. Lesions within the ACA can also produce symptoms of **anomia** (the inability to recall the names of everyday objects), **agraphia** (the inability to write), and **abulia** (lack of will or initiative), as well as emotional and personality changes.

3.2.2 POSTERIOR CIRCULATION STROKES

The vertebral arteries originate from the subclavian arteries and travel upward. Inside the skull, the two vertebral arteries join at the junction between the medulla oblongata and pons to form the basilar artery. The basilar artery contributes to the main blood supply for the brainstem. Several accompanying arteries branch off the basilar artery, including the posterior cerebral arteries, superior cerebellar arteries, and anterior inferior cerebellar arteries, as well as multiple minor paramedian perforating arteries. Strokes involving the posterior circulation account for approximately 20% of all ischemic strokes.[30]

3.2.2.1 Basilar artery stroke

Acute occlusion of the basilar artery has dramatic effects on circulation to the brainstem. They account for 1–4% of all ischemic strokes but are associated with a mortality rate of greater than 85% without intervention.[31] The most common presenting symptoms association with this stroke type is often imprecise on initial evaluation. Prodromal symptoms include nausea, vomiting, headache, and neck pain. If occlusion is located in the mid-basilar region, patients may progress to **locked-in syndrome**, where bilateral ventral pontine ischemia produces full body paralysis, lateral gaze weakness, and aphasia; however, these individuals remain cognitively intact and vertical eye and blink movements are preserved. Occlusion of the distal tip of the basilar artery results in **top of the basilar syndrome**, causing ischemia of the midbrain, thalami, inferior temporal lobes, and occipital lobes (Case 1.3). This can result in decreased alertness, loss of voluntary vertical eye movements, upper eyelid retraction, delayed or absent pupillary reaction to light, or visual hallucinations. In contrast to other syndromes, sensory and motor abnormalities are often absent. Most occlusions of the rostral brainstem are associated with embolic phenomenon and require urgent neurological and neurosurgical evaluation and treatment, given the poor prognosis associated with infarcts in this region.

3.2.2.2 Posterior cerebral artery stroke

Common symptoms of a posterior cerebral artery stroke include dizziness, imbalance, visual deficits (contralateral hemianopia with macular sparing), nausea, and sensory loss affecting the contralateral face and limb. Weakness may be variably present, as the posterior aspect of the internal capsule receives some blood supply from the proximal portions of the posterior cerebral artery.

3.3 Stroke syndromes—medium size vessels

3.3.1 ANTERIOR CHOROIDAL ARTERY STROKE

The anterior choroidal artery originates from the internal carotid artery and travels intracranially to supply portions of the optic tract, thalamus, midbrain, and internal capsule. This rather small-size vessel can nevertheless result in a number of neurological deficits. Infarction of the anterior choroidal artery can produce hemiplegia, sensory deficits of the contralateral body, and homonymous heminanopsia as a result of internal capsule, thalamus, and optic tract impairment. Symptoms are often variable given the presence of adjacent blood supply from lenticulostriate arteries of the MCA.[32]

3.3.2 SUPERIOR CEREBELLAR ARTERY STROKE

The superior cerebellar artery, derived as a branch of the basilar artery, travels posteriorly around the cerebellar peduncle to the surface of the cerebellum, thereby supplying part of the midbrain, cerebellar vermis, and the superior half of the cerebellum. While stroke affecting the cerebellum accounts for less than 2% of all acute ischemic infarcts, nearly half of them involve the superior cerebellar artery.[33] Symptoms associated with cerebellar infarcts are often vague, presenting as poorly defined headache, dizziness, nausea, and vomiting. Signs localizing to the midbrain such as dysarthria, nystagmus, and Horner's syndrome or to the cerebellum (ipsilateral ataxia, intention tremor) may be of diagnostic assistance.

3.3.3 ANTERIOR INFERIOR CEREBELLAR ARTERY STROKE

The anterior inferior cerebellar arteries travel from their origins in the basilar artery posteriorly to the cerebellum, where it supplies the anterior inferior surface of the cerebellum, the middle cerebellar peduncle, and lateral pons. Stroke in this region is somewhat uncommon given anastomoses among the superior cerebellar arteries and posterior inferior cerebellar arteries.[34] When it does occur, multiple nuclei and tracts are affected, producing **lateral pontine syndrome (Marie-Foix Syndrome)**. Symptoms associated with this includes contralateral loss of pain and temperature from the trunk and extremities from spinothalamic tract involvement, contralateral weakness of the upper and lower extremities from corticospinal tract involvement, ipsilateral paralysis of the face secondary to facial nucleus and nerve involvement, and ipsilateral cerebellar ataxia from affected cerebellar peduncles. Descending sympathetic tracts may also be subject to ischemia and result in ipsilateral Horner's syndrome.

3.3.4 POSTERIOR INFERIOR CEREBELLAR ARTERY STROKE

The posterior inferior cerebellar artery is the largest branch of each vertebral artery prior to their confluence to form the basilar artery. This artery travels past the medulla oblongata, over the cerebellar peduncle to the inferior surface of the cerebellum. Occlusion of the posterior inferior cerebellar artery results in a well described syndrome known as **Wallenberg syndrome (lateral medullary syndrome)**. This syndrome classically produces crossed sensory findings of loss of pain and temperature sensation on the contralateral side of the body and ipsilateral side of the face. Multiple cranial nuclei reside in this region and contribute to the other symptomatic findings of this infarction, including gait dysphasia, nystagmus, vertigo, ataxia, and ipsilateral Horner's syndrome (ptosis, miosis, and anihdrosis).

3.3.5 ANTERIOR SPINAL ARTERY STROKE

Infarction of the anterior spinal artery, which branches from each vertebral artery and joins at the level of the medulla oblongata, can result in **Dejerine syndrome (medial medullary syndrome)**. Though extremely infrequent, less than 1% of all vertebrobasilar strokes, it is easily identified with classical clinical characteristics. The presentation usually consists of deviation of the tongue toward the side of the lesion secondary to hypoglossal nerve involvement, contralateral hemiparesis or hemiplegia, and contralateral sensory loss.

3.4 Embolic stroke

Acute ischemia from embolic sources can cause any of the previously mentioned stroke syndromes or a combination of neurological symptoms if emboli travel to multiple vascular territories. Of emboli to the brain, approximately 80% involve the anterior circulation, with the remaining 20% involving the posterior cerebral blood supply.

Cardiogenic embolism accounts for approximately 20% of ischemic strokes in the United States, and nearly 50% of those are related to non-valvular atrial fibrillation.[35,36] Other cardiac sources of emboli include ventricular thrombus, prosthetic valves, acute myocardial infarction, rheumatic heart disease, cardiac tumors, and paradoxical emboli via atrial septal defects such as patent foramen ovale. Atrial fibrillation is present in approximately 1% of the US population and increases in prevalence with age. This arrhythmia is associated with a fivefold increased risk of stroke and often requires extended cardiac workup and electrocardiogram monitoring to uncover.

4 HEMORRHAGIC STROKE

Here we focus our description mainly on intracerebral hemorrhage (ICH), which results from vascular rupture and bleeding directly into brain parenchyma, with possible extension into the ventricles (known as intraventricular extension). Subarachnoid hemorrhage is discussed in the chapters on medical and surgical management of hemorrhagic stroke. Cerebral venous thrombosis shares some features of both ischemic and hemorrhagic stroke. However, given its unique mechanisms and course, cerebral venous thrombosis is a separate category and is reviewed in a separate chapter.

While less frequent than ischemic stroke, ICH encompasses between 10–15%[41] of all strokes, comprising approximately 40,000 to 67,000 cases each year in the United States. The extent of appreciable neurological dysfunction is dependent on several factors, including size and location of the bleed, degree of edema in the surrounding tissue, and compression of surrounding intracranial structures.

The most important risk factor for the development of ICH is hypertension. African Americans, who have a higher frequency of hypertension, have in tandem been noted to have a higher frequency of ICH.[37] Incidence has also been noted to be higher in Asian and Hispanic populations.[38,39] Other risk factors that have been correlated, in varying degrees, with ICH include increasing age, sympathomimetic drug use (cocaine, amphetamines), and high alcohol use. While hypertensive vasculopathy persists as a principal cause of non-traumatic hemorrhages, other etiologies include cerebral amyloid angiopathy, vascular malformations such as arteriovenous malformations and aneurysms, venous sinus thrombosis, vasculitis, coagulopathy, use of anticoagulation medications, and cerebral tumors.

Clinical presentation of ICH is variable but often occurs as an acutely progressive alteration in consciousness, nausea, vomiting, and headache; seizures occur in approximately 6–7% of presenting scenarios. Hemorrhage into a specific cerebral region will likely cause dysfunction of that eloquent tissue and may present as aphasia, hemiplegia, vertigo, diplopia (double vision), or sensory deficits. Hypertension-related ICH occurs predominantly in the basal ganglia, thalamus, pons, and cerebellum, whereas hemorrhage associated with cerebral amyloid angiopathy or cerebral arteriovenous malformations typically appears in a lobar distribution. Large intracranial bleeds may be evident with patients who are comatose at initial presentation, along with markedly high blood pressures >220/170 mm Hg. Rapid computerized tomography (CT) scan and vascular imaging aides significantly in the detection and treatment of these patients, with radiographic variations discussed in the chapter on imaging of acute stroke.

Mortality associated with ICH is significant, with a review from 30 centers reporting a 34% mortality rate at 3 months.[40] Other reviews reported mortality rates of 31% at 7 days, 59% at 1 year, 82% at 10 years, and more than 90% at 16 years.[41,42] To aide in prognostic assessment, an ICH score calculation was developed by JC Hemphill et al. in 2001; it is still an efficient computational tool for all providers. The components of the ICH score are derived from the patient's age, presenting Glasgow Coma Scale, the degree of ICH volume, the presence of intraventricular hemorrhage, and the location of the hemorrhage (infratentorial vs. supratentorial). The corresponding ICH score for these values (between 0–6 points) provides mortality risk at 30 days.

Early assessment and management of intracranial hemorrhage focuses on maintaining hemodynamic stability, airway protection, and correction of any underlying coagulopathy. These patients invariably require intensive care monitoring and often neurosurgical evaluation in the acute phase, given the risk of progression of bleeding, swelling, or herniation syndromes that could necessitate urgent surgical intervention. Diligent correction of fever, hyperglycemia, treatment of seizures with antiepileptic medications, maintenance of systolic blood pressure <180[43] and frequent neurological examinations are vital to the management of ICH in the first few days.

5 CLINICAL CASES

CASE 1.1 Transient ischemic attack

CASE DESCRIPTION
A patient in her 70s with past medical history significant for coronary artery disease and diabetes presented to the ED with a transient episode of word-finding difficulty early in the day, which resolved spontaneously after 30 minutes. The patient's family witnessed the episode and stated that the patient could only answer simple questions with "yes" or "no" answers, but was able to understand most commands. Blood pressure in the ED was 172/95 mm Hg. The patient's neurologic exam, upon evaluation by the emergency room physician, was unremarkable. MRI brain showed no evidence of acute infarction (Figure 1.4).

PRACTICAL POINTS

- This patient's history and presentation are highly suspicious for an episode of TIA. The deficit is best characterized as expressive or Broca's aphasia. Alternative diagnosis, such as complex migraine or a focal seizure, is less likely.

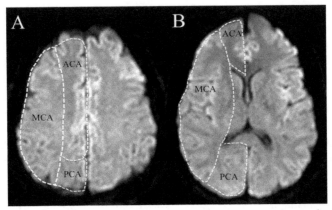

Figure 1.4 Case of a transient ischemic attack. Magnetic resonance imaging brain shows no acute ischemia on the diffusion weighted image sequence, supporting the diagnosis of transient ischemic attack.
(A) Cortical and (B) subcortical regions are shown. The anterior cerebral artery (ACA), middle cerebral artery (MCA), and posterior cerebral artery (PCA) territories are separated by the dotted white lines.

- "Negative" MRI brain imaging helps confirm the diagnosis of a TIA, and the ABCD^2 score can guide the emergency room physician about whether an inpatient admission is indicated. Some hospitals have designated TIA observation units where the minimum required diagnostic TIA workup (such as telemetry, carotid ultrasound, and cardiac echocardiogram) can all be completed within 24 to 48 hours.

CASE 1.2 MCA stroke

CASE DESCRIPTION

A patient was brought to the hospital by the paramedics after a 911 call made by a bystander who witnessed the patient collapsing at the mall. The patient was noted to have deviation of the head and eyes to the right, left-sided hemiplegia (paralysis), and sensory loss. Blood pressure on arrival was 221/112 mm Hg.

PRACTICAL POINTS

- Emergent imaging is required to differentiate between ischemic versus hemorrhagic stroke. This patient's exam fits the description of the right hemispheric syndrome. If intracranial hemorrhage is ruled out, additional imaging is needed to determine if large vessel occlusion is responsible for this patient's neurologic deficits (such as of the proximal right MCA; Figure 1.5).

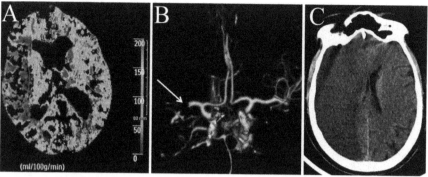

Figure 1.5 Middle cerebral artery stroke.
(A) Computed tomography (CT) perfusion imaging showing an area of decreased cerebral blood flow matching the arterial territory of the right middle cerebral artery (MCA).
(B) Craniocervical CT angiogram demonstrating occluded proximal right MCA (arrow).
(C) Follow-up head CT showing interval development of a large early subacute ischemic infarct with midline shift.

- Depending on prior medical history, timing of symptom onset, and the extent of early ischemic injury on brain imaging, this patient might be a candidate for acute stroke treatment with intravenous thrombolysis and/or endovascular intervention.
- If the deficits are indeed from the occlusion of the proximal MCA, this patient is at risk for malignant infarction with brain herniation (Figure 1.5). Admission to the designated neurointensive care unit is indicated, with close monitoring by the neurosurgery team should this patient require hemicraniectomy.

CASE 1.3 Top of the basilar artery stroke

CASE DESCRIPTION

A patient was brought to the hospital after the family found him unresponsive at home. The patient was very difficult to arouse. While in the ED, he had several episodes of emesis and fluctuating degree of mild bilateral weakness was noted on exam. Initially thought be secondary to intoxication or infectious/metabolic encephalopathy, the patient was subsequently discovered to have an occlusion of the distal basilar artery, requiring endovascular thrombectomy (Figure 1.6).

PRACTICAL POINTS

- This syndrome is often misdiagnosed and is associated with high mortality rates. The clinical presentation can be quite variable and may include

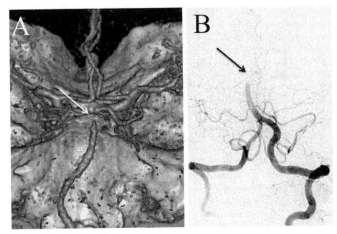

Figure 1.6 Top of basilar syndrome.
(A) Computed tomography angiography and (B) digital subtraction angiography, left vertebral artery injection showing occlusion of the basilar artery at its very distal segment (arrow). This is a classic angiographic appearance of the "top of the basilar" embolic-type occlusion.

one or more of the following: altered level of consciousness, behavioral abnormalities, diplopia, gaze palsy, and pupillary abnormalities.
- Embolic occlusion of the top of the basilar artery is difficult to diagnose on non-contrast CT, thus emergent angiography (either CTA/MRA or catheter digital subtraction angiography) is required to establish the correct diagnosis.

REFERENCES

1. Kochanek KD, Murphy SL, Xu JQ, Arias E. *Mortality in the United States, 2013.* NCHS data brief, no 178. Hyattsville, MD: National Center for Health Statistics. 2014.
2. Talwalkar A, Sayeedha U. *Trends in emergency department visits for ischemic stroke and transient ischemic attack: United States, 2001–2011.* NCHS data brief, no 194. Hyattsville, MD: National Center for Health Statistics. 2015.
3. Albers GW, Caplan LR, Easton JD, et al. Transient ischemic attack—Proposal for a new definition. *New Engl J Med.* 2002;347(21):1713–1716.
4. Sacco RL, Kasner SE, Broderick JP, et al. An updated definition of stroke for the 21st century: a statement for healthcare professionals from the American Heart Association/American Stroke Association. *Stroke.* 2013;44(7):2064–2089.
5. Easton JD, Saver JL, Albers GW, et al. Definition and evaluation of transient ischemic attack: a scientific statement for healthcare professionals from the American Heart Association/American Stroke Association Stroke Council; Council on Cardiovascular Surgery and Anesthesia; Council on Cardiovascular Radiology and Intervention; Council on Cardiovascular Nursing; and the Interdisciplinary Council on Peripheral Vascular Disease: The American Academy of Neurology affirms the value of this statement as an educational tool for neurologists. *Stroke.* 2009;40(6):2276–2293.

6. Johnston SC, Fayad PB, Gorelick PB, et al. Prevalence and knowledge of transient ischemic attack among US adults. *Neurology.* 2003;60(9):1429–1434.

7. Perry JJ, Sharma M, Sivilotti ML, et al. Prospective validation of the ABCD2 score for patients in the emergency department with transient ischemic attack. *Can Med Assoc J.* 2011;183(10):1137–1145.

8. Johnston SC RP, Huynh-Huynh MN, Giles MF, Elkins JS, Sidney S. Validation and refinement of scores to predict very early stroke risk after transient ischemic attack. *Lancet.* 2007;369:283–292.

9. Easton JD, Saver JL, Albers GW, et al. Definition and evaluation of transient ischemic attack: a scientific statement for healthcare professionals from the American Heart Association/American Stroke Association Stroke Council; Council on Cardiovascular Surgery and Anesthesia; Council on Cardiovascular Radiology and Intervention; Council on Cardiovascular Nursing; and the Interdisciplinary Council on Peripheral Vascular Disease: The American Academy of Neurology affirms the value of this statement as an educational tool for neurologists. *Stroke.* 2009;40(6):2276–2293.

10. Saver J. Time is brain—quantified. *Stroke.* 2006;37:263–266.

11. Fisher CM. Lacunes: Small, deep cerebral infarcts. *Neurology.* 1965;15:774–784.

12. Flint Beal M, Williams RS, Pierson Richardson E, Miller Fischer C. Cholesterol embolism as a cause of transient ischemic attacks and cerebral infarction. *Neurology.* 1981(31):860.

13. Fieschi C, Sette G, Fiorelli M, et al. Clinical presentation and frequency of potential sources of embolism in acute ischemic stroke patients: the experience of the Rome Acute Stroke Registry. *Cerebrovascular Dis.* 1995;5:75–78.

14. Hart RG, Catanese L, Perera KS, Ntaios G, Connolly SJ. Embolic stroke of undetermined source. *Stroke.* 2017;48(6).

15. Wardlaw JM, Smith C, Dichgans M. Mechanisms of sporadic cerebral small vessel disease: insights from neuroimaging. *Lancet Neurol.* 2013;12(5):483–497.

16. Sacco S, Marini C, Totaro R, Russo T, Cerone D, Carolei A. A population-based study of the incidence and prognosis of lacunar stroke. *Neurology.* 2006;66(9):1335–1338.

17. Gan R, Sacco RL, Kargman DE, Roberts JK, Boden-Albala B, Gu Q. Testing the validity of the lacunar hypothesis: the Northern Manhattan Stroke Study experience. *Neurology.* 1997;48(5):1204–1211.

18. Chamorro A, Sacco RL, Mohr JP, et al. Clinical-computed tomographic correlations of lacunar infarction in the Stroke Data Bank. *Stroke.* 1991;22(2):175–181.

19. Caplan L. *Basic pathology, anatomy, and pathophysiology of stroke.* 4 ed. Philadelphia: Saunders Elsevier; 2009.

20. Hedna V, Bodhit A, Ansari S, et al. Hemispheric differences in ischemic stroke: is left-hemisphere stroke more common? *J Clin Neurol.* 2013;9(2):97–102.

21. Geschwind N. The apraxias: neural mechanisms of disorders of learned movement: the anatomical organization of the language areas and motor systems of the human brain clarifies apraxic disorders and throws new light on cerebral dominance. *Am Sci.* 1975;63(2):188–195.

22. Gibo H, Carver CC, Rhoton AL, Jr., Lenkey C, Mitchell RJ. Microsurgical anatomy of the middle cerebral artery. *J Neurosurg.* 1981;54(2):151–169.

23. Foix C, Levy M. Les ramollissements sylviens. *Revue Neurologique* 1927;11(51).

24. Hacke W, Schwab S, Horn M, et al. "Malignant" middle cerebral artery territory infarction: clinical course and prognostic signs. *Arch Neurol.* 1996;53:309–315.

25. Lazar RM, Marshall RS, Mohr JP. *Stroke syndromes.* New York: Cambridge University Press; 1995.

26. Brust JC, Shafer SQ, Richter RW, Bruun B. Aphasia in acute stroke. *Stroke.* 1976;7(2):167–174.

27. Russell C, Deidda C, Malhotra P, Crinion JT, Merola S, Husain M. A deficit of spatial remapping in constructional apraxia after right-hemisphere stroke. *Brain* 2010;133:1239–1251.

28. Hollander M, Bots ML, Del Sol AI, et al. Carotid plaques increase the risk of stroke and subtypes of cerebral infarction in asymptomatic elderly: the Rotterdam study. *Circulation.* 2002;105(24):2872–2877.

29. Fischer E. Die Lageabweichungen der vorderen Hirnarterie im Gefässbild. *Zentralbl Neurochir.* 1938;3(300).

30. Nouh A, Remke J, Ruland S. Ischemic posterior circulation stroke: a review of anatomy, clinical presentations, diagnosis, and current management. *Front Neurol.* 2014;5.

31. Devuyst G, Bogousslavsky J, Meuli R, Moncayo J, de Freitas G, van Melle G. Stroke or transient ischemic attacks with basilar artery stenosis or occlusion: clinical patterns and outcome. *Arch Neurol.* 2002;59(4):567–573.

32. Helgason C, Caplan LR, Goodwin J, Hedges T, 3rd. Anterior choroidal artery-territory infarction: Report of cases and review. *Arch Neurol.* 1986;43(7):681–686.

33. Tohgi H, Takahashi S, Chiba K, Hirata Y. Cerebellar infarction: clinical and neuroimaging analysis in 293 patients: the Tohoku Cerebellar Infarction Study Group. *Stroke.* 1993;24(11):1697–1701.

34. Amarenco P, Hauw JJ. Cerebellar infarction in the territory of the anterior and inferior cerebellar artery: a clinicopathological study of 20 cases. *Brain.* 1990;113(Pt 1):139–155.

35. Wolf PA, Abbott RD, Kannel WB. Atrial fibrillation as an independent risk factor for stroke: the Framingham Study. *Stroke.* 1991;22(8):983–988.

36. Wessler BS, Kent DM. Controversies in cardioembolic stroke. *Curr Treat Option N.* 2015;17(1):358.

37. Broderick JP, Brott T, Tomsick T, Huster G, Miller R. The risk of subarachnoid and intracerebral hemorrhages in blacks as compared with whites. *New Engl J Med.* 1992;326(11):733–736.

38. Bruno A, Carter S, Qualls C, Nolte KB. Incidence of spontaneous intracerebral hemorrhage among Hispanics and non-Hispanic whites in New Mexico. *Neurology.* 1996;47(2):405–408.

39. Tanaka H, Ueda Y, Date C, et al. Incidence of stroke in Shibata, Japan: 1976–1978. *Stroke.* 1981;12(4):460–466.

40. Weimar C, Weber C, Wagner M, et al. Management patterns and health care use after intracerebral hemorrhage. a cost-of-illness study from a societal perspective in Germany. *Cerebrovasc Dis.* 2003;15(1–2):29–36.

41. Flaherty ML, Haverbusch M, Sekar P, et al. Long-term mortality after intracerebral hemorrhage. *Neurology.* 2006;66(8):1182–1186.

42. Fogelholm R, Murros K, Rissanen A, Avikainen S. Long term survival after primary intracerebral haemorrhage: a retrospective population based study. *J Neurol Neurosur Ps.* 2005;76(11):1534–1538.

43. Anderson CS, Heeley E, Huang Y, et al. Rapid blood-pressure lowering in patients with acute intracerebral hemorrhage. *New Engl J Med.* 2013;368(25):2355–2365.

2

Stroke Systems of Care

CASEY FREY, LAURA BISHOP, STACEY Q. WOLFE,
AND KYLE M. FARGEN ■

CONTENTS

1 INTRODUCTION

Stroke is the fifth leading cause of death in the United States and accounts for around 1 in every 20 deaths in the United States.[1] Every year approximately 795,000 people experience a stroke; the vast majority (87%) of which are ischemic in nature. For every minute of ischemia, approximately 2 million neurons are irreversibly lost.[2] Therefore, early identification of stroke symptoms, emergency medical services (EMS) activation and transport, rapid imaging and diagnosis, and early initiation of treatment are paramount.

In 1996, after the Food and Drug Administration approval, intravenous (IV) tissue plasminogen activator (alteplase, tPA) was established as the standard of care therapy for patients presenting with acute ischemic stroke within three hours from symptom onset.[3-5] This temporal limitation was later revised after analysis of multiple trials demonstrated benefit of alteplase up to 4.5 hours after onset of symptoms.[6,7]

Recently, seven randomized controlled trials have demonstrated benefit to mechanical thrombectomy for anterior circulation large vessel occlusions.[8-14] These trials have been transformative and have led the American Heart Association (AHA) to update societal guidelines and provide a Class I Recommendation, Level of Evidence A, that thrombectomy be pursued in patients with large vessel occlusions who meet certain criteria, most notably presentation within 6 hours of symptom onset.[15] Accordingly, the last decade has seen a paradigm shift where stroke care has been clustered into highly experienced stroke centers that have the necessary infrastructure, procedural capabilities, and specialized physicians required to manage complex stroke conditions and sequelae. However, large vessel occlusions or severe strokes only account for a small minority of patients presenting with ischemic stroke (24 per 100,000 person-years).[16]

While patient selection and treatments continue to improve, a number of important challenges remain. For instance, reperfusion therapies remain substantially underutilized, as less than 10% of patients presenting with acute stroke actually receive IV alteplase.[17,18] These observations highlight important questions: How do we ensure that as many stroke patients as possible are obtaining the best possible outcomes? How do we ensure that individuals in rural communities without access to large stroke centers continue to receive state-of-the-art stroke care as rapidly as possible? Given the time sensitivity of stroke, is it better to have a greater number of less experienced (lower patient volume) hospitals or triage to a smaller number of hospitals with greater volume and expertise?

This chapter will serve to outline such stroke systems of care and EMS providers and Emergency Department (ED) physicians and personnel in evaluating, managing, and triaging patients with different types stroke (Figure 2.1). We will discuss the reasoning behind the development of stroke centers and provide example cases of patients best managed at the various hospital subtypes.

> **Question 2.1:** How many patients with acute ischemic strokes are treated with revascularization therapies?
>
> **Answer:** The numbers differ significantly depending on geographic location and the time of data capture. It is estimated that more recently, approximately 4–7% of all patients with acute ischemic stroke are treated with IV alteplase, and 2–4% undergo endovascular thrombectomy (EVT).

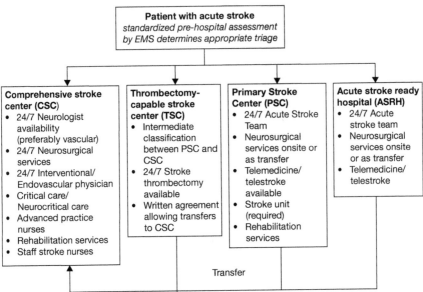

Figure 2.1 Key elements of stroke systems of care.
ABBREVIATIONS: ASRH, acute stroke ready hospital; CSC, comprehensive stroke center; EMS, emergency medical services; PSC, primary stroke center; TSC, thrombectomy-capable stroke center.

2 STROKE VOLUME–OUTCOMES RELATIONSHIP

There is robust literature demonstrating a direct relationship between cerebro-vascular and endovascular patient volume and favorable patient outcomes, both for individual practitioners and for institutions.[19-31] Procedural morbidity and complications have been shown to be lower in patients undergoing endovascular or open cerebrovascular surgery at high-volume centers, including aneurysm coiling and carotid stenting, among others.[19-31] Two Nationwide Inpatient Sample data-base studies have provided evidence of a relationship between higher mechanical thrombectomy volumes and both reduced mortality and increased good clinical out-come rates.[32,33] A multicenter retrospective study comparing high- and low-volume stroke centers demonstrated significantly better angiographic and clinical outcomes for patients treated with thrombectomy at high-volume centers.[34]

Most recently, a Vizient (University HealthSystem Consortium) database study by Rinaldo et al. of over 8500 patients who underwent mechanical thrombectomy admitted to 118 institutions over a 4-year period showed significant indirect associations between mortality and volume for both directly admitted and transferred patients.[35] Using volume criteria, mortality rates were significantly lower for patients admitted to high-volume centers (≥132 procedures per year; 9.8%) compared to medium (27–131 procedures annually; 14.9%) or low (<27 procedures annu-ally; 19.7%) volume centers. In fact, mortality was significantly lower for patients transferred to high-volume centers for thrombectomy compared to those directly admitted to low-volume centers, suggesting the benefit of treatment at a high-volume center may outweigh any detrimental consequences related to transfer delays.[35]

Importantly, the data supporting a volume–outcome relationship transcends patients who are candidates for endovascular procedures. Studies evaluating outcomes at various stroke centers based on volume have strongly suggested that lower-volume stroke centers have lower rates of good outcomes when compared to higher-volume centers.[34,36,37] Generally, the various studies suggest a strong correlation between outcomes of patients with serious cerebrovascular diseases and the expertise of the individuals and hospital stroke systems, using volume as a surrogate marker.

It is worth noting that the recent randomized controlled trials that demonstrated a benefit for EVT over medical management were conducted at high-volume stroke centers. This fact was underscored in an editorial authored by several of the principle investigators that emphasized that the results were only generalizable to other established, efficient stroke systems staffed with highly experienced neurointerventionists, neurologists, intensivists, and supporting staff.[38] The expectation of similar outcomes at low-volume centers with less-experienced physicians and staff is not practical nor reasonable. Therefore, increasing the numbers of low-volume centers to help improve stroke care access, rather than supporting high-volume regionalized systems of care, may potentially be harmful to patients as it may result in a higher percentage of patients with poor outcomes.

3 LESSONS FROM THE ACUTE TRAUMA MODEL

Trauma and stroke systems of care both revolve around timely management of acute and life-threatening injuries. The installment of trauma systems began following the publication of *Accidental Death and Disability: The Neglected Disease of Modern Society* by the National Highway Safety Act of 1966. Following this call to arms, there was an expansion of ambulance and helicopter services for trauma patients, revamping of emergency medical care systems, and the emergence of statewide trauma systems. In 1971, the American Medical Association detailed a hierarchical classification scheme for hospitals based on their size, expertise, and ability to care for trauma patients. Later, trauma hospitals became required to participate in regionalized trauma systems and became regulated under certain requirements proposed by the Committee on Trauma. The emergence and success of trauma systems is largely related to governmental funding and supportive legislation leading to a more structured organization and implementation of detailed systems of care.

Trauma systems of care focus on the principle of timely and appropriate patient triage to facilities that are capable of managing traumatic injuries based on the severity of the injury. In the multitrauma patient, management during the first hour after the acute injury is most critical and aptly referred to as the "golden hour," because failure to implement appropriate life-saving therapies during this time period may be fatal.

In the acute trauma model, trauma patients may be stabilized at lower levels of care and, if the severity of trauma is low, remain at these centers for treatment. Those patients with more severe injuries may either be transported directly to tertiary care centers or may be stabilized at local facilities and then transported to higher-level facilities based on injury severity and complexity. There is robust evidence supporting the importance of regionalized trauma systems in reducing mortality and improving outcomes following traumatic injury.[39–44]

To be effective, regionalized trauma systems require appropriate triage in the field based on easily recognizable and standardized criteria. Field assessment of patients includes evaluation of alertness, vital signs, anatomic factors of injury, mechanism of injury, and individual patient considerations (pregnancy, burns, age). These standardized classifications influence the immediate management of patients and direct transfer by EMS to the appropriate level of care.

3.1 Need for standardized prehospital assessment

Like trauma patients, stroke patients are typically critically ill, need specialized care, and have a finite window for therapeutic measures to be successful. Although the finite time for large vessel occlusions has recently been expanded by randomized controlled trials showing benefit beyond 6 hours, there is a well-described relationship between timely treatment and good outcome. Early recognition in the field is therefore critical (Case 2.1). Standardized prehospital patient assessment tools such as the Los Angeles Motor Scales (LAMS), Rapid Arterial Occlusion Evaluation (RACE) scale, and the Cincinnati Stroke Triage Assessment Tool (C-STAT) screen for cortical symptoms (see Chapter 3 describing clinical stroke detection and severity screens) may help to identify patients with large vessel occlusions that could benefit from EVT. For stroke care to successfully follow a similar model, an organized system of triage revolving around standardized assessment scales must be organized and implemented to guide triage to proper levels of stroke care.

Another important consideration includes the sequelae of stroke, which may require higher levels of care following acute stabilization. For instance, complications following a stroke such as hemorrhagic conversion, hydrocephalus, or malignant intracranial hypertension may require intricate multidisciplinary decision-making best performed by dedicated stroke care teams that include neurointensivists and neurosurgeons.

3.2 Current challenges

Unlike the regionalization of trauma care, the current stroke model is a pseudo-regionalized system that is fragmented and redundant. This is largely due to its development in an uncoordinated manner lacking systemic oversight and control. The current model may lead to patients getting inappropriate care due to lack of expertise in local hospitals or due to inappropriate and arbitrary triage. The establishment and implementation of stroke care requires that governing bodies develop true regionalized care models, proven triage assessment tools, effective means of transportation, and a hierarchal system of care to manage both the acute stroke as well as sequelae from the insult. Fortunately, regionalized care is rapidly evolving through expansion of telestroke, the development of advanced certification for hospitals, and with improved guidelines for stroke care.

Question 2.2: Which organizations offer certification for stroke programs?

Answer: The two main organizations are the Joint Commission and Det Norske Veritas (DNV). Some states also provide local stroke certification programs.

4 DEVELOPMENT OF MODERN STROKE SYSTEMS OF CARE: THE BRAIN ATTACK COALITION

Understanding the need for a hierarchical organization to facilitate stroke patient care, the Brain Attack Coalition (BAC) provided recommendations for the establishment of primary stroke centers (PSCs) in 2000. The BAC itself encompasses of a group of various professional, voluntary, and governmental organizations that work to set direction, advance knowledge, and communicate the best practices to prevent and treat stroke. The group is sponsored by the National Institute of Neurological Disorders and Stroke. The coalition contains members that represent groups like the AHA and the Centers for Disease Control, as well as professionals in the fields of neurosurgery, neurology, diagnostic and interventional neuroradiology, and emergency medicine. Since 2000, the BAC has provided additional recommendations for acute stroke ready hospitals (ASRHs) and comprehensive stroke centers (CSC), as well as a recent proposal for thrombectomy-capable stroke centers (TSC). Certification for each level of stroke care can be achieved via independent groups that offer certification programs, including the Joint Commission.[45] Stroke center organization and implementation can be influenced by city, local, and state authority legislature. For example, laws may require that stroke patients be taken to a certain PSC within a certain distance, providing regulations on where and when to transport patients. In a more tangible example, state legislation has already shown to improve the general availability of stroke centers and leaves room for the standardization of care, which might help to organize transport to and treatment at PSCs.[46]

Collectively, the system continues to evolve based on emerging evidence supporting or disputing aspects at each level of care and will continue to evolve as hierarchal care continues to be implemented. Recommendations from the BAC are derived from evidence-based literature and strive to improve the outcomes for stroke patients throughout all aspects of modern healthcare. In the future, analysis of outcome and performance metrics may be used to compare individual centers and level of certification to optimize patient triage and management.

5 TELESTROKE

Two frequent barriers to stroke care include geographic hurdles and absence of around the clock readily available acute stroke expertise. In a 2009 study of over 4,500 hospitals, 64% of those hospitals reported no IV alteplase administration in the prior two years. Hospitals with no alteplase use were more likely to contain less than 95 beds, be located in a rural setting, and specifically be located in the South or Midwest. Forty percent of the US population lives in a county that treated less than 2.4% of ischemic stroke patients with alteplase.[47] Additionally, alteplase complication rates have been shown to be higher for inexperienced physicians.[48] In recent years, telestroke has become a reliable way to deliver acute stroke care to patients who may not have previously been able to receive it.

In the wake of widespread alteplase use, the late 1990s and early 2000s brought utilization of telestroke. Levine and Gorman coined the term "telestroke" in the 1999 landmark paper and asserted it would bring state of the art neurologic expertise to patients who would not otherwise receive it.[49] Ten years later, the AHA in their 2009 scientific statement recommended a telestroke evaluation to render an opinion in regards to administration of IV altepase in the acute stroke setting in those geographic locations where a physician with acute stroke expertise is not physically available.[50]

A typical telestroke consultation consists of a patient presenting to an ED where vascular neurology expertise is not readily available (Case 2.2). Patients can present via their own vehicle or via EMS in which prehospital notification may occur. On arrival, the patient is evaluated by the ED provider and an acute stroke is suspected with time of onset within the window for acute intervention. A computed tomography (CT) scan is performed, and a telestroke consultation is called. An offsite vascular neurologist or physician with stroke experience then evaluates the patient and imaging remotely via video and audio communication in real-time to confirm the diagnosis of ischemic stroke and determine the patient's candidacy for alteplase. A recommendation is then made to the ED provider. Additionally, if the patient is a potential candidate for EVT, recommendations are made for appropriate further evaluation and/or transfer.

5.1 Models for telestroke

There are two common models for telestroke networks. The first is a distributed model where care is delivered by physicians at multiple distant locations. These physicians are typically employed on a contractual basis, and patients treated who require transfer typically move to an unrelated, geographically close, tertiary care center. The second model is the hub and spoke model in which the hub is typically an academic medical center and the spoke sites are hospitals in the region. If transfer results from these consultations, patients are typically transferred to the hub site.[50]

The AHA recommends that each hub site have a dedicated stroke center medical director as well as a physician and nurse champion.[51]

Question 2.3: How many PSCs and CSCs are in the United States?

Answer: These numbers are constantly growing. The data from 2015 estimated that there were 1197 PSCs and 113 CSCs in the United States.

6 STROKE SYSTEM LEVELS OF CARE

Stroke system levels of care consist of ASRHs, PSCs, and CSCs. Collectively, the BAC created a model to provide an organized and improved methodology for caring for stroke patients everywhere. The highlights of each level of qualification include:

- Available personnel
- Diagnostic techniques
- Surgical/interventional therapies
- Infrastructure
- Educational/research programs

Throughout this section, designations of the three types of stroke centers will be outlined for comparison using the elements previously listed. Importantly, all hospitals with certification are required to collect and report performance metrics (outcomes, complications, etc.) to a national registry.

6.1 Acute stroke ready hospitals

Many hospitals serve areas of the country that have low population densities. Although only <25–75% of stroke patients are admitted to non-PSC-qualifying hospitals like this per year, the cumulative admittance rate for these centers actually comprises a large majority of stroke admissions. In light of this, the BAC created the ASRH designation, which has the capabilities to diagnose, stabilize, treat with alteplase utilizing telestroke expertise, and transfer stroke patients that are not within 60 minutes of a PSC. When directly compared to a PSC (Box 2.1), ASRHs require only 4 annual hours of stroke education in the ED, do not require stroke units unless the patients are admitted, have neurosurgical services available within 3 hours, and require the patient to be transferred to a PSC or CSC within 2 hours or arrival or when medically stable. The BAC requires that certification of an ASRH includes certification by an outside, independent organization with no direct or financial relationship or interest with the ASRH; onsite assessment of the facility, personnel, and protocols; and collection and analysis of >4 disease performance metrics. Certification must

Box 2.1

Selected elements of acute stroke ready hospitals

- Available personnel
  - Designated director training and expertise in cerebrovascular disease
  - Acute stroke team available 24/7 with a minimum of 2 members and a 15-minute response time
  - EMS trained in field assessment tools for stroke
  - Neurosurgical services available within 3 hours—onsite or transfer
  - Initiation of telemedicine link within 20 minutes when deemed medically necessary
  - Telemedicine/teleradiology equipment onsite
- Diagnostic techniques
  - Laboratory testing, electrocardiogram (ECG), and chest radiograph results available within 45 minutes of order
  - Brain imaging tests (non-contrast CT/magnetic resonance imaging [MRI]) completed and read within 45 minutes (60 for MRI) and available 24/7.
- Surgical/interventional therapies
  - IV alteplase door-to-needle time <60 minutes (available 24/7)
- Infrastructure
  - Stroke unit not required unless patients are admitted
  - Transfer of patients to PSC or CSC within 2 hours of ED arrival or once medically stable
- Educational/research programs
  - Written stroke protocol revised annually and including all types of stroke
  - ED with 4 annual hours of stroke education and written protocols for treatment and stabilization
  - EMS with at least 2 hours of stroke-related education annually

be performed at least every two to three years, but with annual data collection and analysis.[52]

6.2 Primary stroke centers

PSCs were the first level of stroke care created to address an overarching problem: patients with an acute stroke were not being treated according to contemporary guidelines.[7,8] The BAC classified recommendations for key elements of PSCs based on high level of evidence literature that could provide information on the benefits of treatments, tests, interventions, or personnel. Recommendations for a PSC can be examined in Box 2.2. The main differences between a PSC and

Box 2.2

- Available personnel
  - Designated director with training and expertise in cerebrovascular disease
  - Acute stroke team available 24/7 with a minimum of two members and a 15-minute response time
  - EMS trained in field assessment tools for stroke
  - Neurosurgical services available within 2 hours—onsite or transfer
  - Initiation of telemedicine link within 20 minutes when deemed medically necessary for CSC consultation and telemedicine/teleradiology equipment onsite and offsite
  - Rehabilitation services (physical, occupational, speech) with early assessment and initiation
- Diagnostic techniques
  - Laboratory testing, ECG, and chest radiograph results available within 45 minutes of order
  - Brain imaging tests (non-contrast CT/MRI) completed and read within 45 minutes (60 for MRI) and available 24/7
  - MRI, magnetic resonance angiography (MRA), or CT angiography (CTA) available, performed within 6 hours, and read within 2 hours of completion
  - At least 1 modality of cardiac imaging available
- Surgical/interventional therapies
  - IV alteplase door-to-needle time <60 minutes (available 24/7)
- Infrastructure
  - Stroke unit required for admitted patients and should include clinical monitoring protocol and multichannel telemetry
- Educational/research programs
  - Written stroke protocol revised annually and including all types of stroke
  - ED with 8 annual hours of stroke education and written protocols for treatment and stabilization
  - EMS with at least 2 hours of stroke-related education annually
  - Stroke registry with outcomes and QI components
  - Professional and public educational programs
  - At least 2 annual programs to educate the public about stroke prevention, diagnosis, and/or the availability of acute therapies
  - Professional staff of the PSC receive at least 8 hours/year of educational credit in areas related to cerebrovascular disease

CSC center around the amount of physician specialists available and the imaging modalities utilized in the hospital (Case 2.2). The BAC mandates that PSC certification requires a certifying body be administratively and financially independent of the hospital; inclusion of an assessment of infrastructure, personnel, protocols, and programs; a site visit at least every 2 years; and a well-defined and quantifiable disease performance measures developed and assessed on a regular basis with mandatory reporting to a stroke data registry.[53]

6.3 Comprehensive stroke centers

CSC level care is meant to benefit patients requiring a multitude of advanced care, including those with hemorrhagic strokes, large ischemic strokes, strokes of unknown or unusual etiology, and those with multisystem involvement. The level of care provided requires highly trained specialty physicians and complex treatment programs, such as neurosurgery, neurocritical care, and neurointerventional physicians. Much of what distinguishes a CSC from a PSC and ASRH includes expertise and infrastructure in diagnostic radiology, EVT, and surgery. These are all vital in the management of large ischemic and hemorrhagic strokes (Cases 2.1 and 2.3). With the advancement of stroke levels of care, more data will become available to determine the efficacy of certain requirements of a CSC and can be adjusted as these come forth. Certification for a CSC requires the same independent process as a PSC, but it is advised by the BAC to include the recommendations listed in Box 2.3. New performance measures for a CSC are currently in development.[54] Similar to PSCs, CSCs require participation in a mandatory stroke data registry.

6.4 Thrombectomy-capable stroke centers

In January 2018, the BAC and the Joint Commission proposed an additional certification entitled the TSC. The TSC Advanced Certification is intended as an intermediate classification between PSC and CSC.[55] Most notably, TSC certification mandates the capacity to perform mechanical thrombectomy 24 hours a day, 7 days a week; the capability for other types of advanced imaging; and a written agreement for transfer with at least one CSC. The Joint Commission has requested comment on minimum thrombectomy volume requirements. Currently, The Joint Commission has suggested TSC certification eligibility mandates that an institution perform a minimum of 12 thrombectomy procedures during the previous year, or 24 procedures over the last 2 years.[55] TSC requirements and their role in stroke systems have yet to be clearly understood or defined.

7 TRIAGING THE STROKE PATIENT

Many strokes are identified by EMS in the prehospital setting. When a potential acute stroke is identified the patient will ideally be taken to the nearest hospital that

Box 2.3

SELECTED ELEMENTS OF COMPREHENSIVE STROKE CENTERS

- Available personnel
    - Center director or his or her designee available 24/7
    - >1 vascular (preferably) neurologist available within 20 minutes for emergency calls and within 45 minutes inhouse
    - Critical care/neurocritical care neurologist, neurosurgeon, anesthesiologist, or internist who cares for >20 patients with acute strokes per year and attends >4 hours per year of continued medical education (CME) activities related to or focused on cerebrovascular disease
    - Neurosurgical expertise available 24/7 within 30 minutes. The hospital must care for >20 subarachnoid hemorrhage patients per year and accomplish >10 craniotomies per year for aneurysm clipping, with each neurosurgeon participating in >10 cases per year.
    - Nurses should attend training sessions sponsored by the CSC >3 times per year, participate in >10 hours of continuing education unit activities related to cerebrovascular disease, and attend >1 national or regional meeting every other year focusing on cerebrovascular disease
    - Advanced practice nurses
    - EMS trained in field assessment tools for stroke who attend initial and ongoing educational programs that focus on cerebrovascular disease
    - Initiation of telemedicine link within 20 minutes when deemed medically necessary
    - Telemedicine/teleradiology equipment onsite and offsite to receive
    - Diagnostic radiology/neuroradiology available 24/7 to read scans within 20 minutes of their completion
    - >1 certified radiology technologist trained in CT techniques inhouse 24/7
    - Magnetic resonance (MR) and cerebral angiogram technologist available on 24/7 basis that can be at hospital within 1 hour of being paged
    - Vascular neurology, neurosurgery, and surgery
    - Interventional/endovascular physician
    - Rehabilitation therapy (physical, occupational, speech therapy), social workers, and nurse case managers must meet state licensure and have > 1 year of experience in the treatment of stroke survivors with consults within 24 hours
    - Staff stroke nurse(s)
    - Respiratory therapist
    - Swallowing assessment
    - Optional—neuroscience intensive care, nursing director for stroke program
- Diagnostic techniques
    - Basic MRI, diffusion MRI, MRA must be available 24/7 and should be completed within 2 hours of the test being ordered

- CTA/CT available on 24/7 basis within 60 minutes of being called
- MR venography
- Digital cerebral angiography
- Transcranial Doppler ultrasound
- Carotid duplex ultrasound
- Transesophageal echo performed and interpreted by technicians and cardiologist with training in these techniques
- Optional—MR perfusion, CT perfusion, Xenon CT, single photon emission computed tomography, positron emission tomography
- Surgical/interventional therapies
  - IV alteplase door-to-needle time <60 minutes (available 24/7)
  - Carotid endarterectomy
  - Clipping of intracranial aneurysm
  - Placement of ventriculostomy
  - Hematoma removal/draining
  - Placement of intracranial pressure transducer
  - Endovascular embolization of aneurysms/AVMs
  - IA reperfusion therapy
  - Endovascular therapy of vasospasm
  - Optional—stenting/angioplasty of extracranial/intracranial vessels
- Infrastructure
  - Stroke unit
  - Intensive care unit (ICU) with director having >8 hours per year of CME related to cerebrovascular disease and physicians with cerebrovascular disease/critical care expertise available 24/7
  - ICU nurses caring for stroke patients who receive >10 hours per year of continuing education unit credit in areas related to cerebrovascular disease
  - Operating room staffed 24/7
  - Interventional services coverage 24/7
  - Optional—stroke clinic, air ambulance, neuroscience ICU
- Educational/research programs
  - Written stroke protocol revised annually and including all types of stroke
  - ED with 8 annual hours of stroke education and written protocols for treatment and stabilization
  - EMS with at least 2 hours of stroke-related education annually
  - At least 2 public activities focused on stroke education and prevention
  - >2 professional education courses per year
  - Patient education
  - Stroke registry with outcomes and QI components
  - Optional—clinical research, laboratory research, fellowship program, presentations at national meetings

has the capabilities to administer thrombolytic therapy, unless the patient is medically unstable. Appropriate facilities for triage include ASRHs, PSCs, or CSCs. After an evaluation by a stroke expert, which may occur in person, remotely via telephone consultation, or remotely via telestroke, the patient may need to be transferred to a higher level of care (CSC) given the outcome of the consultation. Circumstances that would warrant transfer include but are not limited to administration of IV alteplase (which would occur prior to transfer), need for evaluation for EVT, need for neurointensive care unit, need for neurosurgical evaluation, or may be dependent on imaging findings or stroke severity. Concern for a large vessel occlusion would warrant further evaluation for EVT. Signs of a large vessel occlusion warranting EVT include National Institutes of Health Stroke Scale (NIHSS) ≥6, disabling symptom such as dense aphasia, cortical symptoms on exam (aphasia, neglect, etc.) even with NIHSS <6, or posterior circulation symptoms.

8 CLINICAL CASES

Case 2.1 Ischemic stroke from large vessel occlusion

CASE DESCRIPTION
An 84-year-old female with hyperlipidemia was shopping with her daughter when she became acutely hemiplegic. She was able to speak but had neglect and gaze deviation. Given that a CSC was only 10 minutes farther than the PSC and that her Cincinnati Stroke Triage Assessment Tool was 3 (large vessel occlusion likely), EMS contacted the CSC to alert them of the patient's condition and then brought her directly to the CSC for care.

PRACTICAL POINTS

- This patient's initial exam demonstrated a left hemiparesis with neglect and an initial NIHSS 12. Non-contrast CT head (Figure 2.2A) showed no major infarct (Alberta Stroke Program Early CT Score [ASPECTS] = 9) or hemorrhage, and IV alteplase was started 95 minutes from symptom onset.
- CT angiography showed a complete occlusion of the right internal carotid artery with CT perfusion demonstrating a large region of ischemic but potentially salvageable tissue, with prolonged mean transit time in the entire right middle cerebral artery territory and no core infarct on blood volume (Figure 2.2B). This patient underwent emergent mechanical thrombectomy with complete revascularization 3 hours, 4 minutes from symptom onset. (Figures 2.2C and 2.2D) Her strength improved immediately with resolution of the gaze preference. She was discharged home on hospital day 3 with a NIHSS of 2.
- Currently, stroke care lacks a robust regionalized protocol and is fragmented, but improvements to systems continue to occur as stroke

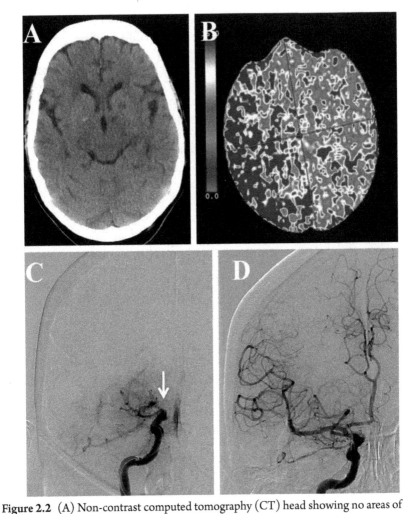

Figure 2.2 (A) Non-contrast computed tomography (CT) head showing no areas of major infarction or hemorrhage. The Alberta stroke program early CT score is 9.
(B) Computed tomography perfusion, mean transit time (MTT) demonstrating slowed mean transit time in the right internal carotid artery distribution.
(C) Digital subtraction angiography (DSA), antero-posterior view demonstrating complete large vessel occlusion of the right supraclinoid internal carotid artery (arrow).
(D) DSA, antero-posterior view demonstrating complete recanalization of the right internal carotid artery thromboembolism.

care evolves. The BAC and Joint Commission have designated advanced certification for hospitals that meet appropriate criteria, which allows for appropriate triage based on stroke severity. Those patients with large vessel occlusions or large territory infarcts require transfer to CSCs, where neurointerventional, neurocritical care, and neurosurgical specialists are present.

Case 2.2 Ischemic stroke without large vessel occlusion and minor symptoms

CASE DESCRIPTION

A 78-year-old female with a history of hypertension and hyperlipidemia called EMS after noticing right-sided weakness and slurred speech. EMS saw no gaze deviation or neglect, calculated her Cincinnati Pre-Hospital Stroke scale to be 2, and alerted a nearby PSC that they were bringing the patient. The patient arrived 4 hours from onset of symptoms and a CT head showed no hemorrhage. The ED paged their Telestroke partners, and a stroke neurologist was able to review the imaging and examine the patient over the next 7 minutes. The patient had a NIHSS score of 6. IV alteplase was given at 4 hours and 20 minutes, and the patient was admitted to the PSC for the rest of her stroke workup. CT angiography showed no large vessel occlusion nor carotid stenosis. The patient spent the night in the medical intensive care unit and was discharged home on aspirin after 4 days with 1-week follow-up with her primary physician for optimization of blood pressure control and follow-up in 2 weeks with stroke neurology.

PRACTICAL POINTS

- Rapid triage and initiation of therapeutic interventions by experienced individuals are critical for patients with stroke. However, not all strokes are equal, as many patients with minor strokes do not require transfer to tertiary care facilities, while those with large vessel occlusions require urgent transfer to facilities capable of performing rescue endovascular therapies or management of malignant intracranial hypertension. Telestroke has also been critical in providing expertise to hospitals receiving acute stroke patients that do not have in-house neurologists or neurosurgeons.
- Patients with minor subcortical symptoms or straightforward diagnoses may be managed at ASRHs or PSCs that have the capability of diagnosing and treating less complex stroke patients. Ultimately, the strengthening of regionalized, evidence-based and protocol-driven stroke care systems will be necessary to further reduce mortality and improve outcomes among stroke patients in the future.

Case 2.3 Hemorrhagic stroke with a large intraparenchymal hematoma/intraventricular hemorrhage

CASE DESCRIPTION

A 67-year-old female with past medical history of hypertension and controlled diabetes mellitus was found unresponsive at home. She had last been seen by her family 3 hours earlier. The patient was found by EMS to have a depressed level of consciousness with a Glasgow Coma Scale of 7 and a RACE score of 6. Upon arrival to a PSC, she had a NIHSS score of 23 with left sided hemiplegia, aphasia, gaze deviation, and eye opening only to pain. Non-contrast CT head showed a 5 cm × 8 cm × 6 cm right

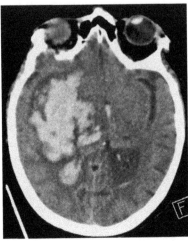

Figure 2.3 Non-contrast computed tomography head showing a large hypertensive intraparenchymal hematoma involving the frontal, temporal and parietal lobe with intraventricular extension into the lateral and third ventricles. There is 8 mm of midline shift with brainstem compression.

intraparenchymal hematoma with intraventricular extension (Figure 2.3). She was transferred to a CSC for emergency neurosurgical evaluation.

PRACTICAL POINTS

- Immediately triage to a CSC for neurosurgical evaluation is indicated. This patient underwent a craniotomy and evacuation of hematoma.
- CSCs offer multidisciplinary care including a team of critical care/neurocritical care neurologists, neurosurgeons, and anesthesiologists required for appropriate management of such challenging cases.

REFERENCES

1. Benjamin EJ, Blaha MJ, Chiuve SE, et al. Heart disease and stroke statistics 2017 update: a report from the American Heart Association. *Circulation.* 2017;135(10):e146–e603.
2. Saver JL. Time is brain—quantified. *Stroke.* 2006;37(1):263–266.
3. National Institute of Neurological Disorders and Stroke rt-PA Stroke Study Group. Tissue plasminogen activator for acute ischemic stroke. *N Engl J Med.* 1995;333(24):1581–1587.
4. Hacke W, Kaste M, Fieschi C, et al. Intravenous thrombolysis with recombinant tissue plasminogen activator for acute hemispheric stroke: the European Cooperative Acute Stroke Study (ECASS). *JAMA.* 1995;274(13):1017–1025.

5. Hacke W, Kaste M, Fieschi C, et al. Randomised double-blind placebo-controlled trial of thrombolytic therapy with intravenous alteplase in acute ischaemic stroke (ECASS II): Second European-Australasian Acute Stroke Study Investigators. *Lancet.* 1998;352(9136):1245–1251.

6. Hacke W, Donnan G, Fieschi C, et al. Association of outcome with early stroke treatment: pooled analysis of ATLANTIS, ECASS, and NINDS rt-PA stroke trials. *Lancet.* 2004;363(9411):768–774.

7. Hacke W, Kaste M, Bluhmki E, et al. Thrombolysis with alteplase 3 to 4.5 hours after acute ischemic stroke. *N Engl J Med.* 2008;359(13):1317–1329.

8. Berkhemer OA, Fransen PS, Beumer D, et al. A randomized trial of intraarterial treatment for acute ischemic stroke. *N Engl J Med.* 2015;372(1):11–20.

9. Campbell BC, Mitchell PJ, Kleinig, TJ, et al. Endovascular therapy for ischemic stroke. *N Engl J Med.* 2015;372(24):2365–2366.

10. Goyal M, Demchuk AM, Menon BK, et al. Randomized assessment of rapid endovascular treatment of ischemic stroke. *N Engl J Med.* 2015;372(11):1019–1030.

11. Jovin TG, Chamorro A, Cobo E, et al. Thrombectomy within 8 hours after symptom onset in ischemic stroke. *N Engl J Med.* 2015;372(24):2296–2306.

12. Saver JL, Goyal M, Diener HC, SWIFT PRIME Investigators. Stent-retriever thrombectomy for stroke. *N Engl J Med.* 2015;373(11):1077.

13. Bracard S, Ducrocq X, Mas JL, et al. Mechanical thrombectomy after intravenous alteplase versus alteplase alone after stroke (THRACE): a randomised controlled trial. *Lancet Neurol.* 2016;15(11):1138–1147.

14. Mocco J, Zaidat OO, von Kummer R, et al. Aspiration thrombectomy after intravenous alteplase versus intravenous alteplase alone. *Stroke.* 2016;47(9):2331–2338.

15. Powers WJ, Derdeyn CP, Biller J, et al. 2015 American Heart Association/American Stroke Association focused update of the 2013 Guidelines for the Early Management of Patients with Acute Ischemic Stroke regarding Endovascular Treatment: a guideline for healthcare professionals from the American Heart Association/American Stroke Association. *Stroke.* 2015;46(10):3020–3035.

16. Rai AT, Seldon AE, Boo S, et al. A population-based incidence of acute large vessel occlusions and thrombectomy eligible patients indicates significant potential for growth of endovascular stroke therapy in the USA. *J Neurointerv Surg.* 2017;9(8):722–726.

17. Adeoye O, Hornung R, Khatri P, Kleindorfer D. Recombinant tissue-type plasminogen activator use for ischemic stroke in the United States: a doubling of treatment rates over the course of 5 years. *Stroke.* 2011;42(7):1952–1955.

18. Adeoye O, Albright KC, Carr BG, et al. Geographic access to acute stroke care in the United States. *Stroke.* 2014;45(10):3019–3024.

19. Brinjikji W, Rabinstein AA, Lanzino G, Kallmes DF, Cloft HJ. Patient outcomes are better for unruptured cerebral aneurysms treated at centers that preferentially treat with endovascular coiling: a study of the national inpatient sample 2001–2007. *AJNR Am J Neuroradiol.* 2011;32(6):1065–1070.

20. Khatri R, Tariq N, Vazquez G, Suri MF, Ezzeddine MA, Qureshi AI. Outcomes after nontraumatic subarachnoid hemorrhage at hospitals offering angioplasty for cerebral vasospasm: a national level analysis in the United States. *Neurocrit Care.* 2011;15(1):34–41.

21. Hoh BL, Rabinov JD, Pryor JC, Carter BS, Barker FG, 2nd. In-hospital morbidity and mortality after endovascular treatment of unruptured intracranial aneurysms in the United States, 1996–2000: effect of hospital and physician volume. *Am J Neuroradiol.* 2003;24(7):1409–1420.

22. Pandey AS, Gemmete JJ, Wilson TJ, et al. High subarachnoid hemorrhage patient volume associated with lower mortality and better outcomes. *Neurosurgery.* 2015;77(3):462–470; discussion 470.

23. Boogaarts HD, van Amerongen MJ, de Vries J, et al. Caseload as a factor for outcome in aneurysmal subarachnoid hemorrhage: a systematic review and meta-analysis. *J Neurosurg.* 2014;120(3):605–611.

24. Jalbert JJ, Gerhard-Herman MD, Nguyen LL, et al. relationship between physician and hospital procedure volume and mortality after carotid artery stenting among medicare beneficiaries. *Circ Cardiovasc Qual Outcomes.* 2015;8(6 Suppl 3):S81–S89.

25. Nallamothu BK, Gurm HS, Ting HH, et al. Operator experience and carotid stenting outcomes in Medicare beneficiaries. *JAMA.* 2011;306(12):1338–1343.

26. Sgroi MD, Darby GC, Kabutey NK, Barleben AR, Lane JS, 3rd, Fujitani RM. Experience matters more than specialty for carotid stenting outcomes. *J Vasc Surg.* 2015;61(4):933–938.

27. Berman MF, Solomon RA, Mayer SA, Johnston SC, Yung PP. Impact of hospital-related factors on outcome after treatment of cerebral aneurysms. *Stroke.* 2003;34(9):2200–2207.

28. Singh V, Gress DR, Higashida RT, Dowd CF, Halbach VV, Johnston SC. The learning curve for coil embolization of unruptured intracranial aneurysms. *Am J Neuroradiol.* 2002;23(5):768–771.

29. Malisch TW, Guglielmi G, Vinuela F, et al. Intracranial aneurysms treated with the Guglielmi detachable coil: midterm clinical results in a consecutive series of 100 patients. *J Neurosurg.* 1997;87(2):176–183.

30. Murayama Y, Vinuela F, Duckwiler GR, Gobin YP, Guglielmi G. Embolization of incidental cerebral aneurysms by using the Guglielmi detachable coil system. *J Neurosurg.* 1999;90(2):207–214.

31. Verzini F, Cao P, De Rango P, et al. Appropriateness of learning curve for carotid artery stenting: an analysis of periprocedural complications. *J Vasc Surg.* 2006;44(6):1205–1211; discussion 1211–1202.

32. Jani VB, To CY, Patel A, Kelkar PS, Richards B, Fessler RD. 116 effect of annual hospital procedure volume on outcomes after mechanical thrombectomy in acute ischemic stroke patients: an analysis of 13,502 procedures. *Neurosurgery.* 2016;63 Suppl 1:149.

33. Adamczyk P, Attenello F, Wen G, et al. Mechanical thrombectomy in acute stroke: utilization variances and impact of procedural volume on inpatient mortality. *J Stroke Cerebrovasc Dis.* 2013;22(8):1263–1269.

34. Gupta R, Horev A, Nguyen T, et al. Higher volume endovascular stroke centers have faster times to treatment, higher reperfusion rates and higher rates of good clinical outcomes. *J Neurointerv Surg.* 2013;5(4):294–297.

35. Rinaldo L, Brinjikji W, Rabinstein AA. Transfer to high-volume centers associated with reduced mortality after endovascular treatment of acute stroke. *Stroke.* 2017;48(5):1316–1321.

36. Saposnik G, Baibergenova A, O'Donnell M, et al. Hospital volume and stroke outcome: does it matter? *Neurology.* 2007;69(11):1142–1151.

37. Vespa P, Diringer MN. High-volume centers. *Neurocrit Care.* 2011;15(2): 369–372.

38. Mocco J, Fargen KM, Goyal M, et al. Neurothrombectomy trial results: stroke systems, not just devices, make the difference. *Int J Stroke.* 2015;10(7):990–993.

39. Cameron PA, Gabbe BJ, Cooper DJ, Walker T, Judson R, McNeil J. A statewide system of trauma care in Victoria: effect on patient survival. *Med J Aust.* 2008;189(10):546–550.

40. Gabbe BJ, Biostat GD, Lecky FE, et al. The effect of an organized trauma system on mortality in major trauma involving serious head injury: a comparison of the United kingdom and victoria, australia. *Ann Surg.* 2011;253(1):138–143.

41. Haas B, Stukel TA, Gomez D, et al. The mortality benefit of direct trauma center transport in a regional trauma system: a population-based analysis. *J Trauma Acute Care Surg.* 2012;72(6):1510–1515; discussion 1515–1517.

42. MacKenzie EJ, Rivara FP, Jurkovich GJ, et al. A national evaluation of the effect of trauma-center care on mortality. *N Engl J Med.* 2006;354(4):366–378.

43. Nathens AB, Brunet FP, Maier RV. Development of trauma systems and effect on outcomes after injury. *Lancet.* 2004;363(9423):1794–1801.

44. Stewart TC, Lane PL, Stefanits T. An evaluation of patient outcomes before and after trauma center designation using Trauma and Injury Severity Score analysis. *J Trauma.* 1995;39(6):1036–1040.

45. Schieb LJ, Casper ML, George MG. Mapping primary and comprehensive stroke centers by certification organization. *Circ Cardiovasc Qual Outcomes.* 2015;8(6 Suppl 3):S193–194.

46. Uchino K, Man S, Schold JD, Katzan IL. Stroke legislation impacts distribution of certified stroke centers in the United States. *Stroke.* 2015;46(7):1903–1908.

47. Kleindorfer D, Xu Y, Moomaw CJ, Khatri P, Adeoye O, Hornung R. US geographic distribution of rt-PA utilization by hospital for acute ischemic stroke. *Stroke.* 2009;40(11):3580–3584.

48. Heuschmann PU, Kolominsky-Rabas PL, Roether J, et al. Predictors of in-hospital mortality in patients with acute ischemic stroke treated with thrombolytic therapy. *JAMA.* 2004;292(15):1831–1838.

49. Levine SR, Gorman M. "Telestroke": the application of telemedicine for stroke. *Stroke.* 1999;30(2):464–469.

50. Schwamm LH, Holloway RG, Amarenco P, et al. A review of the evidence for the use of telemedicine within stroke systems of care: a scientific statement from the American Heart Association/American Stroke Association. *Stroke.* 2009;40(7):2616–2634.

51. Wechsler LR, Demaerschalk BM, Schwamm LH, et al. Telemedicine quality and outcomes in stroke: a scientific statement for healthcare professionals from the American Heart Association/American Stroke Association. *Stroke.* 2017;48(1):e3–e25.

52. Alberts MJ, Wechsler LR, Jensen ME, et al. Formation and function of acute stroke-ready hospitals within a stroke system of care recommendations from the Brain Attack Coalition. *Stroke.* 2013;44(12):3382–3393.

53. Alberts MJ, Latchaw RE, Jagoda A, et al. Revised and updated recommendations for the establishment of primary stroke centers: a summary statement from the Brain Attack Coalition. *Stroke.* 2011;42(9):2651–2665.

54. Alberts MJ, Latchaw RE, Selman WR, et al. Recommendations for comprehensive stroke centers: a consensus statement from the Brain Attack Coalition. *Stroke.* 2005;36(7):1597–1616.

55. Proposed requirements for the New Thrombectomy-Capable Stroke Center Certification Program. Field Reviews. The Joint Commission. 2017; https://www.jointcommission.org/standards_information/field_reviews.aspx. Accessed April 19, 2017.

3

Prehospital Triage of Stroke

Clinical Evaluation

VERA SHARASHIDZE, CLARA BARREIRA,
DIOGO HAUSEEN, AND RAUL G. NOGUEIRA ■

CONTENTS

1 INTRODUCTION

Timely recognition is one of the most critical steps in the prehospital care of a stroke patient because the treatment effect of commonly used early interventions such as intravenous (IV) alteplase and endovascular thrombectomy (EVT) is highly time-sensitive and any delays may significantly worsen clinical outcomes.[1,2] Emergency medical services (EMS) play a pivotal role in stabilizing the patient, recognizing an acute stroke, collecting important information (e.g., time last known normal, medications), and providing rapid transport to the most appropriate healthcare facility.

Proper identification of patients with acute ischemic stroke (AIS) in the prehospital setting can be challenging. The field triage to stroke centers has become considerably more complex with demonstration of the dramatic benefit of EVT in recent randomized clinical trials.[3] Acute stroke ready hospitals (ASRH), primary stroke centers (PSCs), and comprehensive stroke centers (CSCs) are required to perfom quickly clinical and imaging evaluation and administer IV alteplase. However, only CSCs have the capability of providing 24/7 emergent EVT and appropriate postinterventional care. Therefore, simple, reproducible, easily adoptable stroke screening and severity tools with good performance are imperative to accurately triage suspected stroke victims to the most appropriate facilities. Figure 3.1 and Table 3.1 describe and compare the role of these tools in stroke recognition and triage.

Question 3.1: What is the "best" prehospital stroke scale?

Answer: There are no data to suggest superiority of one scale over another. Each EMS region should choose a single screening and severity scale for prehospital stroke triage.

2 STROKE SCREENING TOOLS

Stroke screens are intended to serve as simple and straightforward tools to distinguish stroke patients from those with non-stroke events such as encephalopathy, hypoglycemia, or seizure. They are intended to be highly sensitive but not necessarily specific to diagnose acute stroke to ensure that all patients with acute stroke are appropriately triaged by EMS.

2.1 Cincinnati Prehospital Stroke Scale

The Cincinnati Prehospital Stroke Scale (CPSS) is a three-item (facial palsy, motor arm, and dysarthria) screen developed at the University of Cincinnati (Box 3.1).[4,5] It is an abbreviated version of the National Institutes of Health Stroke Scale (NIHSS) for identification of patients with stroke. This screen has good

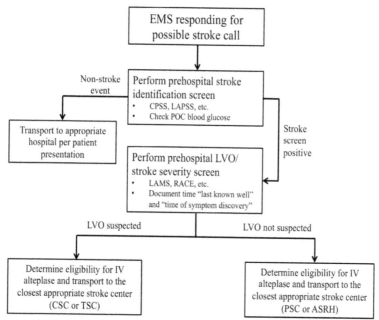

Figure 3.1 Stroke triage algorithm using stroke screening and stroke severity tools.
ABBREVIATIONS: ASRH, acute stroke ready hospital; CSC, comprehensive stroke
center; CPSS, Cincinnati Prehospital Stroke Scale; EMS, emergency medical services;
IV, intravenous; LAMS, Los Angeles Motor Scale; LAPSS, Los Angeles Prehospital
Stroke Screen; LVO, large vessel occlusion; POC, point of care; PSC, primary stroke
center; RACE, Rapid Arterial oCclusion Evaluation; TSC, thrombectomy-capable
stroke center.

agreement with on-the-scene assessments and can be correctly administered and
interpreted over the phone, making it a useful tool in early prehospital detection of
stroke by dispatchers.[6,7]

2.2 Los Angeles Prehospital Stroke Screen

The Los Angeles Prehospital Stroke Screen (LAPSS) is another screening tool to
identify stroke patients (Box 3.2). In addition to those criteria tested for in CPSS,
LAPSS also includes four history items and a blood glucose measure to exclude likely
stroke mimics.[8,9] CPSS and LAPSS have been validated in the prehospital setting.

2.3 Face Arm Speech Time test

The Face Arm Speech Time (FAST) test contains items that measure unilateral facial
droop (F), arm drift (A), and speech problems (S); (T) means "time to call 911." In

Table 3.1 COMPARISON OF STROKE TRIAGE SCREENING AND STROKE
SEVERITY SCREENS

Screening tool	Main goals	Advantages	Disadvantages
Cincinnati Prehospital Stroke Scale (CPSS)	• To identify stroke patients	• Fast and easy to administer • Validated in prehospital setting	• Fails to recognize importance of cortical signs
Face Arm Speech Test (FAST)	• To identify stroke patients • Designed for public, less so for clinicians/ EMS	• Simple, easy-to-use stroke recognition score	• The scale in insensitive to isolated stroke-related visual or sensory impairments, vertigo and gait disturbances
Rapid Arterial oCclusion Evaluation scale (RACE)	• To identify stroke patients with LVO	• Has been validated in the prehospital setting • Balanced points for left as well as right hemispheric strokes	• Validated in a population where most of patients were diagnosed with Transcranial Doppler • Higher chance of misdiagnosing pure motor stroke as LVO
Los Angeles Prehospital Stroke Screen (LAPSS)	• To identify stroke patients	• Includes four history items and a blood glucose measure to exclude stroke mimics	• Low sensitivity and non-recognition of young patients with stroke by the lower age limit
The Recognition of Stroke in the Emergency Room (ROSIER)	• To identify stroke patients	• To reduce significant number of non-stroke referrals to stroke teams that would result in a more targeted use of imaging and resources	• Cannot confidently rule out stroke as a diagnosis • Designed for use in ED

Table 3.1 CONTINUED

Screening tool	Main goals	Advantages	Disadvantages
Los Angeles Motor Scale (LAMS)	• To identify stroke patients with LVO	• Can be quickly performed • Sevenfold increased incidence of LVO with LAMS>4 points	• Does not incorporate an assessment of cortical function • High chance of misdiagnosing pure motor stroke as LVO
3-Item Stroke Scale (3I-SS)	• To identify stroke patients with LVO	• Simplicity and good overall accuracy	• Scoring items not selected based on comprehensive analysis of the predictive value of NIHSS items
Cincinnati Stroke Triage Assessment Tool (C-STAT)	• To identify stroke patients with LVO	• Brevity, incorporation of gaze abnormalities	• Only computes aphasia if global and does not include neglect
Vision, Aphasia Neglect (VAN) screening tool	• To identify stroke patients with LVO	• Has been demonstrated to perform well when applied by NIHSS certified emergency room triage nurses	• Complex and time consuming to be performed by emergency medical system personnel
Field Assessment Stroke Triage for Emergency Destination (FAST-ED)	• To identify stroke patients with LVO	• Simple and has high accuracy • Balanced point distribution of motor and cortical signs	• Still needs to be prospectively tested among emergency medical personnel system
National Institutes of Health Stroke Scale (NIHSS)	• To identify stroke patients with LVO • Most commonly used in the hospital	• Excellent predictor of outcome • Has been repeatedly validated as a tool for assessing stroke severity	• Complex scoring system • Necessitates regular training

NOTES: ED = emergency department. LVO = large vessel occlusion.

contrast to the CPSS, speech assessment is based on the entire conversation with the patient, not on repeating a given sentence. The FAST acronym is easy to remember, and it has been used in multiple public education campaigns to improve knowledge of stroke signs and symptoms.

Box 3.1

CINCINNATI PREHOSPITAL STROKE SCALE (CPSS)

- Facial droop
  - Normal: both sides of face move equally
  - Abnormal: one side of face does not move
- Arm drift
  - Normal: both arms move equally or not at all
  - Abnormal: one arm drifts
- Speech
  - Normal: correct words with no slurring
  - Abnormal: slurred, inappropriate words or mute

SOURCE: Adapted with permission from Elsevier. Kothari, Rashmi U et al. "Cincinnati Prehospital Stroke Scale: Reproducibility and Validity." Ann Emerg Med. 1999 Apr;33(4):373–8.

2.4 Recognition of Stroke in the Emergency Room scale

The Recognition of Stroke in the Emergency Room (ROSIER) scoring system consists of facial palsy, hemiparesis, speech disturbances, and visual field defects

Box 3.2

LOS ANGELES PREHOSPITAL STROKE SCREEN (LAPSS)

- Screening criteria
  1. Age > 45 (Yes/No)
  2. No history of seizure or epilepsy (Yes/No)
  3. Symptom duration < 24 hours (Yes/No)
  4. At baseline, patient is not wheelchair bound or bedridden (Yes/No)
  5. Blood glucose between 60 and 400 (Yes/No)
- Exam—look for obvious asymmetry
  - Facial smile/grimace
    - Normal/right droop/left droop
  - Grip
    - Normal/right weak grip/right no grip/left weak grip/left no grip
  - Arm strength
    - Normal/right drifts down/right falls rapidly/left drifts down/left falls rapidly
  6. Based on exam, patient has only unilateral and not bilateral weakness
- If "yes" (or "unknown") to all items 1–6 then LAPPS screening criteria are met. Call receiving hospital with "code stroke."

SOURCE: Adapted with permission from Wolters Kluwer Health, Inc.. Kidwell CS, Starkman S, Eckstein M, Weems K, Saver JL. "Identifying stroke in the field. Prospective validation of the Los Angeles prehospital stroke screen (LAPSS)." Stroke 2000 Jan;31(1):71–6.

Table 3.2 THE RECOGNITION OF STROKE IN THE EMERGENCY ROOM
(ROSIER) SCALE

Question	Score description
Has there been loss of consciousness or syncope?	Yes (–1 point)
	No (0 point)
Has there been seizure activity?	Yes (–1 point)
	No (0 point)
Is there a **new acute** onset (or on awakening from sleep)?	
I. Asymmetric facial weakness	Yes (+1 point)
	No (0 point)
II. Asymmetric arm weakness	Yes (+1 point)
	No (0 point)
III. Asymmetric leg weakness	Yes (+1 point)
	No (0 point)
IV. Speech disturbance	Yes (+1 point)
	No (0 point)
V. Visual field defect	Yes (+1 point)
	No (0 point)
Total score	

NOTE: Total score: stroke is unlikely but not completely excluded if total score is 0 or less.

Adapted from Nor AM, Davis J, Sen B, et al. The Recognition of Stroke in the Emergency Room (ROSIER) scale: development and validation of a stroke recognition instrument. *Lancet Neurol.* 2005;4(11):727–734.

(Table 3.2).[10] In addition, blood glucose must be measured, and in case of hypoglycemia, assessment is postponed until blood glucose has risen above 62 mg/dL. As loss of consciousness and seizure activity are scored as –1 (if present) or 0 (if absent), the scale score can range between –2 and +5. If the total score is negative or zero, then stroke is unlikely and alternative diagnoses should be considered.[11,12] This screen was designed for the Emergency Department (ED) personnel to differentiate acute stroke from stroke mimics in the ED.

> **Question 3.2:** What is the correct way to document the time of unwitnessed stroke onset?
>
> **Answer:** The term "time of symptom discovery" refers to the time the symptoms were first discovered. Time "last known well" describes when the patient was last seen at baseline.

3 LARGE VESSEL OCCLUSION DETECTION TOOLS

Accurate identification of stroke patients with high probability of having a large vessel occlusion (LVO) is of cardinal importance considering the limited availability of CSCs and the time sensitivity of both IV alteplase and EVT (11). Clinically based LVO detection screens (sometimes referred to as "stroke severity scales") were developed to identify patients harboring LVO once the diagnosis of stroke is suspected.

3.1 Los Angeles Motor Scale

The Los Angeles Motor Scale (LAMS) is a 3-item, motor stroke-deficit screen (Table 3.3).[13] The LAMS was constructed by assigning point values to the LAPSS items of facial weakness, arm strength, and grip. While the LAPSS targets unilateral weakness only, LAMS also addresses bilateral weakness, resulting in a total score of 0–10 in bilateral weakness and 0–5 in unilateral weakness.[14]

The LAMS can be quickly performed, taking about 20–30 seconds. Although the LAMS does not incorporate an assessment of cortical function, a sevenfold increased incidence of LVO was found with LAMS ≥4 points. The disadvantage of this screen is that all patients with dense hemiplegia including those with pure motor syndrome would be directed to CSC, whereas many of these patients may actually have had a lacunar or subcortical non-LVO stroke.

3.2 3-Item Stroke Scale

The 3-Item Stroke Scale (3I-SS) is a 0–6-point screen that scores points for disturbance of consciousness, gaze/head deviation, and hemiparesis (Table 3.4).[15] The strength of this screen is its simplicity and the high overall accuracy for detection

Table 3.3 LOS ANGELES MOTOR SCALE (LAMS)

Category	Score description
Facial smile/grimace	0 – Normal
	1 – Droop, right
	1 – Droop, left
Grip	0 – Normal
	1 – Weak grip, right
	2 – No grip, right
	1 – Weak grip, left
	2 – No grip, left
Arm strength	0 – Normal
	1 – Drift, right
	2 – Falls rapidly, right
	1 – Drift, left
	2 – Falls rapidly, left

SOURCE: Adapted with permission from Wolters Kluwer Health, Inc. Nazliel et al. "A Brief Prehospital Stroke Severity Scale Identifies Ischemic Stroke Patients Harboring Persisting Large Arterial Occlusions" Stroke. 2008 Aug; 39(8): 2264–2267.

Table 3.4 3-ITEM STROKE SCALE (3I-SS)

Category	Score description
Consciousness disturbance	0 – None
	1 – Mild
	2 – Severe
Gaze and head deviation	0 – Absent
	1 – Incomplete
	2 – Complete
Hemiparesis	0 – Absent
	1 – Moderate
	2 – Severe

Adapted with permission from Wolters Kluwer Health, Inc. Singer OC et al. "A simple 3-item stroke scale: comparison with the National Institutes of Health Stroke Scale and prediction of middle cerebral artery occlusion." Stroke. 2005 Apr;36(4):773–6. Epub 2005 Feb 24.

of proximal middle cerebral artery occlusions, especially in patients with low (0–1 point) or high (≥4 points) likelihood of LVO (7).

3.3 Cincinnati Stroke Triage Assessment Tool

The Cincinnati Stroke Triage Assessment Tool (C-STAT) was developed to optimize the identification of LVO in severe anterior ischemic strokes (Box 3.3). The CPSSS is a relatively simple screen incorporating gaze, speech, and motor components of the NIHSS.[16] The advantages associated with this screen include its brevity, use of less subjective dichotomous responses, and incorporation of gaze abnormalities. The limitations to this screen are that it only computes global aphasia, thus patients do not get any points for isolated expressive or receptive aphasia. Also, the CPSSS does not specifically assess neglect; therefore, it is theoretically inferior for the detection of right-sided LVO.[17]

Box 3.3

CINCINNATI STROKE TRIAGE ASSESSMENT TOOL (C-STAT)

- Conjugate gaze deviation (2 points)
- Incorrectly answers at least one question (age, current month) **and** does not follow commands (1 point)
- Cannot hold arm up (either right, left or both) for 10 seconds (1 point)

Adapted with permission from Elsevier. Katz, BS et al. "Design and validation of a prehospital scale to predict stroke severity: Cincinnati Prehospital Stroke Severity Scale." Stroke. 2015 Jun;46(6):1508–12. doi: 10.1161/STROKEAHA.115.008804. Epub 2015 Apr 21.

3.4 Rapid Arterial oCclusion Evaluation scale

The Rapid Arterial oCclusion Evaluation (RACE) screen incorporates motor function with assessment of cortical function of each hemisphere: aphasia assessment for the left hemisphere and agnosia (the loss of the ability to recognize objects, faces, voices, places, etc.) assessment for the right hemisphere (Table 3.5).[18] When validated prospectively in the field by the EMS, the screen showed a strong correlation with the NIHSS ($r = 0.76$; $P < 0.001$). A RACE scale ≥5 had 85% sensitivity, 68% specificity, 42% positive predictive, and 94% negative predictive value for detecting LVO.[18]

There are some disadvantages to RACE including the fact that overemphasizes motor function, which, in fact, is a poor discriminator of LVO. As such, the RACE scale has a higher chance of misdiagnosing a pure motor stroke as having an LVO. This is an important issue since pure motor strokes represent approximately 13% of all strokes, and about 85% of pure motor strokes have a lacunar etiology.[19] Moreover, it gives less weight to gaze deviation, which was shown to be one of the best predictors of LVO.[16,20] Finally, while the RACE scale computes 2 points for receptive aphasia, it computes no points for expressive aphasia.

Table 3.5 RAPID ARTERIAL OCCLUSION EVALUATION (RACE) SCALE

Category	Score description
Facial palsy	0 – Absent
	1 – Mild
	2 – Moderate to severe
Arm motor function	0 – Normal
	1 – Moderate
	2 – Severe
Leg motor function	0 – Normal
	1 – Moderate
	2 – Severe
Head and gaze deviation	0 – Absent
	1 – Present
Aphasia (if right hemiparesis)	0 – Performs both tasks correctly
	1 – Performs 1 task correctly
	2 – Performs neither tasks
Agnosia (if left hemiparesis)	0 – Patient recognizes his/her arm and the impairment
	1 – Does not recognize his/her arm or the impairment
	2 – Does not recognize his/her arm nor the impairment

SOURCE: Adapted with permission from Wolters Kluwer Health, Inc. Pérez de la Ossa N et al. "Design and validation of a prehospital stroke scale to predict large arterial occlusion: the rapid arterial occlusion evaluation scale." Stroke. 2014 Jan;45(1):87–91. doi: 10.1161/STROKEAHA.113.003071. Epub 2013 Nov 26.

3.5 Vision, Aphasia Neglect scale

The Vision, Aphasia, Neglect (VAN) screening tool incorporates assessment of vision, aphasia, and neglect with motor assessment of arm strength (Box 3.4).[21] It is a dichotomous tool rather that a numeric scale, with the overall screen considered positive for weakness combined with any positive vision, aphasia, or neglect screen.

Box 3.4

VISION, APHASIA NEGLECT (VAN) SCREENING TOOL

- Part 1: How weak is the patient? Raise both arms up
  - If the patient has mild, moderate, or severe weakness—continue to Step 2.
    - Mild (minor drift)
    - Moderate (severe drift)
    - Severe (flaccid or no antigravity)
  - Patient shows no weakness—patient is VAN "negative."
- Part 2
  - Visual disturbance
    - Field cut (which side) (4 quadrants)
    - Double vision (ask patient to look to right then left; evaluate for uneven eyes)
    - New onset blindness
    - None
  - Aphasia
    - Expressive (inability to speak or paraphasic errors); do not count slurring of words
    - Receptive (not understanding or following commands)
    - Mixed
    - None
  - Neglect
    - Forced gaze or inability to track to one side
    - Unable to feel both sides at the same time or unable to identify own arm
    - Ignoring one side
    - None
- If the patient has weakness and any other positive finding among the vision, aphasia, or neglect categories, he or she is considered VAN "positive"

SOURCE: Adapted from Teleb MS, Ver Hage A, Carter J, et al Stroke vision, aphasia, neglect (VAN) assessment—a novel emergent large vessel occlusion screening tool: pilot study and comparison with current clinical severity indices Journal of NeuroInterventional Surgery Published Online First: 17 February 2016. doi: 10.1136/neurintsurg-2015-012131.

The initial and essential action of the VAN examination is to perform a motor function assessment. Patients are asked to raise both arms up and hold them up for 10 seconds. If the patient has mild drift, severe weakness, or paralysis, the assessment continues. In their absence, the patient is VAN "negative" and the assessment ends. If any motor weakness (mild drift, severe weakness, or paralysis) is observed, the VAN assessment is continued. If the patient has weakness and any other positive finding among the vision, aphasia, or neglect categories, they are considered VAN "positive" and, as such, having a high likelihood of an LVO.

The main disadvantage of the VAN screen is that, in comparison with other screens, it requires EMS personnel to become familiar with and be able to perform many additional tests including detailed visual field examination, which can be difficult to accomplish on many stroke patients.

3.6 Field Assessment Stroke Triage for Emergency Destination scale

The Field Assessment Stroke Triage for Emergency Destination (FAST-ED) screen is based on items of the NIHSS with higher predictive value for LVO (Table 3.6).[22] In a study of 727 patients who underwent computed tomographic angiography (CTA) within the first 24 hours of stroke onset, FAST-ED demonstrated comparable accuracy in predicting LVO to the NIHSS.[22] In the same cohort, the FAST-ED showed higher accuracy than the RACE and CPSS screens in predictive LVO. A score of ≥4 had sensitivity of 0.60, specificity of 0.89, positive predictive value of 0.72, and negative predictive value of 0.82 for predicting LVO.

The FAST-ED screen was further tested in the Bernese Stroke cohort of 1,085 patients with anterior circulation strokes who underwent CTA or magnetic resonance angiography within 6 hours of symptom onset.[23] FAST-ED showed the best performance when compared to other prehospital scales (area under the curve FAST-ED = 0.847; NIHSS = 0.846; RACE = 0.831; CPSS = 0.802).[24] These scores likely reflect the more balanced point distribution across motor and other better discriminative cortical functions within the scale.

3.7 FAST-ED Smartphone app

The FAST-ED app is a smartphone application that assists EMS professionals to make decisions regarding the most appropriate destination for any given stroke patient in the field (Case 3.1). The application is based on an algorithm that comprises a brief series of questions including the patient's age, time last known normal, anticoagulant usage, and stroke symptoms.[25] The system also includes information about the different regional stroke centers according to their capability

Table 3.6 FIELD ASSESSMENT STROKE TRIAGE FOR EMERGENCY DESTINATION (FAST-ED) SCALE

Category	Score description
Facial palsy	0 – Normal or minor paralysis
	1 – Partial or complete paralysis
Arm weakness	0 – No drift
	1 – Drift or some effort against gravity
	2 – No effort against gravity or no movement
Speech changes	0 – Absent
	1 – Mild to moderate
	2 – Severe, global aphasia or mute
Eye deviation	0 – Absent
	1 – Partial
	2 – Forced deviation
Denial/neglect	0 – Absent
	1 – Extinction to bilateral simultaneous stimulation in only 1 sensory domain
	2 – Does not recognize own hand or orients only to one side of the body

SOURCE: Published with permission from Wolters Kluwer Health, Inc. Lima, FO et al. "Field Assessment Stroke Triage for Emergency Destination." Stroke. 2016; STROKEAHA.116.013301

to provide endovascular treatment as well as Global Positioning System (GPS) technology with real-time traffic information for the accurate calculation of transportation times.

3.8 National Institutes of Health Stroke Scale

The NIHSS is the most commonly used in-hospital acute stroke severity score (Table 3.7).[26] There is a strong relationship between the neurological deficit as measured by the NIHSS and the presence of a proximal arterial occlusion.[27,28] Although the NIHSS has proven useful in the context of clinical trials and in-hospital care, it remains a complex scoring system necessitating regular training and deeper medical knowledge for its accurate application.

For prehospital assessment of stroke severity, shortened versions of the NIHSS (sNIHSS) have been developed, using 8 (sNIHSS-8) or 5 (sNIHSS-5) items of the NIHSS that were found to be most predictive of outcome at 3 months. The items on the sNIHSS-5 are gaze, visual field, motor function of the right and left leg, and

Table 3.7 The National Institutes of Health Stroke Scale (NIHSS)

Category	Score description
Level of consciousness (LOC)	0 – alert 1 – easily arousable by minor stimulation 2 – not alert, requires repeated stimulation; 3 – unresponsive/flaccid
LOC questions (current month and patient's age)	0 – answers both questions correctly 1 – one question correctly 2 – answers neither question correctly
LOC one-step commands	0 – performs both tasks correctly 1 – preforms one command correctly 2 – performs neither command correctly
Gaze	0 – normal gaze 1 – partial gaze palsy 2 – forced deviation or total palsy
Vision (visual fields)	0 – no visual loss 1 – partial hemianopia 2 – complete hemianopia 3 – bilateral hemianopia or cortical blindness
Face	0 – normal 1 – minor paralysis 2 – partial paralysis (lower face) 3 – complete paralysis (of one or both side)
Motor arm	0 – no drift 1 – drift 2 – some effort against gravity 3 – no effort against gravity 4 – no movement
Motor leg	0 – no drift 1 – drift 2 – some effort against gravity 3 – no effort against gravity 4 – no movement
Limb ataxia	0 – absent 1 – present in one limb 2 – present in two limbs
Sensory	0 – normal 1 – mild or moderate sensory loss 2 – severe or total sensory loss
Language	0 – normal 1 – mild or moderate aphasia 2 – severe aphasia 3 – global aphasia or patient is mute

Table 3.7 CONTINUED

Category	Score description
Dysarthria	0 – normal
	1 – mild or moderate dysarthria;
	2 – severe dysarthria
	UN – intubate
Extinction and inattention	0 – normal
	1 – deficit in one modality
	2 – deficit in more than one modality or profound deficit

Adapted from https://stroke.nih.gov/resources/scale.htm

language, with the sNIHSS-8 additionally assessing the level of consciousness, facial paresis, and dysarthria.[29,30]

4 PREHOSPITAL STROKE ASSESSMENT TOOLS— SIGNIFICANCE AND IMPLEMENTATION

There is currently insufficient evidence to define which screen is best for recognizing acute stroke and identifying LVO in patients with a suspected stroke. The American Heart Association (AHA) recommends that each EMS region choose a single screening tool and severity tool for use across all EMS providers. It is important for EMS medical directors and stroke specialists involved in prehospital stroke care to understand and compare these tools so that they can identify the tool that performs optimally for their individual needs.

5 CLINICAL CASE

Case 3.1 Acute stroke with high likelihood of LVO

CASE DESCRIPTION

A 74-year-old man with a past medical history of hypertension and ischemic cardiomyopathy was found by the daughter at home and unable to move the left side of the body. The daughter recalled seeing signs of a stroke on a FAST billboard and called 911. When the paramedics arrived, they found the patient to have right gaze deviation and left hemiplegia. Time "last known well" was 5 hours earlier. The patient was outside the time window for IV thrombolysis. The FAST-ED score was calculated to be 6 (indicating 60–85% probability of LVO), and using the FAST-ED app (Figure 3.2), the team transported the patient to the nearest CSC for possible thrombectomy. On arrival at the ED, the patient's NIHSS score was 17. Non-contrast computed tomography (CT) ruled out intracerebral hemorrhage.

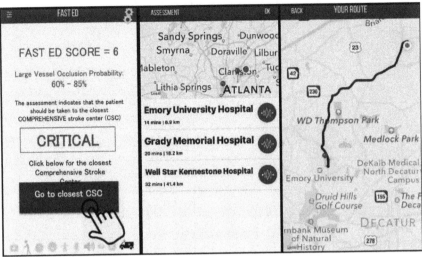

Figure 3.2 Acute stroke with high likelihood of large-vessel occlusion—Field Assessment Stroke Triage for Emergency Destination (FAST-ED) application. The screenshots showing the FAST-ED application.

(Left) The application calculates the probability of large vessel occlusion and assists emergency medical services in identify the most appropriate level of care, depending on patient's eligibility for intravenous alteplase and/or endovascular thrombectomy. The decision-making algorithm relies on a series of questions including patient's anticoagulant usage, time last known well, and symptoms.

(Middle) The application also includes the database of all regional stroke centers.

(Right) The application provides real-time traffic information to the different neighboring stroke centers.

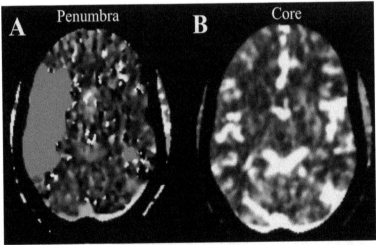

Figure 3.3 Acute stroke with high likelihood of large vessel occlusion—computed tomography perfusion.

(A) Computed tomography perfusion (CTP) showing an area of ischemic penumbra within the right middle cerebral artery territory.

(B) No significant ischemic core is present on CTP.

The Alberta Stroke Program Early CT score was above 5. CT perfusion revealed large area of ischemic penumbra (Figure 3.3). The patient was immediately taken for endovascular thrombectomy, resulting in successful recanalization of the right middle cerebral artery occlusion.

PRACTICAL POINTS

- In this case, a family member correctly recognized signs of acute stroke using the FAST tool. Because of its simplicity, this tool is commonly utilized in awareness campaigns to help the public recognize and seek immediate help if stroke is suspected.
- The FAST-ED app was used in this case to help the paramedics identify the most appropriate level of care. The application considers multiple different scenarios. If the patient is not a likely candidate for either IV alteplase or EVT based on the time from symptom onset, stroke severity, and certain contraindications, that individual is preferentially referred to the closest stroke center (either PSC, ASRH, or CSC). If the patient is likely a candidate for both IV alteplase and EVT, the algorithm takes into consideration the likelihood of LVO and the additional transportation time from the closest center to CSC.
- At the time of preparing this chapter, the AHA, in its severity-based stroke triage algorithm, recognized the lack of randomized trial data to support a firm recommendation on the acceptable delay when considering re-routing a patient to CSC for possible EVT.[31] The AHA committee agreed on setting the additional time delay to 15 minutes, however, adding that longer delays of up to 30 minutes may be reasonable in rural communities.

REFERENCES

1. Lees KR, Bluhmki E, von Kummer R, et al. Time to treatment with intravenous alteplase and outcome in stroke: an updated pooled analysis of ECASS, ATLANTIS, NINDS, and EPITHET trials. *Lancet.* 2010;375(9727):1695–1703.
2. Saver JL, Goyal M, van der Lugt A, et al. Time to treatment with endovascular thrombectomy and outcomes from ischemic stroke: a meta-analysis. *JAMA.* 2016;316(12):1279–1288.
3. Goyal M, Menon BK, van Zwam WH, et al. Endovascular thrombectomy after large-vessel ischaemic stroke: a meta-analysis of individual patient data from five randomised trials. *Lancet.* 2016;387(10029):1723–1731.
4. Kothari RU, Pancioli A, Liu T, Brott T, Broderick J. Cincinnati Prehospital Stroke Scale: reproducibility and validity. *Ann Emerg Med.* 1999;33(4):373–378.
5. Kothari R, Hall K, Brott T, Broderick J. Early stroke recognition: developing an out-of-hospital NIH Stroke Scale. *Acad Emerg Med.* 1997;4(10):986–990.
6. Liferidge AT, Brice JH, Overby BA, Evenson KR. Ability of laypersons to use the Cincinnati Prehospital Stroke Scale. *Prehosp Emerg Care.* 2004;8(4):384–387.

7. De Luca A, Giorgi Rossi P, Villa GF, Stroke Group Italian Society Pre Hospital Emergency Services. The use of Cincinnati Prehospital Stroke Scale during telephone dispatch interview increases the accuracy in identifying stroke and transient ischemic attack symptoms. *BMC Health Serv Res.* 2013;13:513.

8. Kidwell CS, Starkman S, Eckstein M, Weems K, Saver JL. Identifying stroke in the field: prospective validation of the Los Angeles prehospital stroke screen (LAPSS). *Stroke.* 2000;31(1):71–76.

9. Kidwell CS, Saver JL, Schubert GB, Eckstein M, Starkman S. Design and retrospective analysis of the Los Angeles Prehospital Stroke Screen (LAPSS). *Prehosp Emerg Care.* 1998;2(4):267–273.

10. Nor AM, Davis J, Sen B, et al. The Recognition of Stroke in the Emergency Room (ROSIER) scale: development and validation of a stroke recognition instrument. *Lancet Neurol.* 2005;4(11):727–734.

11. Whiteley WN, Wardlaw JM, Dennis MS, Sandercock PA. Clinical scores for the identification of stroke and transient ischaemic attack in the Emergency Department: a cross-sectional study. *J Neurol Neurosurg Psychiatry.* 2011;82(9):1006–1010.

12. Mingfeng H, Zhixin W, Qihong G, Lianda L, Yanbin Y, Jinfang F. Validation of the use of the ROSIER scale in prehospital assessment of stroke. *Ann Indian Acad Neurol.* 2012;15(3):191–195.

13. Llanes JN, Kidwell CS, Starkman S, Leary MC, Eckstein M, Saver JL. The Los Angeles Motor Scale (LAMS): a new measure to characterize stroke severity in the field. *Prehosp Emerg Care.* 2004;8(1):46–50.

14. Kim JT, Chung PW, Starkman S, et al. Field Validation of the Los Angeles Motor Scale as a tool for paramedic assessment of stroke severity. *Stroke.* 2017;48(2):298–306.

15. Singer OC, Dvorak F, du Mesnil de Rochemont R, Lanfermann H, Sitzer M, Neumann-Haefelin T. A simple 3-item stroke scale: comparison with the National Institutes of Health Stroke Scale and prediction of middle cerebral artery occlusion. *Stroke.* 2005;36(4):773–776.

16. Katz BS, McMullan JT, Sucharew H, Adeoye O, Broderick JP. Design and validation of a prehospital scale to predict stroke severity: Cincinnati Prehospital Stroke Severity Scale. *Stroke.* 2015;46(6):1508–1512.

17. Kummer BR, Gialdini G, Sevush JL, Kamel H, Patsalides A, Navi BB. External validation of the Cincinnati Prehospital Stroke Severity Scale. *J Stroke Cerebrovasc Dis.* 2016;25(5):1270–1274.

18. Perez de la Ossa N, Carrera D, Gorchs M, et al. Design and validation of a prehospital stroke scale to predict large arterial occlusion: the Rapid Arterial Occlusion Evaluation scale. *Stroke.* 2014;45(1):87–91.

19. Arboix A, Padilla I, Massons J, Garcia-Eroles L, Comes E, Targa C. Clinical study of 222 patients with pure motor stroke. *J Neurol Neurosurg Psychiatry.* 2001;71(2):239–242.

20. Heldner MR, Hsieh K, Broeg-Morvay A, et al. Clinical prediction of large vessel occlusion in anterior circulation stroke: mission impossible? *J Neurol.* 2016;263(8):1633–1640.

21. Teleb MS, Ver Hage A, Carter J, Jayaraman MV, McTaggart RA. Stroke vision, aphasia, neglect (VAN) assessment: a novel emergent large vessel occlusion screening tool:

pilot study and comparison with current clinical severity indices. *J Neurointerv Surg.* 2017;9(2):122–126.

22. Lima FO, Silva GS, Furie KL, et al. Field Assessment stroke triage for emergency destination: a simple and accurate prehospital scale to detect large vessel occlusion strokes. *Stroke.* 2016;47(8):1997–2002.

23. Heldner MR, Mattle HP, Fischer U. Letter by Heldner et al regarding article, "Field Assessment Stroke Triage for Emergency Destination: a simple and accurate prehospital scale to detect large vessel occlusion strokes." *Stroke.* 2016;47(12):e274.

24. Lima FO, Silva GS, Nogueira RG. Response by Lima et al to letter regarding article, "Field Assessment Stroke Triage for Emergency Destination: a simple and accurate prehospital scale to detect large vessel occlusion strokes." *Stroke.* 2016;47(12):e275–e276.

25. Nogueira RG, Silva GS, Lima FO, et al. The FAST-ED App: a smartphone platform for the field triage of patients with stroke. *Stroke.* 2017;48(5):1278–1284.

26. Brott T, Adams HP, Jr., Olinger CP, et al. Measurements of acute cerebral infarction: a clinical examination scale. *Stroke.* 1989;20(7):864–870.

27. Heldner MR, Zubler C, Mattle HP, et al. National Institutes of Health stroke scale score and vessel occlusion in 2152 patients with acute ischemic stroke. *Stroke.* 2013;44(4):1153–1157.

28. Fischer U, Arnold M, Nedeltchev K, et al. NIHSS score and arteriographic findings in acute ischemic stroke. *Stroke.* 2005;36(10):2121–2125.

29. Demeestere J, Garcia-Esperon C, Lin L, et al. Validation of the National Institutes of Health Stroke Scale-8 to detect large vessel occlusion in ischemic stroke. *J Stroke Cerebrovasc Dis.* 2017;26(7):1419–1426.

30. Tirschwell DL, Longstreth WT, Jr., Becker KJ, et al. Shortening the NIH Stroke scale for use in the prehospital setting. *Stroke.* 2002;33(12):2801–2806.

31. Association AH. Mission: Lifeline Stroke—Severity-based stroke triage algorithm for EMS. 2017; http://www.heart.org/HEARTORG/Professional/MissionLifelineHomePage/Mission-Lifeline-Stroke_UCM_491623_SubHomePage.jsp.

4

Prehospital Assessment of Stroke

Mobile Stroke Units

ANDREW BLAKE BULETKO, JASON MATHEW,
TAPAN THACKER, LILA SHEIKHI, ANDREW RUSSMAN,
AND M. SHAZAM HUSSAIN ■

CONTENTS

1 INTRODUCTION

Mobile stroke units (MSUs) are a major advancement in prehospital stroke treatment. Through performance of in-field computed tomography (CT) imaging and physician presence, either in person or through telemedicine, administration of intravenous (IV) alteplase and other acute therapies can be performed. Since the first MSU was launched in 2008, there has been an increasing number of MSUs around the world. Compared to standard care, current evidence shows MSUs are able to deliver IV alteplase faster, have higher rates of treatment with IV alteplase, and transport patients more often to appropriate levels of care. Studies are also ongoing to establish benefit in clinical outcomes and cost-effectiveness. Though still in its early stages, prehospital stroke assessment with a MSU is becoming more widely recognized as an efficient, feasible, and integral component of acute advanced stroke systems of care. We will cover important concepts in the advent and growth of MSUs including time-based treatment benefit, clinical process efficiency, application of telemedicine, imaging capabilities, transport destination and triage, cost effectiveness, and clinical outcomes (Figure 4.1).

2 HISTORY OF MOBILE STROKE UNITS

In May 2003, the specific characteristics of a MSU were proposed by Dr. Klaus Faßbender and colleagues from the University of Saarland (Homburg,

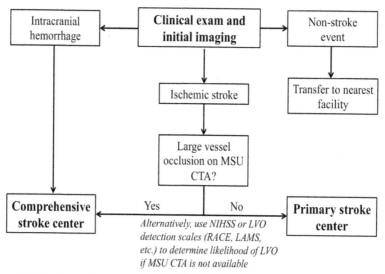

Figure 4.1 Mobile stroke unit triage algorithm.
ABBREVIATIONS: CTA, computed tomography angiography; LAMS, Los Angeles motor scale; LVO, large vessel occlusion; MSU, mobile stroke unit; NIHSS, National Institutes of Health stroke scale; RACE, Rapid arterial occlusion evaluation.

Germany).[1] Dr. Faßbender and colleagues then launched the first MSU in 2008, operating within a mixed, but predominantly urban environment, around Homburg, Germany. In 2011, Dr. Heinrich Audebert and colleagues at Charité Hospital (Berlin, Germany) began to operate the second MSU under the STEMO program in the Berlin, Germany area in cooperation with the Berlin Fire Brigade. The MSU concept then spread to the United States in 2014, with the launching of MSUs at both the University of Texas (Houston, Texas) and the Cleveland Clinic (Cleveland, Ohio). Growth of MSU programs have increased exponentially with more than 15 programs currently operational at the time of this publication and dozens of programs in various stages of development worldwide.

3 "TIME IS BRAIN" IS ACUTE STROKE

Currently, IV alteplase and endovascular thrombectomy (EVT) for large vessel occlusions (LVO) are the only Food and Drug-approved therapies for acute ischemic stroke (AIS). Both therapies rely on rapid recognition of acute stroke symptoms and administration of IV alteplase or EVT, according to national and international guidelines.[2,3] Favorable outcomes at 3 months were more likely achieved when IV alteplase was given earlier (OR 2.55 within 0–90 minutes, 1.64 within 91–180 minutes, 1.34 within 180–270 minutes).[4]

Unfortunately, many patients arrive either late or outside the time window for treatment. In an analysis of the American Heart Association Get with the Guidelines Stroke program from 2002 to 2009, only 25.1% of patients arrived within the 3-hour time window for IV alteplase, and upon extension of the time window to 4.5 hours the percentage of eligible patients only increased by 6.3%. Moreover, patients treated within 60 minutes of symptom onset (termed the "golden hour") were more likely to be discharged home and free from disability, but only about 1.3% of all stroke patients are treated within this timeframe with conventional, Emergency Department (ED) care.[4]

This was further supported by the American Heart Association "Target: Stroke Initiative" data, which showed that implementation of a quality improvement program directed toward achieving administration of IV alteplase within 60 minutes resulted in lower in-hospital mortality, increased percentage of patients discharged home, and lower rates of intracranial hemorrhage.[5]

Question 4.1: What are the barriers to a wider use of MSU?

Answer: High start-up and maintenance costs of MSU, lack of IV alteplase reimbursement when given in the prehospital environment, licensing, and radiation safety.

4 MOBILE STROKE UNIT PERSONNEL AND PROCESS

The key components of MSUs include on-board CT scanner, laboratory equipment and personnel, including physician presence either in person or via telemedicine. Figure 4.2 shows the Cleveland Clinic MSU. The exact size of vehicle, crew, and presence of physician varies depending on local factors. The Cleveland emergency medical services (EMS) utilizes a 4-person crew, including an emergency medical technician (EMT),

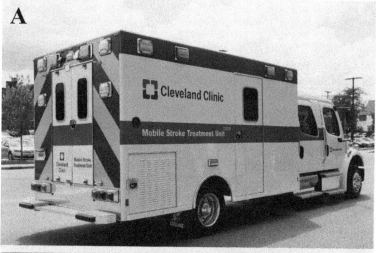

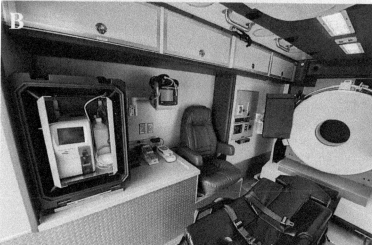

Figure 4.2 Mobile stroke unit at the Cleveland Clinic.
(A) Outside and (B) inside views are shown.

paramedic, critical care nurse, and CT technologist who is also cross trained as EMT. Physician presence on the vehicle is provided via telemedicine, though the majority of MSUs worldwide still have a physician directly on the vehicle. In the German system, direct physician presence on MSU is in keeping with their present prehospital system of care, due to all prehospital Advanced Life Support responses requiring physician presence. In other countries, where direct physician presence is not the norm in the prehospital setting, such as the United States, having a physician on board is a significant resource to add, and it is likely that most systems will incorporate telemedicine.

4.1 Utilization of mobile stroke units

Utilization of a MSU relies on early recognition of stroke symptoms. In Cleveland, the MSU is dispatched simultaneously with municipal EMS for all presumed AIS patients according to an algorithm utilized by the dispatching center. Municipal EMS is usually the first-responder and performs the initial assessment including prehospital stroke scale (e.g., Cincinnati Stroke Scale), then transitions care to the MSU upon their arrival if AIS is still suspected. If AIS is not suspected, MSU activation is cancelled and the ambulance returns to its base station.

Of the first 317 activations of the Cleveland Clinic MSU, 217 (68%) resulted in cancellations.[6] According to the PHANTOM-S study, a large randomized controlled trial comparing MSU and standard emergency services, only 56 dispatches out of 208 (27%) were cancelled.[7] Of note, their MSU is deployed simultaneously with conventional EMS. Thus, the variability in cancellation rates may be a reflection of different dispatch algorithms or prehospital stroke scales, but limited data exist comparing various cancellation rates among MSUs. Of all patients transported by MSUs, 50–70% are ultimately diagnosed with stroke.[8,9]

Once care is assumed by MSU, the patient is placed on monitors to obtain vital signs, blood is drawn and analyzed for prothrombin time/international normalized ratio (INR; Coagucheck®, Roche, Indianapolis, Indiana), CBC (POCH-100i™, McKesson, Lincolnshire, Illinois), and BMP (i-STAT, Abbott, Princeton, New Jersey), and CT scanning is completed while ambulance remains stationary at the site. Once the CT scan is complete, the crew with the stroke neurologist via telemedicine assesses the patient and makes a determination for alteplase if the patient is a candidate. The patient is then triaged to the most appropriate center. In selected cases, CT angiography (CTA) can be performed on the vehicle prior to triage determination to assess the presence of emergent LVO, so that the patient can be transferred to an interventional capable center immediately, rather than taking the patient to the closest non-interventional center, thereby avoiding a secondary transfer.

4.2 Role of telemedicine

The Cleveland Clinic was the first MSU to solely utilize telemedicine (audio and video connection plus CT image transfer) for assessment by a stroke physician prior to treatment with IV alteplase. Prior to this, few studies looked at the feasibility of telemedicine on ambulances. Liman et al. tested the feasibility of telestroke based ambulances in Berlin, Germany, and reliability of the National Institutes of Health Stroke Scale (NIHSS) assessment.[10] However, the telestroke system utilized a third-generation commercial cellular network, and more than half of the assessments were incomplete due to absence or loss of audio video signal.[10] With the improvement of cellular network transmission, the feasibility of telestroke on specialized ambulances became clearer.

Analysis of the first 100 patients treated on the Cleveland Clinic MSU revealed telemedicine utilization on the MSU yielded shorter door to IV alteplase times compared to traditional EMS with low rates of technical failure.[6] More specifically, 93% of the telemedicine encounters were executed without disruptions. The low rate of disruptions that occurred were secondary to areas of poor network reception and did not result in significant treatment delays.

Similarly, Wu et al., using a fourth-generation network connection, concluded that telemedicine in Houston MSU was feasible with 85% of encounters conducted without disruption.[11] The Houston MSU has the unique capability of telestroke assessment, as well as an on-site vascular neurologist. Wu et al. showed that telemedicine-based MSU had an 88% agreement in IV alteplase decision making with on-site vascular neurologists, thereby supporting the reliability and accuracy of telemedicine on MSU.[11] Telestroke evaluation would be incomplete without access to CT scans. It is important to note, in addition to the low likelihood of technical failure during encounters, CT was fully completed in 99/100 cases in Cleveland MSU. However, in 5 of the cases, there were short delays in image transfer due to poor connectivity.[6]

Telemedicine and teleradiology in the field will rely on advanced cellular networks (4G/LTE) at present, and their usefulness in areas with poor cellular coverage (especially remote rural areas) may be limited. However, as cellular networks advance, the speeds of transmission of imaging (including larger data sets seen with CTA/CT profusion) and reliability of telemedicine interactions will only continue to improve.

4.3 Imaging capabilities

The on-board CT scanner can perform non-contrast CT head, CTA of the intracranial vessels allowing for detection for LVO (Case 4.1, Figure 4.3; Case 4.2, Figure 4.4), and has the capability to perform CT perfusion.[12] There are several portable CT scanners on the market, including the CereTom (Neurologica Samsung, Danvers, Maine), the Tomoscan (Phillips Medical Systems, Best, the Netherlands), and the xCAT ENT (Xo-ran technologies, Ann Arbor, Michigan) each varying in their designs, imaging capabilities, and intended uses.[13] Siemens has also developed a mobile stroke solution, with a 16-slice CT scanner with a full bore and ability to perform CT and full CTA from the aortic arch to the intracranial vasculature. However, the CT scanner requires a larger truck to house it due to its size, and this MSU is presently the largest unit to date.

4.3.1 PORTABLE CT SCANNERS

Portable scanners have smaller gantry aperture, which allows for smaller size and reduced power requirements making them suitable for use in the MSU.[15] The smaller gantry aperture remains adequate for brain, affording an image field of view (FOV) of 25 cm versus 22 cm FOV used for our conventional fixed CT brain scanner. A distinct disadvantage for smaller bore scanners is the potential for truncation artifact when the subject is not centered. Furthermore, slower gantry motion and absence of gantry tilt leads to reduced temporal resolution especially with motion and increased artifacts from the dental amalgams or skull base, respectively.[12]

When comparing images obtained from portable CT scanners and standard CT scanner in 60 patients, image quality was reported to be inferior in portable CT imaging, including decreased contrast between gray and white matter, higher level of noise, and increased artifacts. However, all the images obtained were still considered to be of adequate diagnostic quality on direct comparisons allowing for accurate diagnosis and treatment decisions.[13] There have been case reports with successful use of CTA on MSU enabling rapid detection and triaging of patients with LVO to thrombectomy-capable centers allowing for reduced time to endovascular treatment, but larger scale studies regarding feasibility of CTA on MSU are lacking.[14]

Due to the resolution differences between the portable and fixed CT scanners, safety concerns are raised with the possibility of missing subtle hemorrhages in patients being considered for IV alteplase. Review of the literature did not show any differences in the sensitivity of detecting hemorrhages in stroke patients between portable and fixed CT scanners. A large randomized trial showed a trend toward lower rates of post-IV alteplase hemorrhage in MSU-treated patients compared to conventionally treated IV alteplase patients though this was not statistically significant (3.5% in MSU vs. 6.8% in conventional treatment; $p = 0.06$).[15]

4.4 Destination determination

The need for a prehospital system for destination and transfer is crucial in delivering "the right patient, to the right hospital, the first time." A well-designed system should minimize delays in the chain of survival beginning with EMS dispatch.

Non-contrast head CT remains one of the key components in the hyperacute stroke treatment decision-making process. Along with a non-contrast head CT, CTA capabilities, and laboratory testing equipment, primary stroke centers should also be equipped to complete NIHSS, administer IV alteplase, and ultimately use clinical and diagnostic information to triage patients for possible endovascular therapy. Additional considerations include therapies for the management of other acute neurologic emergencies, such as reversal of anticoagulation with prothrombin concentrate complex (PCC) in the event of identification of a hemorrhagic stroke or antiepileptic therapies.

Using these components, a MSU should function as an on-scene primary stroke center. Once the initial diagnosis and treatment decision is made, the patient should be triaged to the most appropriate center able to care for his or her condition, and if multiple centers are presence, patient or family preference should be taken into account.

Wendt et al. showed that patients with ischemic stroke transported by conventional methods were taken to hospitals without a stroke unit 10.1% of the time compared with 3.9% in patients evaluated by a MSU. In the same study, MSU patients with intracranial hemorrhages were taken to hospitals without a neurosurgery department in 43% of the conventional care group compared to 11.3% in the MSU group.[16] This finding emphasizes both the importance and the feasibility of appropriately triaging patients with acute strokes.

In Cleveland, patients are first triaged to the appropriate level of care and then are taken to the patient's choice hospital regardless of affiliation as long as that hospital meets level-appropriate care. The neurologist assessing the patient through telemedicine calls the ED of the destination hospital and gives a report to an ED physician or neurologist. In addition, the MSU crew gives report to accepting facility about history, exam, and any known past medical history along with physician and nurse documentation, lab results obtained on MSU, and with a CD containing the initial CT imaging.

4.4.1 MOBILE STROKE UNITS AND ENDOVASCULAR THERAPY

Triage for EVT has been shown to benefit from initial evaluation by a MSU. Substantial reductions in times have been described in door to initial CT, door to departure to CSC, and CT time to endovascular treatment.[6,17] MSUs are now recognized as part of advanced stroke systems of care and allow for prehospital clinical efficiency unmatched by traditional ED evaluation, especially for patients presenting within an IV alteplase or endovascular treatment window or with intracranial hemorrhage. It is crucial that MSUs optimize the transport of patients to hospital destinations that provide appropriate level of care (Case 4.1; Figure 4.3; Case 4.2; Figure 4.4; Case 4.3).

5 EFFECT ON TIME TO TREATMENT

In an analysis of the first 100 patients managed on the Cleveland Clinic MSU, median alarm to CT completion (33 minutes, interquartile range [IQR] 29–41) was shorter in the MSU group compared to traditional EMS (56 minutes, IQR 47–68).[18] Similarly, median MSU alarm to CT completion times in Berlin and Homberg, Germany, were 35 minutes (IQR 30–42) and 34 minutes (IQR 30–38), respectively.[8,9] Dispatch to IV alteplase time for Cleveland MSU was 38.5 minutes shorter (median 55.5 minutes, IQR 46–65) in comparison to controls.[18]

The PHANTOM-S study in Germany also showed similar dispatch to IV alteplase reductions compared to controls of 24 minutes and 34 minutes, respectively, with median dispatch to IV alteplase time in PHANTOM-S of 48 minutes.[8] The rate of IV alteplase among MSUs varies between 16–30%, whereas conventional IV alteplase rates for AIS range from 3.4–9.1%.[8,9,17,18]

6 EFFECT ON CLINICAL OUTCOMES

Meta-analyses have shown that effects of IV alteplase in patients with AIS depend on when it is administered in relation to time of stroke onset. If administered in less than 90 minutes, the numbers needed to treat (NNT) were 4–5 compared to a NNT of 9 for those treated within 91–180 minutes and 14 if treated within 181–270 minutes. Median onset-to-drug treatment times of 144 minutes and 140 min have been described in the United States and Europe, respectively.[19,20]

Better short-term outcomes have been reported when IV alteplase is administered within 60 minutes from time of onset. In the Target: Stroke quality improvement initiative published by Fonarow et al., modeling best practices in prehospital and ED care reduced median door-to-needle time for IV alteplase administration from 77 minutes to 67 minutes and increased the percentage of patients receiving IV alteplase within 60 minutes from 26.5% to 41.3%. Improving door-to-needle times by 10 minutes result in reduced in-hospital mortality, fewer symptomatic intracranial hemorrhages, fewer alteplase-related complications, increased stroke discharges to home, and higher rates of ambulatory independence at discharge.[5] In another comparison, a MSU was able to administer IV alteplase within 60 minutes, sixfold more often than conventional care. Though long-term outcomes were not observed, stroke patients were more likely to be discharged home and had no increased treatment risks.[21]

At the time of this review, there has only been one published observational study looking at 90-day functional outcomes of patients treated with prehospital IV alteplase in a MSU (n = 305) compared with conventional care (n = 353).[22] MSU care resulted in no difference in the proportion of patients living without disability at 90-days. Secondary outcomes analysis showed the proportion of patients with a modified Rankin scale score 0–3 (83% vs. 74%, p = 0.004) and mortality at 90 days (6% vs. 10%, p = 0.022) were more favorable in patients treated in a MSU than a traditional ED. Intracranial hemorrhage due to thrombolytic therapy and 7-day mortality did not differ between the two groups.

Two prospective studies are ongoing at the time of this review investigating 90-day functional outcomes, with the blinded outcome assessment by Ebinger et al.[23] and a randomized control trial by Yamal et al.[24] with additional evaluation on quality of life and post stroke costs. With the increasing numbers of MSUs being utilized throughout the world, along with follow-up treated patients over longer periods of time, further studies are in progress to explore clinical outcome data, specifically with regards to functional outcomes.

Question 4.2: What is the cost of operating an MSU?

Answer: Excluding staff costs, it is estimated that a single MSU costs approximately $600,000 in the first year, and $80,000/year in the subsequent years.

7 COST-EFFECTIVENESS

The average annual direct cost of stroke in the United States was $17.2 billion from 2011 to 2012, and mean expense per patient for direct care was $4,830. These direct medical stroke-related costs are projected to triple by 2030.[25] Though specific studies have not been published to compare cost-effectiveness of MSU to conventional care, there have been publications looking at MSU cost-effectiveness.

Looking at prehospital direct costs, Dietrich et al. reported a 1-year benefit–cost ratio of 1.96 with possibility of further MSU direct cost reduction with use of reduced MSU crew and through telemedicine utilization. This benefit was positively related to population density but was also greater than unity in rural settings (defined as 79 inhabitants per square kilometer or 202 inhabitants per square mile).[26]

Cost effectiveness in MSU was also analyzed in the PHANTOM-S study with net annual cost of MSU of €963,954. MSU-treated patients were treated earlier and more frequently with IV alteplase than conventional care leading to an annual health gain of avoidance of 18 patients with disability (29.7 quality-adjusted life-years) and an incremental cost-effectiveness ratio of €32,456 per quality-adjusted life-year.[27]

Future studies dedicated to assessing cost-effectiveness of MSUs, both short- and long-term, will provide better insight into the benefits and challenge from a societal and institutional planning perspective. Early studies have shown that MSUs have the potential of providing cost-effective, prehospital care to acute stroke patients, especially in densely populated areas.

8 LESSONS LEARNED

The creation of a MSU program is a difficult challenge, requiring the input of multiple, important stakeholders including city officials, EMS providers, transport teams, emergency and intensive care units and EDs, hospital administration, competing hospitals, and state and national regulators, to name a few. It is critically important to engage these stakeholders early and acquire their support and input, as each group will bring unique perspectives to ensure the success of the program. Training of multiple groups who will contact these patients on the care continuum is also important, including but not limited to EMS dispatchers, EMS personnel, hospital critical care transport personnel, and the receiving teams at each hospital to ensure they understand the role and benefits of MSU is helpful.

As MSU remains a relatively new concept, there is ample space for continued refinement and improvement in processes and procedures. As an example, we noted certain artifacts in the CT scans of our first patients, but through work with our radiologist and CT technologists aboard the vehicle, we were able to refine the CT acquisition to provide substantial improvement. New equipment such as better head-holders, which can attach to ambulance stretchers have been developed uniquely to aid in patients treated on MSUs.

Finally, it is important to note that MSU is a great advancement in stroke care, but this does not replace systems continuing to work on their basic infrastructure for stroke care, including prenotification of the ED for incoming patients and ED processes to ensure rapid assessment, administration of acute stroke therapies, and triage in the system of stroke care locally. MSU should be considered at present as an addition to an advanced system of stroke, though ongoing studies may change this outlook.

9 CONCLUSIONS

The advent and rapid growth of MSUs has changed prehospital stroke evaluation and treatment. It is clear that MSUs reduce time to deliver acute stroke treatment through earlier prehospital stroke assessment and imaging. In addition, MSU patients are more effectively triaged within advanced systems of stroke care. It has also been shown that use of telemedicine in MSUs is feasible and when discussing long term cost effectiveness, this will be an important component to lower operational costs and make widespread adoption of MSUs feasible. Though still in early stages, MSUs appear to be an important advancement in stroke and will drive prehospital stroke care in the near future.

10 CLINICAL CASES

Case 4.1 Rapid thrombolysis on mobile stroke unit

CASE DESCRIPTION

A 43-year-old man develops sudden onset of dense left-sided weakness. The family found him down shortly after and called 911. The dispatcher, following their algorithm, identified a possible stroke situation and dispatched a local EMS vehicle and the MSU. The MSU arrived 19 minutes after dispatch (40 minutes after symptom onset). NIH stroke scale was performed via telemedicine and measured at 20. Noncontrast CT revealed no hemorrhage, but a right hyperdense middle cerebral artery (MCA; Figure 4.3A). Within 11 minutes from MSU door time, IV alteplase was initiated on site. The patient was then brought to the closest comprehensive stroke center with prenotification performed en route, and he was taken directly to the ED for CTA, which confirmed a right M1 MCA occlusion (Figure 4.3B). The patient was immediately directed to the angiography suite, where the occluded M1 MCA was recanalized in 38 minutes (Figure 4.3 and Figure 4.3D). Symptom onset to M1 recanalization was 2 hours and 50 minutes. The patient improved immediately, and by next day only facial droop remained (NIHSS score 1). He was discharged home on hospital day 4.

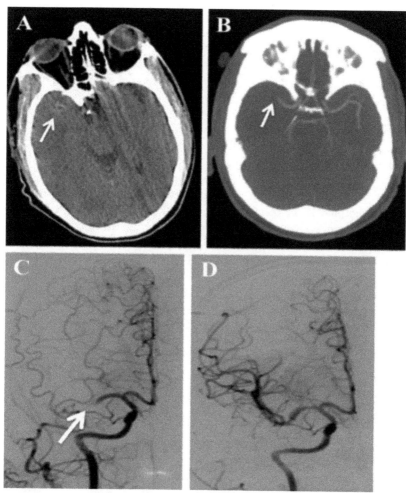

Figure 4.3 (A) Non-contrast computed tomography (CT) head showing no areas of major infarction or hemorrhage. Hyperdense (bright) appearance of the proximal right middle cerebral artery (MCA) is shown (arrow).
(B) Computed tomography angiography confirming the right MCA occlusion (arrow).
(C) Digital subtraction angiography (DSA), antero-posterior view demonstrating the right MCA occlusion (arrow).
(D) After successful thrombectomy, normal blood flow has been restored.

PRACTICAL POINTS

- This case illustrates the critical role MSUs play in optimizing the transport of patients to hospital destinations that provide appropriate level of care.

Case 4.2 CTA on mobile stroke unit

CASE DESCRIPTION

A 47-year-old man presented as a wake-up stroke with right-sided weakness and aphasia. He fell onto the floor while he tried to get out of bed alerting his family who called 911. A MSU was dispatched. Rapid evaluation with telemedicine on the MSU revealed NIHSS score of 14. Non-contrast head CT performed 15 minutes after patient aboard vehicle was negative for acute ischemic or hemorrhagic processes (Figure 4.4A). Labs including blood glucose, complete blood count, basic metabolic panel, and prothrombin time resulted within 15 minutes. CTA was then performed on MSU (28 minutes after aboard vehicle), revealing a left M1 occlusion (Figure 4.4B). He was then transported to Cleveland Clinic (arrival at hospital 47 minutes after being placed on MSU). Due to presentation as a wake-up stroke, he was taken for a hyperacute magnetic resonance imaging, and then transferred for emergent thrombectomy, with a groin puncture time at 107 minutes after being placed on the MSU. He was recanalized at 30 minutes after groin stick. The patient continued to improve through his hospital stay and was discharged to acute rehab with resolution of all cortical signs but residual right hemiparesis (NIHSS of 8).

PRACTICAL POINTS

- The performance of CTA on MSU can shorten time to groin puncture in cases of emergent LVO.[14]

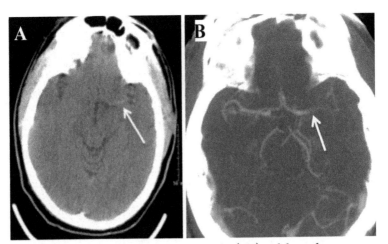

Figure 4.4 (A) Non-contrast computed tomography (CT) with hyperdense appearance of the left middle cerebral artery (MCA) M1 segment (arrow). This suggests an acute thrombus within the left MCA.

(B) CT angiography showing a filling defect within the left MCA M1 segment (arrow).

Case 4.3 Anticoagulation reversal

CASE DESCRIPTION

A 93-year-old woman with known atrial fibrillation on warfarin was found by her family with dense right-sided weakness and aphasia. MSU was dispatched and patient was placed on the MSU 7 minutes after dispatch. NIHSS performed via telemedicine was 19. Non-contrast CT head performed aboard MSU revealed a left thalamic ICH. Point of care INR was measured to be 2.2. Anticoagulation reversal with 4-factor PCC (Kcentra, CSL Behring) was given. The patient was then transported to the neurological intensive care unit of the closest comprehensive stroke center. There, the INR sent upon hospital arrival (106 minutes after dispatch) to the laboratory showed an INR of 1.1.

PRACTICAL POINTS

- This case illustrates the acute care of other conditions besides AIS and particularly the ability to rapid reverse anticoagulation.[28] Four-factor PCC can be stored at room temperature and is a useful medication to include in the armamentarium of treatment options of the MSU.

REFERENCES

1. Fassbender K, Walter S, Liu Y, et al. "Mobile stroke unit" for hyperacute stroke treatment. *Stroke.* 2003;34(6):e44.
2. Jauch EC, Saver JL, Adams HP, Jr., et al. Guidelines for the early management of patients with acute ischemic stroke: a guideline for healthcare professionals from the American Heart Association/American Stroke Association. *Stroke.* 2013;44(3):870–947.
3. Powers WJ, Derdeyn CP, Biller J, et al. 2015 American Heart Association/American Stroke Association focused update of the 2013 Guidelines for the Early Management of Patients with Acute Ischemic Stroke regarding Endovascular Treatment: a guideline for healthcare professionals from the American Heart Association/American Stroke Association. *Stroke.* 2015;46(10):3020–3035.
4. Kim JT, Fonarow GC, Smith EE, et al. Treatment with tissue plasminogen activator in the golden hour and the shape of the 4.5-hour time-benefit curve in the national United States Get with the Guidelines-Stroke population. *Circulation.* 2017;135(2):128–139.
5. Fonarow GC, Zhao X, Smith EE, et al. Door-to-needle times for tissue plasminogen activator administration and clinical outcomes in acute ischemic stroke before and after a quality improvement initiative. *JAMA.* 2014;311(16):1632–1640.
6. Itrat A, Taqui A, Cerejo R, et al. Telemedicine in prehospital stroke evaluation and thrombolysis: taking stroke treatment to the doorstep. *JAMA Neurol.* 2015:1–7.
7. Weber JE, Ebinger M, Rozanski M, et al. Prehospital thrombolysis in acute stroke: results of the PHANTOM-S pilot study. *Neurology.* 2013;80(2):163–168.

8. Ebinger M, Winter B, Wendt M, et al. Effect of the use of ambulance-based thrombolysis on time to thrombolysis in acute ischemic stroke: a randomized clinical trial. *JAMA*. 2014;311(16):1622–1631.

9. Walter S, Kostopoulos P, Haass A, et al. Diagnosis and treatment of patients with stroke in a mobile stroke unit versus in hospital: a randomised controlled trial. *Lancet Neurol*. 2012;11(5):397–404.

10. Liman TG, Winter B, Waldschmidt C, et al. Telestroke ambulances in prehospital stroke management: concept and pilot feasibility study. *Stroke*. 2012;43(8):2086–2090.

11. Wu TC, Parker SA, Jagolino A, et al. Telemedicine can replace the neurologist on a mobile stroke unit. *Stroke*. 2017;48(2):493–496.

12. John S, Stock S, Cerejo R, et al. Brain imaging using mobile CT: current status and future prospects. *J Neuroimaging*. 2016;26(1):5–15.

13. Rumboldt Z, Huda W, All JW. Review of portable CT with assessment of a dedicated head CT scanner. *Am J Neuroradiol*. 2009;30(9):1630–1636.

14. John S, Stock S, Masaryk T, et al. Performance of CT Angiography on a mobile stroke treatment unit: implications for triage. *J Neuroimaging*. 2016;26(4):391–394.

15. Fakhraldeen M, Segal E, de Champlain F. Effect of the use of ambulance-based thrombolysis on time to thrombolysis in acute ischemic stroke: a randomized clinical trial. *CJEM*. 2015;17(6):709–712.

16. Wendt M, Ebinger M, Kunz A, et al. Improved prehospital triage of patients with stroke in a specialized stroke ambulance: results of the pre-hospital acute neurological therapy and optimization of medical care in stroke study. *Stroke*. 2015;46(3):740–745.

17. Bowry R, Parker S, Rajan SS, et al. Benefits of stroke treatment using a mobile stroke unit compared with standard management: the BEST-MSU study run-in phase. *Stroke*. 2015;46(12):3370–3374.

18. Taqui A, Cerejo R, Itrat A, et al. Reduction in time to treatment in prehospital telemedicine evaluation and thrombolysis. *Neurology*. 2017;88(14):1305–1312.

19. Saver JL, Fonarow GC, Smith EE, et al. Time to treatment with intravenous tissue plasminogen activator and outcome from acute ischemic stroke. *JAMA*. 2013;309(23):2480–2488.

20. Wahlgren N, Ahmed N, Davalos A, et al. Thrombolysis with alteplase for acute ischaemic stroke in the Safe Implementation of Thrombolysis in Stroke-Monitoring Study (SITS-MOST): an observational study. *Lancet*. 2007;369(9558):275–282.

21. Ebinger M, Kunz A, Wendt M, et al. Effects of golden hour thrombolysis: a Prehospital Acute Neurological Treatment and Optimization of Medical Care in Stroke (PHANTOM-S) substudy. *JAMA Neurol*. 2015;72(1):25–30.

22. Kunz A, Ebinger M, Geisler F, et al. Functional outcomes of pre-hospital thrombolysis in a mobile stroke treatment unit compared with conventional care: an observational registry study. *Lancet Neurol*. 2016;15(10):1035–1043.

23. Ebinger M, Harmel P, Nolte CH, Grittner U, Siegerink B, Audebert HJ. Berlin prehospital or usual delivery of acute stroke care: study protocol. *Int J Stroke*. 2017;12(6):653–658.

24. Yamal JM, Rajan SS, Parker SA, et al. Benefits of stroke treatment delivered using a mobile stroke unit trial. *Int J Stroke*. 2017. doi:10.1177/1747493017711950

25. Mozaffarian D, Benjamin EJ, Go AS, et al. Executive summary: heart disease and stroke statistics—2016 update: a report from the American Heart Association. *Circulation*. 2016;133(4):447–454.

26. Dietrich M, Walter S, Ragoschke-Schumm A, et al. Is prehospital treatment of acute stroke too expensive? An economic evaluation based on the first trial. *Cerebrovasc Dis*. 2014;38(6):457–463.

27. Gyrd-Hansen D, Olsen KR, Bollweg K, Kronborg C, Ebinger M, Audebert HJ. Cost-effectiveness estimate of prehospital thrombolysis: results of the PHANTOM-S study. *Neurology*. 2015;84(11):1090–1097.

28. Gomes JA, Ahrens CL, Hussain MS, et al. Prehospital reversal of warfarin-related coagulopathy in intracerebral hemorrhage in a mobile stroke treatment unit. *Stroke*. 2015;46(5):e118–120.

5

Evaluation of Stroke in the Emergency Department

ROBERT SAWYER AND EDWARD C. JAUCH ■

CONTENTS

1 INTRODUCTION

This chapter discusses the Emergency Department (ED) evaluation and treatment of stroke, the structure required to support the stroke program in the ED and the types of stroke cases to be treated. Using the fundamental classification of stroke subtypes based on pathophysiology, strokes can be classified as ischemic (87% of all strokes) or hemorrhagic (13% of all strokes). Figure 5.1 summarizes an algorithm for the initial evaluation and management of stroke patients in the ED.

Aggressive management of acute ischemic stroke with intravenous (IV) thrombolysis and endovascular thrombectomy (EVT) can result in rapid resolution of clinical symptoms or reduction in the amount of brain involved in the stroke.[1,2]

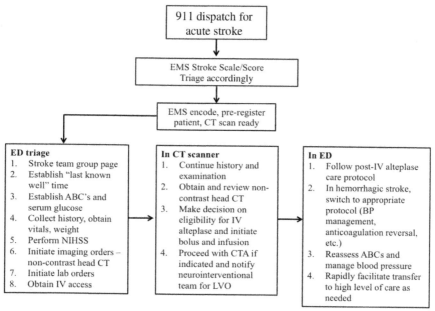

Figure 5.1 Basic algorithm for the initial evaluation and management of stroke patients in the Emegency Department.

ABBREVIATIONS: ABC, airway, breathing, circulation; BP, blood pressure; CT, computed tomography, CTA, computed tomography angiography; ED, emergency department; EMS, emergency medical services; IV, intravenous; LVO, large vessel occlusion; NIHSS, National Institutes of Health Stroke Scale.

Emergency management of hemorrhagic strokes involves controlling blood pressure, reversal of any coagulopathies, deciding if neurosurgical intervention is appropriate, and providing optimal supportive care. All interventions must be delivered in a very timely fashion if the morbidity and mortality of the stroke are to be mitigated. Thus, emergent diagnosis and imaging are imperative as both ischemic and hemorrhagic strokes can have similar clinical presentations but require distinct management and treatment approaches.

Question 5.1: How can I get "NIHSS trained"?

Answer: An online training course is available on the American Heart Association website https://learn.heart.org/nihss.aspx.

2 INITIAL EMERGENCY DEPARTMENT EVALUATION AND ASSESSMENT

2.1 Organizing the Emergency Department for acute stroke

The care of a potential stroke patient precedes their arrival. As noted in Chapter 3 on the prehospital evaluation of stroke, advanced notification by the emergency medical services (EMS) personnel can help speed the triage, evaluation, and treatment of stroke patients. With advanced notification, additional medical history may be obtained from the health record, activation of the stroke team and pharmacy facilitates rapid assessment, and the patient, assuming they are hemodynamically stable, may be transported directly to the computed tomography (CT) suite.

A prospective interventional trial conducted in Helsinki focused on 12 tenets for reducing time between onset of symptoms and time to IV alteplase administration ("door to needle" [DTN] time).[3,4] The three most notable recommendations were (i) ambulance prenotification with patient details so the stroke team meets the patient on arrival; (ii) patients are transferred directly from triage onto the CT table from the ambulance stretcher; and (iii) alteplase is delivered in the CT room immediately after imaging is interpreted.

More recently, the American Heart Association (AHA) Target Stroke I and II programs, implementing best practices across over a thousand stroke centers resulted in faster door-to-CT times, improved rates of alteplase use, shorter DTN times, more patients ambulatory at discharge, and more patients being discharged home (Box 5.1).[5] These processes do not require additional staff or resources, rather, organizing existing processes to be more efficient.

Implementation of Target Stroke Best Practices in 1030 Get with the Guidelines-Stroke participating hospitals of varying capabilities led to statistically and clinically significant improvements in DTN times, alteplase administration under 60 minutes from arrival, rates of symptomatic hemorrhage, rates of patients being discharged home, and all-cause in-hospital mortality.[6]

Box 5.1

TARGET STROKE BEST PRACTICES

- Hospital prenotification by EMS
- Rapid triage protocol and stroke team notification
- Single call/paging activation system for entire stroke team
- Use of a stroke toolkit containing clinical decision support, stroke-specific order sets, guidelines, hospital-specific algorithms, critical pathways, NIHSS, and other stroke tools
- Rapid acquisition and interpretation of brain imaging
- Rapid laboratory testing (including point-of-care testing) if indicated
- Pre-mixing alteplase ahead of time for high likelihood candidates
- Rapid access to IV alteplase in the ED/brain imaging area
- Team-based approach
- Rapid data feedback to stroke team on each patient's DTN time and other performance data

Based on the success of Target Stroke Phase I, Target Stroke Phase II was initiated, again emphasizing the previous best practices but adding EMS transfer directly to CT/MRI. The national goals of Target: Stroke Phase II are:

- Primary Goal: Achieve DTN times within 60 minutes in 75% or more of acute ischemic stroke patients treated with IV alteplase.
- Secondary Goal: Achieve DTN times within 45 minutes in 50% or more of acute ischemic stroke patients treated with IV alteplase.

These best practices are applicable to all facilities caring for acute stroke patient and, implemented nationally, lead to major reductions in morbidity and mortality.

> **Question 5.2:** What is the first step in evaluating the patient with a suspected stroke in the ED?
> **Answer:** Evaluate the ABCs—airway, breathing, and circulation first.

2.2 Initial assessment of potential stroke patients

As with all potentially critically ill patients, the initial assessment of a potential stroke patient begins with the ABCs—airway, breathing, and circulation. Fortunately, with the exception of intracerebral hemorrhage (ICH) and vertebrobasilar strokes, most stroke patients do not require emergent airway management, respiratory assistance, or circulatory support. Airway assessment is typically straightforward; breathing is assessed by auscultation and pulse oximetry.

Supplement oxygen is recommended to maintain oxygen saturations >94%. Circulation rarely requires intervention unless the patient is clinically hypotensive, hypertensive in the setting of an ICH, or is a potential candidate for IV alteplase. Current blood pressure recommendations for patients with ICH can be found in the ICH chapter. For patients being considered for alteplase use, blood pressure before alteplase should be below 185 mmHg systolic and 105 mmHg diastolic. For patients with acute ischemic stroke not undergoing reperfusion therapies, mild hypertension is acceptable to maintain adequate penumbral perfusion. Unless there are active comorbidities which require acute blood pressure management, current guidelines do not recommend intervention unless the patient's blood pressure is in excess of 220 mm Hg systolic or 120 mm Hg diastolic. A patient's clinical status may deteriorate so frequent reassessment is critical.

2.3 Recognizing a potential stroke patient

Recognition of a potential stroke patient ideally begins in the prehospital setting. Yet, nearly 25% of stroke patients arrive by means other than EMS. ED triage nurses must be keenly sensitive to potential stroke patients arriving through the lobby. Delays to recognition, CT, first physician contact, and alteplase administration all occur when patients do not arrive by EMS.

2.3.1 NATIONAL INSTITUTES OF HEALTH STROKE SCALE

Fundamental to identification of stroke is the ability to localize symptoms to the brain (a hemisphere) or brainstem. Additionally, for treatment decision, risk stratification, and outcome prognosis, quantifying the neurologic deficits with the National Institutes of Health Stroke Scale (NIHSS) is essential. Refer to Chapter 3 for the description of the NIHSS. Initially designed for research purposes, the NIHSS is now widely used among the ED and stroke physicians and is a critical component when determining the appropriate treatment strategy. Parietal strokes can be challenging to recognize when the patient may only present with complete denial of symptoms and few language deficits. Posterior circulation strokes are particularly difficult to identify, as there are so many signs and symptoms in common with more benign etiologies, and the NIHSS does not fully assess posterior circulation neurologic functions.

2.3.2 ISCHEMIC VERSUS HEMORRHAGIC STROKE

Analysis of 19 prospective studies with a total of 6,438 patients who presented to EDs with a diagnosis of stroke showed that no bedside finding or combination of clinical findings were definitively able to discriminate between ischemic and hemorrhage strokes, and diagnostic certainty requires emergent brain imaging.[7] Still, some clinical findings increase the probability of a hemorrhagic stroke and can be utilized in certain clinical scenarios before definitive imaging data become available. Specifically, coma, neck stiffness, seizures, diastolic blood pressure greater than

110 mm Hg, vomiting, and headache on admission increase the likelihood of hemorrhagic stroke.

2.3.3 STROKE MIMICS

Up to 20% of suspected strokes can present as stroke mimics.[8] Listed from most to least common, these include seizures, systemic infection, toxic-metabolic disorders such as hyponatremia and hypoglycemia, conversion disorder, positional vertigo, and brain tumors. Additional neurologic examinations and diagnostic modalities may be required when a stroke mimic is being considered.

2.4 Evaluation

The history and physical examination should be thorough, directed and performed rapidly. Alteplase is administered based on the time last known well (LKW) and yet is often confused with time when patient was found with stroke symptoms—time found with stroke symptoms is not the same as LKW. Do not accept a reported time of onset that matches the time the patient was found by family/bystander or time EMS arrived. When available, family members or witnesses provide the most accurate LKW time. The circumstances of the patient's onset of symptoms are key—was there associated trauma, seizure activity, or other medical complaint prior to onset of symptoms? Many patients present with either rapidly improving symptoms or waxing and waning symptoms so details of the onset of symptoms are essential.

Obtaining a detailed past medical history is equally key. Patients with a history of atrial fibrillation, valvular disorders, or other indications for anticoagulation need to be identified early in the course of evaluation since use of anticoagulation is a critical factor in determining eligibility for alteplase. Recent illness, trauma, new medications, or surgery are also critical historical elements when deciding upon optimal reperfusion options. The history and physical can be initiated while the patient is being prepared for brain imaging and done concurrently with other ongoing assessments.

Once a stroke is suspected, the ED-based stroke protocol should be initiated. The protocol should be a consensus-based approach to emergency stroke evaluation and treatment, which treats the stroke team as a team who works in parallel with one another given the local resources. Similar to trauma, each member should have a well-defined role and function. Establishing such a team-based approach has demonstrated real clinical benefit to stroke patients. Actions should be based on priorities, with a special emphasis on performing only those tasks required to stabilize the patient and determine eligibility for reperfusion strategies. A limited number of hematologic, coagulation, and biochemistry test are recommended in the emergency evaluation. In those patients with no significant comorbidities, of the recommended diagnostic tests, only a serum glucose is required before IV alteplase use. Box 5.2 highlights required diagnostic testing.

Box 5.2

DIAGNOSTIC TESTING IN POTENTIAL STROKE PATIENTS

Required
- Cerebral imaging
- Complete blood count with platelets
- Electrocardiograph
- Serum electrolytes
- Serum glucose
- Serum troponin

Consider as indicated
- Arterial blood gas
- Coagulation parameters (INR, PT, PTT)
- Chest radiograph
- CSF analysis
- Ethanol level
- Pregnancy test
- Urine analysis
- Urine toxicology screen

2.5 Brain imaging

The vast majority of stroke patients undergo brain imaging using CT scans, although magnetic resonance imaging (MRI) use from the ED is possible. Imaging, typically a non-contrast head CT, should be completed within 25 minutes of arrival to the ED. A CT angiogram (CTA) can be generated shortly thereafter, but the initial decision to initiate alteplase is based on LKW time, physical examination, and non-contrast CT results, and performing the CTA should not delay administration of alteplase. In patients suspected of harboring emergent LVO, CTA can be performed immediately after alteplase infusion is initiated.

Any imaging beyond a non-contrast head CT is not required to give alteplase. Careful consideration must be given to sending the patient for any additional imaging, such as MRI brain to "rule out stroke" beyond what has already been obtained. Most hospital EDs are not capable of completing MRI studies within 5–10 minutes. It is often less important to have imaging confirmation of a stroke prior to administration of alteplase than to deliver alteplase in a timely manner.

2.6 Additional diagnostic considerations

Many if not most potential stroke patients have morbidities that may require evaluation. Additional testing may be indicated to evaluate the cause of the patient's stroke symptoms, as well as to consider active comorbidities, which may require emergent management.

3 THERAPY SELECTION

Once brain imaging is performed and the history and physical suggest the patient is experiencing an ischemic stroke, the focus turns to determining eligibility for reperfusion strategies.

3.1 Intravenous alteplase

IV alteplase remains recommended for all patients meeting current eligibility requirements. The stroke community has learned a great deal regarding the use of alteplase over the past 20 years, and based on these experiences, the number of stroke patients eligible for alteplase have increased through an expanded time window for select patients and through relaxation of originally absolute contraindications to now relative contraindications, summarized in Box 5.3. While alteplase is considered standard of care, informed decision-making should include the patient and their family in the decision. Through the expansion of eligibility and the development

---

Box 5.3

UPDATED 2015 FDA PRODUCT INSERT FOR ALTEPLASE USE IN ACUTE ISCHEMIC STROKE

Absolute contraindications
- Current intracranial hemorrhage
- Subarachnoid hemorrhage
- Recent (within 3 months) intracranial or intraspinal surgery or serious head trauma
- Current severe uncontrolled hypertension
- Bleeding diathesis
- Active internal bleeding
- Presence of intracranial conditions that may increase the risk of bleeding (e.g., some neoplasms, arteriovenous malformations, or aneurysms)

Relative contraindications
- Recent major surgery or procedure
- Recent gastrointestinal or genitourinary bleeding
- Recent trauma
- Hemostatic defects including those secondary to severe hepatic or renal disease
- Acute pericarditis
- Pregnancy
- Septic thrombophlebitis or occluded AV cannula at seriously infected site
- Recent intracranial hemorrhage
- High likelihood of left heart thrombus
- Diabetic hemorrhagic retinopathy, or other hemorrhagic ophthalmic conditions
- Hypertension
- Subacute bacterial endocarditis
- Advanced age
- Patients currently receiving anticoagulants
- Any other condition in which bleeding constitutes a significant hazard or would be particularly difficult to manage because of its location

---

of systems of care, recent experience with alteplase use have replicated the original National Institutes of Neurological Disorders and Stroke (NINDS) data, and based on the Get with the Guidelines data, administration of alteplase remains safe and effective across a wide range of hospital settings.[9,10]

Based on subanalyses of larger alteplase trials, anecdotal evidence and, importantly, the European Cooperative Acute Stroke Study (ECASS) III study, the window from LKW to alteplase administration was formally expanded for carefully selected patients in a scientific advisory by the AHA.[11] This scientific advisory stated "alteplase should be administered to eligible patients who can be treated in the time period of 3 to 4.5 hours after stroke" (Class I Recommendation, Level of Evidence B).

The eligibility criteria for treatment in this time period are similar to those for persons treated at earlier time periods, with the additional exclusion criteria: (i) patients older than 80 years, (ii) those taking oral anticoagulants with an international normalized ratio (INR) <1.7, (iii) those with a baseline NIHSS >25, or (iv) those with both a history of stroke and diabetes. Therefore, for the 3- to 4.5-hour window, all patients receiving an oral anticoagulant are excluded regardless of their international normalized ratio. Patients who possess one or more of these exclusion criteria were not involved in the ECASS III study thus the efficacy of alteplase in this group is not well established. The use of alteplase in this group of patients must be weighed against potential harm and should be studied further.

Alteplase administration remains the same as utilized in the original NINDS tPA trials.[12] Despite several clinical trials of other fibrinolytic agents, alteplase remains the only agent approved for use in acute stroke. Dosing remains weight based at 0.9 mg/kg up to a maximum of 90 mg (10% as a bolus; the remainder administered over 1 hour). Administration can begin as soon as the brain imaging does not reveal a contraindication to alteplase, such as ICH. The bolus and infusion should begin prior to additional cerebrovascular imaging.

Careful monitoring is essential during the administration of alteplase. Scheduled neurologic and physiologic monitoring remains prescriptive, every 15 minutes for the first 2 hours after bolus, then every 30 minutes for 6 hours, and finally every hour until 24 hours from bolus administration. Strict blood pressure management is critical to minimizing the chance of developing a symptomatic ICH, blood pressure criteria for alteplase eligibility are a systolic BP <185 mmHg and diastolic BP <110 mmHg, after administration, the blood pressure must be maintained below a systolic BP of 180 mmHg and a diastolic BP of 105 mmHg.

Sudden neurologic deterioration during alteplase use should immediately lead to stopping the infusion, repeating a brain non-contrast CT, drawing critical labs for possible alteplase reversal, and strict blood pressure control. Other adverse events associated with alteplase use include bleeding, both intracranial and extracranial; transient hypotension; and angioedema. Observation for these adverse events must occur regardless of patient location, whether in the ED, stroke unit, neurointerventional suite, or especially during institutional transfer.

3.2 Endovascular thrombectomy

Endovascular therapies for emergent large vessel occlusion (LVO) represent a major advance in acute stroke care since the approval of alteplase. Patient selection continues to evolve with more recent studies suggesting even longer time from LKW based on penumbral selection strategies. Chapter 9 on EVT details selection consideration and the actual performance of EVT. Since EVT is just as time dependent as alteplase, the same system must ensure not only timely alteplase use if indicated but also timely cerebrovascular and perfusion imaging as well as internal or external transfer to a capable center that can both perform EVT and as importantly care for these potentially more critically ill patients.

3.3 Supportive therapy

Physiologic optimization may be appropriate for some stroke patients. Hyperthermia is detrimental in the setting of acute brain injury. Treatment of the febrile stroke patient should begin immediately if temperatures exceed >38°C. Induced hypothermia has yet to demonstrate clinical benefit in the setting of acute stroke. Hypoxia can exacerbate cerebral injury. Supplemental oxygen should be provided if oxygen saturations are below 95%. Supplemental normobaric oxygen or hyperbaric oxygen for patients without an oxygen requirement has not shown clinical effectiveness. Hyperglycemia, similar to hyperthermia, is detrimental in the setting of acute brain injury. Current targets for hyperglycemic control remain based on consensus opinion with the most recent AHA guidelines recommending glycemic control with a target range of 140 to 180 mg/dL. Ongoing studies of aggressive glycemic control, such as the Stroke Hyperglycemia Insulin Network Effort (SHINE) study, may provide evidence that even lower levels of glucose intervention are beneficial.[13] Hypoglycemia should be avoided as well, and treatment initiated if patients are symptomatic or serum glucose levels drop below 60 mg/dL.

Adjunct therapies for acute ischemic stroke, such as neuroprotectants or antiplatelet agents, have yet to demonstrate clinical efficacy. Two decades of negative neuroprotection trials have not stopped these efforts. Several ongoing trials are investigating neuroprotection in the setting of alteplase use and EVT.[14,15] Phase II studies of combination therapy with alteplase and IV GP IIb/IIIa inhibitors or argatroban are encouraging, and it is likely a definitive Phase III study will be initiated in the coming year.

Not all patients are eligible for reperfusion strategies, but they too require attention. The patients' neurologic condition may wax and wane, and where they may not have been eligible for reperfusion at initial assessment, deterioration now require new consideration. All patients should be started on a stroke protocol that emphasizes early attention to complication prevention, such as aspiration pneumonia, and early secondary prevention, such as antiplatelet therapy. The stroke protocol must be started in the ED and continued to the stroke unit or floor.

Education of all healthcare providers, physicians and nurses in particular, is critical to ensure optimal implementation of the protocols and management of all stroke patients.

Eligibility for IV thrombolysis with alteplase and EVT, as well as safety and efficacy of these life-saving treatments, can be greatly improved by adherence to the recommended metrics. Avoiding common mistakes leading to erroneous exclusion of patients or delays to treatment is critically important. At the same time, failure to recognize major contraindications to these therapies can result in devastating events. The following discussion provides common scenarios that are frequently encountered when evaluating patients with acute stroke.

4 HEMORRHAGIC STROKE

Once a non-contrast CT shows the presence of intracranial hemorrhage and the patient is no longer eligible for alteplase or EVT, the level of "acuteness" needs to remain high. Patients with hemorrhagic strokes can deteriorate rapidly and required more aggressive management of their ABCs. Blood pressure targets for patients with ICH remain uncertain but most physicians caring for these patients routinely work to achieve systolic blood pressure below 150 mmHg or less. Large hemispheric hemorrhages and those located within the posterior fossa (cerebellum, brainstem) should be monitored closely, including emergent evaluation by a neurosurgeon.

Increasingly, ICH is associated with anticoagulation use. Specific reversal protocols for warfarin and the factor Xa inhibitors and direct thrombin inhibitors must be developed and well known to the ED staff; failure to reverse anticoagulation allows continued bleeding with significant increase in mortality and morbidity. Since many centers do not have the necessary neurosurgical or neurointensive care expertise necessary for these patients, transfer to a higher level of care is recommended. As with patients who received alteplase prior to facility, stabilization of blood pressure, reversal of anticoagulation, repeat assessment of the patient's ABCs must occur prior to transfer to minimize deterioration en route.

5 QUALITY ASSURANCE AND FEEDBACK

No matter what the local protocol for delivering alteplase, best results are derived by reviewing each individual case for performance errors or system problems that led to delays in recognizing stroke or administering treatment. Problems and potential solutions are briefly discussed, and the team leader can improve provider knowledge in real time and note any issues to be solved at a later time. This is the time to congratulate the entire team, from EMS through discharge, on a good performance. Perform systemic review of each case in a delayed fashion, ensuring that all parties involved in the stroke protocols are informed and any system problems are addressed in a timely manner.

5.1 Get with the Guidelines-Stroke

Get with the Guidelines-Stroke is a program supported by the AHA with the goal of improving stroke care by promoting consistent adherence to the latest scientific treatment guidelines. Participating hospitals can submit their data and receive feedback on adherence to the current guideline on the treatment of both ischemic and hemorrhagic stroke including its early diagnosis and treatment provided in the ED.

An ideal time for alteplase administration is 25 minutes from patient's arrival to the ED. The AHA demands less than 60 minutes and prefers less than 45 minutes. Get with the Guidelines-Stroke criteria for performance are summarized in Box 5.4. DTN times like these require crew resource commitments that are best addressed at the system level. Written protocols must specify the person and time to complete a particular task. The ability to surge healthcare workers is essential and unfortunately one of the most difficult challenges to convince hospital systems to fund. A protocol overview listed in Box 5.5 may be adapted to any hospital, depending on capabilities.

6 CONCLUSIONS

A carefully planned, aggressive and in-depth response to stroke will reduce time to treatment for acutely ill stroke patients presenting to the ED and expand opportunities for patients to make a meaningful recovery. Engaging all stakeholders and preparing comprehensive and rehearsed protocols will ensure consistency, quality, and effectiveness. The clinical science of stroke care is changing rapidly and will have profound impact on both early hospital and prehospital treatment of stroke.

Box 5.4

GET WITH THE GUIDELINES®-STROKE TIME INTERVAL GOALS FOR INTRAVENOUS THROMBOLYSIS IN ACUTE ISCHEMIC STROKE

- Door to MD 10 minutes: perform an initial patient evaluation within 10 minutes of arrival in the ED
- Notify the stroke team within 15 minutes of arrival
- Initiate a CT scan within 25 minutes of arrival
- Interpret the CT scan within 45 minutes of arrival
- Ensure a DTN time for IV alteplase within 60 minutes from arrival

SOURCE: Association AH. Target: Stroke Phase II Campaign. http://www.strokeassociation.org/STROKEORG/Professionals/TargetStroke/Target-Stroke_UCM_314495_SubHomePage.jsp

---

Box 5.5

A PROTOCOL FOR EVALUATION OF STROKE IN THE EMERGENCY DEPARTMENT

(This general protocol is tailored towards evaluation of ischemic stroke for IV thrombolysis and thrombectomy but can be also applied to hemorrhagic strokes).

ED triage
- Notify essential personnel (ED physician and/or stroke team)
- Evaluate the ABCs
- Establish the time LKW
- Obtain minimum required patient demographics
- Obtain vital signs, estimated weight, anticoagulant use, and allergies (including to iodine contrast)
- Obtain stroke assessment to include NIHSS, Glasgow coma scale, and need for immediate intubation
- Initiate imaging orders to include non-brain CT scan, and when applicable CT angiogram, CT perfusion, and/or MRI
- Initiate laboratory orders to include: prothrombin time (PT), partial thromboplastin time (PTT), INR complete blood count including platelets, renal function, and electrolytes. Some tests, including PT, INR, blood glucose, and creatinine may be obtained at point of care rather than sending to the lab
- Attach cardiac, blood pressure and pulse oximeter monitors if not already present
- Obtain IV access if not already completed in the field. Consider a proximal IV suitable for contrast administration to perform CTA/CTP
- Obtain a limited medical history, including contraindications to alteplase. Page the stroke team
- Review the electronic medical record for medical history and contraindications to alteplase
- Note: The patient is not actually transferred to an ED room at this time, but ideally patients are taken by EMS directly to the CT scanner.

CT scanner
- Obtain an actual patient weight, ideally before they are loaded onto the scanner
- Continue the examination and history
- Obtain and review a non-contrast CT head in real time to rule out blood, subacute stroke, and acute hypodensity. The Alberta Stroke Program Early CT Score (ASPECTS) may be calculated at this time.
- If the patient meets criteria for alteplase administration, give bolus, and initiate infusion at this point. If NIHSS is >6 or there is a suspicion for a LVO, obtain CTA to determine if LVO is present and endovascular treatment is required

- If the patient does **not** meet criteria for alteplase administration, evaluate if CTA with/without CT perfusion is indicated to screen for LVO for possible thrombectomy (typically, in patients with NIHSS of 6 or above and symptom onset up to 24 hours)
- If clinical suspicion for stroke from LVO is high (based on severity of NIHSS score, or prehospital LAMS, C-STAT, or RACE LVO screening scales), neurointerventional team should be notified before results of non-contrast CT or CTA are available

Emergency Department

- When applicable, complete alteplase infusion with careful attention of vitals (especially systolic/diastolic blood pressure) and any worsening of neurological exam
- Achieve nurse-to-nurse communication and transfer the patient from the ED to the neurointerventional suite, neurocritical care unit, step-down unit, or stroke floor depending on diagnosis

7 CLINICAL CASES

Case 5.1 Acute ischemic stroke with large vessel occlusion

CASE DESCRIPTION

A 63-year-old patient with a history of hypertension and recent diagnosis of localized colon cancer with subsequent colon resection >3months ago arrives to the ED with dysarthria, gaze preference to left, right facial droop, and severe right arm and leg weakness (NIHSS score >20). Patient is not on any form of anticoagulation and has had no recent trauma. Non-contrast CT is performed (Figure 5.2). The following information is recorded by the triage nurse:

- LKW: Patient's family describes the patient as completely normal at 21:00 and was found with symptoms at 22:32
- ED arrival at 00:06
- VS: Heart rate 82 and regular, BP 156/76 mm Hg, SaO$_2$ 97%, temp 98.6°C
- Non-contrast CT read completed at 00:26

PRACTICAL POINTS

- This patient presented with a high NIHSS score within the alteplase time "window." The CT did not show a major hypodensity or bleed. The time of onset seemed to be reasonably well described by the family. Alteplase infusion was started since the patient met ECASS III inclusion criteria, and CTA showed a proximal left middle cerebral artery occlusion, followed by

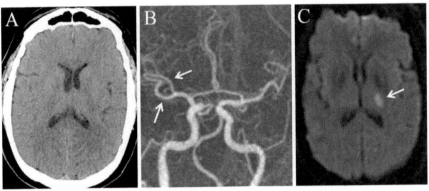

Figure 5.2 Acute ischemic stroke with large vessel occlusion.
(A) Non-contrast head computed tomography (CT), axial view, shows no significant acute intracranial pathology. Based on this study, there are no contraindications to alteplase.
(B) CT angiography, 3D reconstruction, shows a single left M2 branch. The other M2 branch is occluded. For comparison, note two distinct M2 branches originating at the right middle cerebral artery bifurcation (arrows).
(C) Magnetic resonance imaging brain, diffusion weighted imaging repeated at approximately 24 hours after onset of symptoms. The study shows acute 3.8 cm infarct involving the left basal ganglia.

     successful intra-arterial clot extraction. MRI brain obtained the following day showed a very small final infarct.

- The family confirmed patient had not been taking any anticoagulants at home. To ensure alteplase could be started before the 4.5 hour-mark, the bolus was administered before INR and platelet count results were available for review. Extremely high severity the patient's deficits justified why some relatively exclusion criteria for thrombolysis were weighed against the potential benefit and harm if treatment was not initiated.

- High NIHSS score also accurately predicted a proximal occlusion. While there is indirect evidence that thrombectomy may be equally effective without prior administration of alteplase, the current guidelines do not recommend withholding alteplase in patients who are eligible for both types of treatment.

- Based on the initial presentation and the final stroke located in the basal ganglia (seen on follow-up MRI), the occlusion likely initially involved M1 segment of the middle cerebral artery. Partial clot lysis with alteplase or distal migration of the clot may explain why M2 rather than M1 branch occlusion was seen on CTA.

Case 5.2 Stroke with rapidly improving symptoms

CASE DESCRIPTION

A patient with a history of chronic kidney disease is admitted after significant difficulty with speech, discovered upon waking from up after a nap. His symptoms

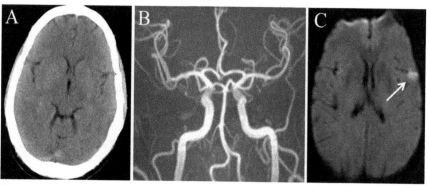

Figure 5.3 Stroke with rapidly improving symptoms.
(A) Non-contrast head computed tomography axial view, shows no significant acute intracranial pathology.
(B) Magnetic resonance angiography, 3D reconstruction, shows no significant intracranial stenosis or occlusion.
(C) Magnetic resonance imaging brain, diffusion weighted imaging, axial view shows a small acute left frontal lobe infarct (arrow) confirming that the patient indeed had a stroke.

partially resolve upon arrival to the ED. The NIHSS score obtained by the ED physician is 2, and blood pressure is 156/83 mm Hg. The family arrives shortly and reports the patient was seen normal 1 hour before taking the nap. Also, they inform the ED physician that the patient is a high school teacher.

The following information is available to the ED physician (Figure 5.3):

- LKW—13:05 when went to sleep
- Discovery of symptoms—14:21
- ED arrival—15:11
- Non-contrast CT head—15:23

PRACTICAL POINTS

- About half of all strokes are of mild severity.[16] Patients can present with rapidly improving deficits with a NIHSS that is 0 or at least non-disabling. About 29% of these patients will go on to have worsening of their symptoms with discharge to acute rehabilitation, a skilled nursing facility, and not to home.[17] The risk of symptomatic bleeding after alteplase administration to these types of patients is low, about 2.4%, compared to the NINDS trial experience of 6.4%.[18] An observational study of 1386 patients demonstrated better outcomes with alteplase therapy than not receiving IV alteplase.[19] A recent randomized, prospective trial, Patients with Mild Stroke (PRISMS) was stopped before it could be completed. Given the risk versus benefit, it would seem reasonable to discuss the use of alteplase with the patient with intent to consent and treat with alteplase rather than assuming the patient will recover spontaneously and have no disability.[20]

- In this particular case, the patient was still within the 4.5-hour window for alteplase, and his professional occupation (teacher) was one of the key reasons in support of thrombolysis when discussing benefits versus risks of alteplase with the family. Patient's deficit (aphasia) made this case even more challenging, as the patient himself had limited ability to comprehend the situation. Fortunately, the family was immediately available for discussion and consent.
- These are difficult decisions, and this case emphasizes the need for a consistent clinical approach to patients with rapidly improving or non-disabling strokes based on risks, benefits, and pre-existing functional status. Patients with mild symptoms should not be excluded from a standardized protocol to ensure all time metrics are met if treatment is indicated.
- Given low NIHSS score, there was a very low likelihood of LVO in this case; thus, the risk of performing emergent CTA in a setting of chronic renal failure likely outweighed the benefit.
- Magnetic resonance angiography was done later and showed patent vessels. MRI of the brain showed a left frontal stroke explaining the symptoms.

Case 5.3 Intracranial hemorrhage in a setting of anticoagulation

CASE DESCRIPTION

A nursing home resident was found down after sustaining a fall. The patient's medical history is significant for atrial fibrillation, for which she takes warfarin. Upon arrival to the ED, she was lethargic and required intubation. The blood pressure was 187/112 mm Hg and a non-contrast CT head was done and showed a large parenchymal hemorrhage (Figure 5.4). INR was 3.8.

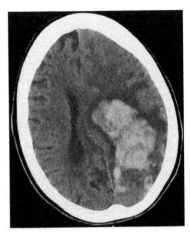

Figure 5.4 Intracranial hemorrhage in a setting of anticoagulation.
Non-contrast head computed tomography, axial view, shows acute left fronto-parietal hemorrhage. Localized mass effect and edema with midline shift is present.

PRACTICAL POINTS

- This patient has suffered an ICH in a setting of anticoagulation. The fall was likely a result of the hemorrhage because traumatic hemorrhages typically present with a subdural or subarachnoid type, which is not seen on head CT in our case. Elevated INR would explain the mechanism of the hemorrhage.
- Treatment of ICH is strongly protocol driven. Construct protocols prior to patient presentation so that rapid implementation is possible.[21] Protocols should address the following: blood pressure control, reversal of anticoagulation with vitamin K antagonists (warfarin) and PCCs for novel oral anticoagulants, and reversal of anticoagulation induced by alteplase.
- Patients presenting with ICH require essential services such as neurology, neurosurgery, neuroradiology, and neurocritical care to optimally manage. Those emergency facilities without requisite resources should transfer patients appropriately.
- In this case, prompt reversal of anticoagulation and control of intracranial pressure followed by emergent neurosurgical to evaluate for possible hematoma evacuation is warranted.

REFERENCES

1. Goyal M, Menon BK, van Zwam WH, et al. Endovascular thrombectomy after large-vessel ischaemic stroke: a meta-analysis of individual patient data from five randomised trials. *Lancet.* 2016;387(10029):1723–1731.
2. Lansberg MG, Bluhmki E, Thijs VN. Efficacy and safety of tissue plasminogen activator 3 to 4.5 hours after acute ischemic stroke: a metaanalysis. *Stroke.* 2009;40(7):2438–2441.
3. Puolakka T, Kuisma M, Lankimaki S, et al. Cutting the prehospital on-scene time of stroke thrombolysis in Helsinki: a prospective interventional study. *Stroke.* 2016;47(12):3038–3040.
4. Meretoja A, Weir L, Ugalde M, et al. Helsinki model cut stroke thrombolysis delays to 25 minutes in Melbourne in only 4 months. *Neurology.* 2013;81(12):1071–1076.
5. American Heart Association/American Stroke Association. Target: Stroke Phase II campaign. http://www.strokeassociation.org/STROKEORG/Professionals/TargetStroke/Target-Stroke_UCM_314495_SubHomePage.jsp.
6. Fonarow GC, Zhao X, Smith EE, et al. Door-to-needle times for tissue plasminogen activator administration and clinical outcomes in acute ischemic stroke before and after a quality improvement initiative. *JAMA.* 2014;311(16):1632–1640.
7. Runchey S, McGee S. Does this patient have a hemorrhagic stroke? clinical findings distinguishing hemorrhagic stroke from ischemic stroke. *JAMA.* 2010;303(22):2280–2286.
8. Huff JS. Stroke mimics and chameleons. *Emerg Med Clin North Am.* 2002;20(3):583–595.

9. Romano JG, Smith EE, Liang L, et al. Outcomes in mild acute ischemic stroke treated with intravenous thrombolysis: a retrospective analysis of the Get with the Guidelines-Stroke registry. *JAMA Neurol.* 2015;72(4):423–431.

10. Schwamm LH, Ali SF, Reeves MJ, et al. Temporal trends in patient characteristics and treatment with intravenous thrombolysis among acute ischemic stroke patients at Get with the Guidelines-Stroke hospitals. *Circ Cardiovasc Qual Outcomes.* 2013;6(5):543–549.

11. Del Zoppo GJ, Saver JL, Jauch EC, Adams HP, Jr., American Heart Association Stroke C. Expansion of the time window for treatment of acute ischemic stroke with intravenous tissue plasminogen activator: a science advisory from the American Heart Association/American Stroke Association. *Stroke.* 2009;40(8):2945–2948.

12. National Institute of Neurological Disorders and Stroke rt-PA Stroke Study Group. Tissue plasminogen activator for acute ischemic stroke. *N Engl J Med.* 1995;333(24):1581–1587.

13. Bruno A, Durkalski VL, Hall CE, et al. The Stroke Hyperglycemia Insulin Network Effort (SHINE) trial protocol: a randomized, blinded, efficacy trial of standard vs. intensive hyperglycemia management in acute stroke. *Int J Stroke.* 2014;9(2):246–251.

14. Tymianski M. Combining Neuroprotection with endovascular treatment of acute stroke: is there hope? *Stroke.* 2017;48(6):1700–1705.

15. Lapchak PA. Critical early thrombolytic and endovascular reperfusion therapy for acute ischemic stroke victims: a call for adjunct neuroprotection. *Transl Stroke Res.* 2015;6(5):345–354.

16. Reeves M, Khoury J, Alwell K, et al. Distribution of National Institutes of Health stroke scale in the Cincinnati/Northern Kentucky Stroke Study. *Stroke.* 2013;44(11):3211–3213.

17. Khatri P, Conaway MR, Johnston KC, Acute Stroke Accurate Prediction Study I: ninety-day outcome rates of a prospective cohort of consecutive patients with mild ischemic stroke. *Stroke.* 2012;43(2):560–562.

18. Greisenegger S, Seyfang L, Kiechl S, Lang W, Ferrari J, Austrian Stroke Unit Registry Collaborators. Thrombolysis in patients with mild stroke: results from the Austrian Stroke Unit Registry. *Stroke.* 2014;45(3):765–769.

19. Choi JC, Jang MU, Kang K, et al. Comparative effectiveness of standard care with IV thrombolysis versus without IV thrombolysis for mild ischemic stroke. *J Am Heart Assoc.* 2015;4(1):e001306.

20. Balucani C, Levine SR. Mild stroke and rapidly improving symptoms: it's not always a happy ending. *Stroke.* 2011;42(11):3005–3007.

21. Hemphill JC, 3rd, Greenberg SM, Anderson CS, et al. Guidelines for the management of spontaneous intracerebral hemorrhage: A guideline for healthcare professionals from the American Heart Association/American Stroke Association. *Stroke.* 2015;46(7):2032–2060.

6

Imaging of Acute Stroke

MAXIM MOKIN ■

CONTENTS

1 INTRODUCTION

The goal of initial imaging performed in the Emergency Department (ED) is to rapidly and reliably establish whether the patient with a suspected acute stroke is suffering from an ischemic or a hemorrhagic event or whether there is an alternative diagnosis, which could present as stroke mimics. Once this critical judgment is made, patients with ischemic stroke need to be rapidly evaluated to determine eligibility for intravenous (IV) alteplase or endovascular thrombectomy (EVT). Some patients may be eligible for only one therapy, whereas others will benefit from both. Timing and imaging criteria defining eligibility for treatment vary between the medical and endovascular therapies. The decision on ordering a particular study is based on several basic rules, which will be discussed in this chapter.

For patients with a hemorrhagic stroke, depending on the type, size, and location of the bleed, further emergent imaging may be required. Some types of hemorrhages need immediate medical or surgical treatment. This chapter explains the value of imaging modalities available for the evaluation of patients with a suspected stroke. Figure 6.1 summarizes the basic algorithm for emergent evaluation of patients with a suspected acute stroke.

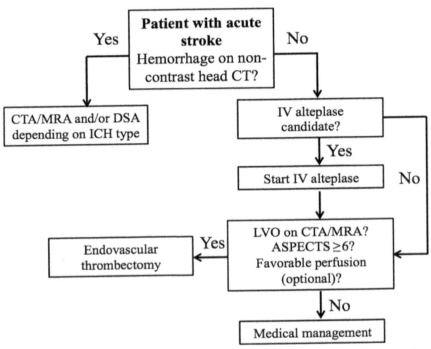

Figure 6.1 Basic algorithm for emergent evaluation of patients with a suspected acute stroke. Abbreviations: ASPECTS, Alberta Stroke Program Early CT Score; CT, computed tomography; CTA, computed tomography angiography; ICH, intracranial hemorrhage; IV, intravenous; LVO, large vessel occlusion; MRA, magnetic resonance angiography.

Question 6.1: Should a computed tomography (CT) with contrast be ordered in acute stroke?

Answer: Whether an ischemic or hemorrhagic stroke is suspected, a non-contrast head CT scan should be ordered. A contrast-enhanced head CT is rarely needed, such as when an intracranial mass lesion (tumor) is suspected. Magnetic resonance imaging (MRI) with contrast rather than CT is the preferred imagining modality in such cases.

2 COMPUTED TOMOGRAPHY

For initial evaluation of patients with acute stroke, non-contrast head CT remains the most commonly utilized imaging modality. The main advantage of CT over MRI is that MRI cannot be performed in patients with imaging-incompatible implanted devices. If there is a limited past medical history, which physicians often encounter when evaluating patients with a suspected acute injury, CT is a great initial imaging study, can be performed in seconds, and does not require "clearance for MRI."

Non-contrast head CT is highly sensitive in identifying acute hemorrhages. Based on the distribution and pattern of blood, an accurate distinction can be made using a head CT between a subarachnoid and intraparenchimal hemorrhage and epidural and subdural hematomas (Box 6.1).[1,2] Cases of intracerebral hemorrhage (ICH) are often triaged based on the size of the hematoma. The ABC/2 method allows quick estimation of the size of the clot, and it can help the neurologist and neurosurgeon decide on the type of treatment (Case 6.1).[3]

The decision about whether to proceed with treatment of ischemic stroke hinges on the results of an initial brain scan that excludes acute hemorrhage. Next, the extent of ischemic burden must be evaluated from the imaging. Depending on the severity, treatment could be futile or even harmful; furthermore, unlike in hemorrhagic stroke, non-contrast CT has rather limited sensitivity in identifying early ischemic changes in patients with hyperacute stroke.[4,5] Head CT can often be read as "normal" in a patient with a hyperacute ischemic stroke (Case 6.2). This commonly happens when the study was performed early, and there were minimal or no early ischemic changes detectable by non-contrast CT at that time in a patient with suspected acute stroke.

When selecting patients for IV alteplase in the early years of thrombolysis, clinicians were originally advised to utilize the "1/3 rule," which identifies large multilobar infarctions with hypodensity over one third of middle cerebral artery (MCA) territory. These patients were thought to be at increased risk of intracranial hemorrhage. In the revised criteria for IV alteplase in acute stroke, the "hypodensity >1/3 cerebral hemisphere" as a neuroimaging criterion was removed.[6] Instead, the guidelines warned against the use of IV alteplase to patients whose CT brain imaging exhibits extensive regions of clear hypodensities ("dark" regions on CT) (Case 6.3). The change was made due to insufficient evidence for identifying a threshold of hypoattenuation severity or the extent that affects treatment response to alteplase (Boxes 6.2 and 6.3).

Box 6.1

IMAGING FINDINGS OF DIFFERENT TYPES OF HEMORRHAGIC STROKE

Intracerebral hemorrhage
- Focal or multifocal parenchymal hyperdense ("bright") lesions on non-contrast CT
- ABC/2 method allows quick calculation of hematoma volume. A: largest diameter of hemorrhage; B: largest diameter 90° to A; and C: total thickness of CT slices with hemorrhage
- CTA "spot sign" from contrast enhancement indicates high risk for hematoma expansion
- MRI appearance varies on stages of hemorrhage (hyperacute, acute, subacute, chronic) due to different phases of blood on MRI sequences (T1, T2, gradient echo)

Subarachnoid hemorrhage
- Blood products are seen in subarachnoid space, commonly within the circle of Willis
- Requires CT, MR, and catheter angiography to rule out ruptured aneurysms

Subdural hematoma
- Crescent-shaped extra-axial (outside of brain) collection of blood

Epidural hematoma
- Bi-convex extra-axial collection of blood

Intraventricular hemorrhage
- Often accompanies intracerebral or subarachnoid hemorrhages
- Blood present in the ventricular system
- Can cause hydrocephalus (enlargement of ventricular size)

Box 6.2

IMAGING FINDINGS IN ACUTE ISCHEMIC STROKE

Early ischemic changes

- Include loss of grey–white matter differentiation, sulcal effacement (swelling), hypoattenuation of deep nuclei
- Can be difficult to detect, especially in hyperacute stages (first few hours) of stroke
- ASPECTS can improve diagnostic accuracy of early ischemic findings
- As infarction progresses, areas with ischemic findings will expand and become more obvious on serial imaging

Hyperdense vessel sign

- Suggests presence of acute arterial occlusion within the corresponding vessel segment
- Most commonly described in cases of proximal MCA occlusion
- Can also be seen with ICA, basilar artery, or proximal posterior cerebral artery occlusion

---

Box 6.3

KEY IMAGING CRITERIA FOR TREATMENT OF ACUTE ISCHEMIC STROKE

Intravenous alteplase

- IV alteplase is not recommended in patients with CT with extensive regions of clear hypoattenuation (hypodensities)
- ASPECTS scoring system is not recognized in the guidelines as a selection criterion

Endovascular thrombectomy

- By contrast to IV alteplase, ASPECTS is a major imaging selection criterion for EVT
- Recommended in patients with ASPECTS range 6–10 and evidence of LVO on CTA/MRA
- Best available evidence supports endovascular therapy for MCA M1 and intracranial ICA occlusion
- Other occlusion sites, such as basilar artery and MCA M2 segment, are likely to benefit, but direct evidence is lacking (no randomized trials)

Question 6.2: How quickly should CT scan be obtained in the ED?

Answer: Based on the American Heart Association metrics, CT scan should be initiated within 25 minutes, and interpretation of the scan should be completed within 45 minutes of arrival to the ED.

2.1 Alberta Stroke Program Early CT Score

The Alberta Stroke Program Early CT Score (ASPECTS) is a grading scale designed to measure and quantify the burden of early ischemic changes in patients with acute stroke.[7] This score is widely used in clinical trials as an imaging criterion for screening and selection of patients. The score is considered a fundamental selection criterion endorsed by the American Heart Association guidelines on endovascular treatment of ischemic stroke and therefore requires detailed description of its measure and interpretation. While ASPECTS can be applied to selection of patients for IV thrombolysis as well, the current guidelines have not officially incorporated this score as an imaging criterion. For IV alteplase, ASPECTS remains more of a tool for clinical research studies than a guideline in the clinic.

ASPECT score ranges from 0 to 10, with each point applied to the territory of the MCA without the evidence of early ischemic changes. Points are subtracted from territories where early ischemic changes can be seen, such as focal swelling or parenchymal hypoattenuation. Therefore, the score of 10 is assigned to a brain CT with no evidence of early ischemic changes within the MCA territory, whereas the score of 0 corresponds to diffuse ischemia throughout the entire MCA territory.

ASPECTS has higher accuracy in detecting early ischemic changes with longer time from stroke onset. In cases of ultra-early stroke, such as within the first 3 hours of onset, the sensitivity and observer agreement in the overall score results decreases. Therefore, some clinicians advocate for the use of MRI or CT with perfusion sequences to improve diagnostic accuracy of initial imaging in patients with acute stroke. Attempts have been made to develop software that would assist the reader with automatic or semiautomatic interpretation of the score.[8,9] Such technology is still at early stages of development and has not become a routine tool in clinical practice.

Question 6.3: How can I improve my ability to read ASPECTS?

Answer: A free online course can be found at http://www.aspectsinstroke.com. The course includes technical details on the optimal window settings, as well as multiple case examples.

2.1.1 DETERMINING ELIGIBILITY FOR ACUTE TREATMENT BASED ON ASPECTS

The guidelines for selection of patients for IV alteplase do not use any specific range of ASPECTS as a part of imaging selection criteria. The guidelines acknowledge lack of strong evidence in support of a specific "ASPECTS threshold" at which systemic thrombolysis becomes futile. On the contrary, ASPECTS is highly important for selection of patients for catheter-based therapies.

For EVT, the majority of randomized trials that were used to establish the guidelines on the management of acute stroke selected patients according to ASPECTS. Thus, ASPECTS is a key imaging criterion endorsed by the major clinical societies; they recommend that patients with acute ischemic stroke with ASPECTS of 6 and above should be considered for EVT, assuming other selection criteria are met. The decision to proceed with endovascular therapy in patients with poor baseline ASPECTS should be made on a case by case basis after consideration of the severity of neurological deficits and prognosis for recovery. Indirect evidence suggests that patients with a higher ischemic burden, corresponding to ASPECTS <6, can sometimes be safely and effectively treated with EVT. The data come from meta-analysis of the randomized endovascular trials (the HERMES collaboration), where patients with ASPECTS ranging from 0 to 5 showed a trend in higher rates of good clinical outcomes when treated with EVT, when compared to control subjects (OR 1.24, 95% CI 0.62–2.49).[10] A study from Emory University, that included primarily young patients (mean age 67) with high National Institutes of Health Stroke Scale (NIHSS) severity (average NIHSS = 20) showed a lower degree of disability and fewer patients requiring hemicraniectomy with endovascular therapy compared to medical therapy alone.[11] It remains to be determined whether this population of patients is best selected with the use of non-contrast CT ASPECTS only or with perfusion imaging, which offers an additional advantage by identifying large ischemic scores or large mismatches in the imaging profile. The role of advanced perfusion imaging in selection of patients for revascularization is discussed in next chapter.

2.1.2 ASPECTS FOR OTHER VASCULAR TERRITORIES

The majority of ischemic strokes occur within the MCA territory. The original ASPECTS score was intended to measure the extent of early ischemic signs in this territory. Other vascular territories that are not included in the initial scoring system are the anterior cerebral artery (ACA) and the posterior circulation. ACA strokes are quite rare, accounting for only 1–2% of all strokes.[12] Presently, there are no standardized, commonly accepted regions, although attempts have been made to introduce ACA ASPECTS territories in pediatric stroke.[13]

Stroke within the posterior circulation, such as from occlusion of the basilar or posterior circulation arteries and its branches, is more common, representing 10–20% of ischemic strokes. The posterior circulation score for measurement of ischemic changes (named pcASPECTS) has been proposed and used by some centers. The structures that are used in pcASPECTS when evaluating the extent of ischemic include the midbrain, pons, bilateral thalami, cerebellum, and the occipital regions. pcASPECTS has failed to become widely accepted as a primary tool to select patients for acute treatment.[14]

A major limitation of applying ASPECTS to the posterior circulation structures is the artifact produced by the adjacent bony structures, which restricts the ability of non-contrast CT to accurately show the extent of early stroke. MRI provides a much more accurate assessment of early ischemia in patients with posterior circulation strokes. Presently, there is no agreement on the best imaging predictors for guiding clinicians when selecting patients with posterior circulation strokes for acute treatments.

2.1.3 ASPECTS DECAY AND ITS SIGNIFICANCE

Because of infarct growth over time, ASPECTS values change with time after symptom onset, a phenomenon known as ASPECTS "decay."[15] This phenomenon is not well understood; however, evidence suggests that initial stroke severity, baseline blood pressure and glucose, and the degree of collaterals might influence the rate of infarct progression.[16,17] Because of this phenomenon, a repeat imaging study can be required before considering a patient for treatment in cases where initial imaging was performed several hours earlier. This often applies to patients who experience significant delays during inter-hospital transfer. In one study that compared CT findings on initial imaging with repeat CT at accepting hospital, 1 out of 3 patients became ineligible for thrombectomy because of unfavorable ASPECTS "decay" following inter-hospital transfer.[18]

2.2 Hyperdense vessel sign

A hyperdense vessel sign is a fresh clot within the vessel seen on non- contrast CT; most commonly referred to as the "hyperdense MCA" sign. It can also be seen in strokes with acute occlusion of the internal carotid artery (ICA) or basilar artery (Case 6.2).[19-21] Its presence warns a physician of a high likelihood of acute large vessel occlusion (LVO). While specific, it is not a sensitive marker and should not be considered a replacement for angiography.[22] It can also be mistaken for focal dense calcifications or Herpes simplex viral encephalitis.[23-25] In such cases, measurement of Hounsfield units (HU) values can help establish the correct diagnosis.

One intriguing, growing area of stroke research involves the role of clot characteristics in predicting the success of IV alteplase and EVT.[26,27] Depending on the appearance of the clot on CT or MRI, it can help distinguish between red blood cell versus fibrin-reach clots. Researchers are trying to improve the efficacy of currently available devices as well as develop new "clot-specific" tools and treatment protocols.

3 MAGNETIC RESONANCE IMAGING

This imaging modality has excellent sensitivity in early detection of acute ischemic stroke. MRI can also distinguish between acute versus chronic hemorrhage. Unfortunately, MRI is often not readily available in the ED, and it requires prolonged scanning time and clearance to exclude the presence of certain implantable devices and metal foreign bodies. To reduce the time it takes to complete the study and to avoid treatment delay, hospitals that utilize MRI as the primary screening test utilize specific MRI stroke protocols that include only the minimal number of sequences; these include diffusion-weighted imaging and fluid attenuated inversion recovery for detection of ischemia and gradient recalled echo for detection of hemorrhage. Additional MRI sequences and administration of gadolinium contrast require more time. Contrast-enhanced complete MRI is necessary to evaluate for secondary causes of ICH such as brain tumors, amyloid angiography, and vascular malformations.

Several issues arise with the use of MRI for selection of patients for IV alteplase. While alteplase is contraindicated in the presence of acute hemorrhage, there are no established guidelines on its safety in patients with incidental findings of chronic cerebral microbleeds, cerebral amyloid angiopathy or cavernous malformations.[28-30] Also, no data-driven guidelines exist on the size of ischemic stroke at which alteplase becomes unsafe and should not be administered. To put it simply, while non-contrast head CT often does not provide "enough" information, MRI gives "too much information" beyond what is required by acute stroke guidelines. In addition, in the hyperacute stage of ischemic stroke, MRI can still provide false-negative results.[31,32] Such findings can prompt a physician to mistakenly exclude patients from treating with IV alteplase (Case 6.4).

For selection of patients for EVT, the burden of ischemic core can be measured by calculating the number of ASPECTS regions.[33] An alternative strategy is to measure the volume of ischemic lesion.[34,35] However, there is great variability in how to interpret MRI findings in patients with ischemic strokes because of studies suggesting that MRI markers of acute ischemia, specifically diffusion-weighted imaging sequence, can be reversible in patients who achieve successful reperfusion with IV alteplase or EVT.[36] Thus, many centers that utilize MRI for screening of stroke patients also rely on the results of perfusion imaging for selection of patients for stroke therapies; this combination more reliably defines the extent of irreversible ischemic brain damage.

Question 6.4: What is the risk of acute kidney injury with CTA?

Answer: The estimated incidence of acute contrast-induced neuropathy with CTA is very low (2–3%). Emergent CTA is not associated with subsequent chronic kidney disease or hemodialysis.

4 CT AND MR ANGIOGRAPHY

In patients with acute ischemic stroke these tests help distinguish between a complete occlusion, stenosis or patency of cervical and intracranial vessels. In hemorrhagic stroke, CT angiography (CTA) and magnetic resonance angiography (MRA) are critical in detecting vascular lesions such as aneurysms and vascular malformations (arteriovenous malformations and fistulas). The decision to proceed with catheter angiography as a diagnostic modality in ICH is rarely required emergently and is typically left to the discretion of a neurosurgeon or vascular neurologist. In spontaneous ICH without an underlying vascular lesion, both CTA and MRA are expected to be "negative." However, CTA offers an advantage by identifying patients with high risk for hematoma expansion. CTA can identify foci with contrast enhancement and extravasation; this radiographic finding is known as the "spot sign."[37,38] Early recognition of the "spot sign" can alert a physician for closer monitoring of such patients, who could benefit from more aggressive blood pressure control and other therapeutic interventions.[39]

In acute ischemic stroke, CTA or MRA is typically not required to determine eligibility for IV alteplase. With the recognition of EVT as another recommended treatment of ischemic stroke, it is not uncommon to face the following dilemma in the emergency room—should the patient who is a candidate for both therapies have CTA or MRA performed first, followed by administration of IV alteplase *or* should EVT be performed after the alteplase drip has been started? The dilemma comes from conflicting recommendations, which state that both therapies should be initiated without a delay because the success rate of both systemic and endovascular therapies is time-dependent. The use of standardized protocols allows improved workflow and minimizes delays to baseline imaging and initiation of both treatments.[40,41,42] Such protocols should be tailored toward an individual hospital based on the performance of the following metrics: door to CT time, door to needle time (IV alteplase metric), and door to puncture time (endovascular therapy metric). Hospitals that chose to perform angiography together with non-contrast CT typically establish an NIHSS cut-off to avoid unnecessary testing in patients who are less likely to harbor an LVO. Many centers now choose the NIHSS cutoff of 6 because this number is recommended by the American Heart Association as the lower threshold for selection of patients for endovascular therapy.

Angiography not only detects the presence and location of occlusion but also helps the neurointerventionalist with planning of the procedure. Many factors, such as aortic arch anatomy, cervical tortuosity, severe stenosis or occlusion, and the extent of thrombus will affect the choice of vascular access, thrombectomy devices, and adjunct tools. MRA can be of benefit in patients who have serious allergies to iodine contrast, which is required to perform CTA. While emergent premedication with steroid, antihistamine, and H2-receptor antagonist can be performed, concern for such allergies often significantly delays performance of CTA.

It should be emphasized that while there is a body of literature describing clot characteristics that are associated with higher rates of IV alteplase "failure"—such as clot length exceeding 8 mm and certain locations of occlusion including the ICA terminus—in patients who are eligible for both therapies, IV alteplase should be administered first, followed by EVT.[43,44] For ischemic stroke, there has been no direct comparison of EVT as the sole treatment with the combined IV alteplase + EVT, and such trials are currently at the early stages of design.

4.1 Multiphase CT angiography (mCTA)

Often termed "dynamic CTA," multiphase CT angiography (mCTA) is a modification of the conventional (single-phase) CTA that allows a more detailed evaluation of the degree of intracranial collaterals. These collaterals are networks of vessels that redirect blood in a retrograde fashion to allow reperfusion of the brain area affected by arterial occlusion. They have a strong effect on neurologic recovery in patients who undergo EVT. This approach to patient selection was utilized in the ESCAPE randomized trial of endovascular stroke therapy.[45] mCTA uses a single-time administration of contrast, but it requires repeat scanning of intracranial circulation several seconds after the initial scan to image the contrast distribution within the collateral circulation during the capillary and venous phases. It is proposed that additional information obtained with mCTA can better assist with selection of patients for endovascular therapy, as well as improve identification of smaller, more distal occlusions, which can be challenging to recognize with conventional CTA.[46,47]

5 PERFUSION IMAGING

Both CT and MR-based perfusion imaging can be applied to the evaluation of patients with acute ischemic stroke. Because of the widespread use of CT tomography in the emergency setting, most clinical centers utilize CT rather than MR-based perfusion. There is great variability among stroke centers regarding which patients undergo perfusion imaging. Some centers apply perfusion imaging only to "challenging" stroke cases such as wake-up strokes, cases with limited clinical information, or when CT ASPECTS cannot be reliably interpreted. Other centers use perfusion imaging on all patients with suspected ischemic stroke. In such cases, computed tomography perfusion is performed simultaneously with CTA head/neck. Perfusion imaging is rarely used for the evaluation of hemorrhagic stroke.

In ischemic stroke, perfusion imaging helps determine the extent of irreversibly infracted brain tissue (called ischemic "core") and of potentially salvageable tissue at risk (called ischemic "penumbra"). Various fully automated software processing packages are currently available that provide clinicians with easy-to-interpret color maps, as well as quantitative data on the volume of infarcted tissue and tissue at risk. There is no uniform agreement on which perfusion map parameters best define ischemic "core" and "penumbra." Critics of perfusion imaging argue that it might overcall the degree of ischemic burden and thus mistakenly deny treatment to patients who might still benefit from reperfusion.[48] The proponents of perfusion imaging believe that it allows more accurate selection of patients for acute reperfusion therapies, when compared to non-contrast CT alone. An example of perfusion imaging generated with RAPID automated software is shown in Case 6.5.

6 CLINICAL CASES

Case 6.1 Hypertension-related intracranial hemorrhage

CASE DESCRIPTION

A patient presented to the ED with acute onset of headache and right hemiparesis 2 hours prior to admission. Systolic blood pressure was 240 mm Hg and non-contrast head CT showed a parenchymal hemorrhage. CTA of head was unremarkable (Figure 6.2).

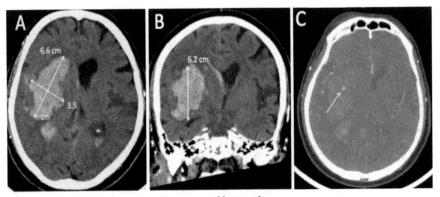

Figure 6.2 Hypertension-related intracranial hemorrhage.
(A,B) Non-contrast head computed tomography, axial and coronal views, showing a large intraparenchymal hematoma. Intraventricular blood and hydrocephalus is also present. Using the ABC/2 method, the estimated size of the hematoma is 72 ml (6.6 × 3.5 × 6.2/ 2 = 72).
(C) CT angiography shows the spot sign (arrow), representing extravasation of contrast within the hematoma.

PRACTICAL POINTS

- Elevated blood pressure, "negative" CTA, and location of the hemorrhage suggest hypertension as the primary etiology of this ICH. However, elevated blood pressure could be the brain's secondary physiologic response to regulate cerebral perfusion pressure. Therefore, other potential causes of ICH such as an underlying tumor (primary or metastatic) or amyloid angiography need to be rule out, which is done using MRI brain with gadolinium.
- Approximately 1 in 3 patients with ICH will develop hematoma growth. The dot sign on CTA can help identify patients who are at risk for hematoma expansion. However, in a general population of patients with ICH, trials have failed to demonstrate the benefit of aggressive lowering of blood pressure in the acute phase of the hemorrhage.
- Minimally invasive surgical approaches to hematoma removal, such as stereotactic aspiration, are being tested in this population of patients.[49]

Case 6.2 Acute ischemic stroke, left MCA occlusion

CASE DESCRIPTION
A patient with acute onset of global aphasia, left gaze deviation, and dense right hemiparesis witnessed by a coworker 90 minutes prior to arrival to the ED. Patient's NIHSS score was above 20. Non-contrast head CT showed no hemorrhage and a

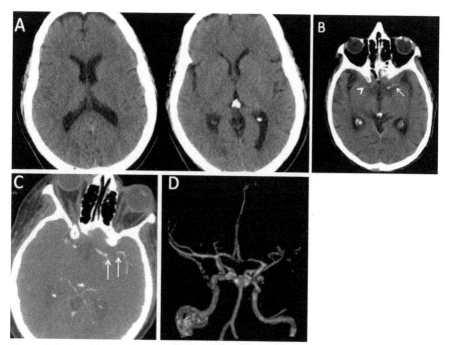

Figure 6.3 Acute ischemic stroke, left middle cerebral artery occlusion.
(A) Non-contrast head computed tomography with no evidence of hemorrhage or major areas of hypoattenuation. ASPECTS of 10.
(B) Hyperdense appearance of the horizontal segment (M1 segment) of the left middle cerebral artery is seen (arrow). The appearance of the right middle cerebral artery (MCA) is "normal" (arrowhead).
(C) Computed tomography angiography, axial cut, and 3D reconstruction (D) shows a filling defect within the left MCA M1 segment, confirming its occlusion. The occluded segment measures >8 mm in length, which is best appreciated on the axial image (indicated by the two arrows). Distal MCA branches fill in a retrograde fashion via the collaterals.

bright appearance of the left MCA M1 segment. CTA head and neck demonstrated occlusion of the left M1 segment (Figure 6.3).

PRACTICAL POINTS

- ASPECTS is calculated by scoring the number of regions with signs of early ischemic changes. These regions are assigned within two axial cuts: one at the level of the thalamus and basal ganglia structures and one at the level above the ganglionic structures. Manually adjusting window settings to 40 HU width and 40 HU level provides an optimal view to score ASPECTS.
- Based on the severity of stroke symptoms (NIHSS >20), time of arrival to the ED within 4.5 hours and non-contrast CT results, the patient is a

candidate for IV thrombolysis. CTA confirmed presence of LVO, making the patient eligible for EVT. Once IV alteplase (bolus, followed by a drip for 60 minutes) infusion is started, the patient should be immediately taken to the angiography suite for EVT. Waiting for a clinical response from the alteplase is not recommended, because delaying EVT can greatly reduce the patient's chances of a good clinical outcome.

Case 6.3 "Wake-up" stoke and LVO

CASE DESCRIPTION

A patient was found in the morning by a family member to have decreased level of consciousness, right gaze deviation, and left hemiplegia. Patient was last known to be "well" before going to bed the night before. Non-contrast CT head showed a large area of hypodensity within the right hemisphere. Right ICA occlusion was diagnosed on MRA (Figure 6.4).

PRACTICAL POINTS

- This scenario is frequently referred to as a "wake-up" stroke. The exact time of stroke onset is unknown, and the time of last known well is used instead. Most patients present well outside of the 4.5-hour window for IV alteplase. EVT, based on favorable non-contrast CT ASPECTS or perfusion, can

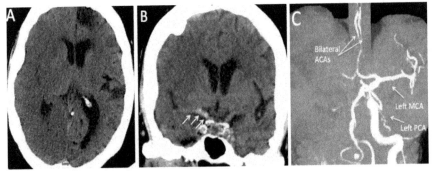

Figure 6.4 Wake-up stoke and large vessel occlusion.
(A) Non-contrast head computed tomography (CT), axial view, shows a large area of hypodensity involving the majority of the right middle cerebral artery (MCA) territory, as well as of the right posterior cerebral artery (PCA) territory. (B) Non-contrast head CT, coronary view, a hyperdense vessel sign including the proximal MCA as well as the distal internal carotid artery (ICA) can be seen (arrows). This indicates a possibility of a large clot within the affected arterial segments.
(C) MR angiography, 3D reconstruction, confirms presence of intracranial right ICA occlusion. NOTE the lack of opacification of the right PCA, which explains the extent of stroke seen on non contrast CT. This is often seen in cases of "fetal" PCA variant.

be considered. Perfusion-based selection of wake-up strokes for EVT has been proven highly effective in the latest randomized trial (DAWN), which enrolled patients up to 24 hours of stroke onset.

- Unfortunately, in this case, the patient arrived with evidence of major infarct seen on the initial CT. Such low ASPECTS indicates futility of revascularization with high risk for reperfusion hemorrhage.
- The term "malignant MCA infarct" refers to large infarction with acute brain edema and elevated intracranial pressure. Medical management involves the use of osmotic agents, such as mannitol or hypertonic saline.[50] Decompressive hemicraniectomy performed within the first 48 hours of stroke onset is indicated in carefully selected patients due to the risk of brain herniation.[50] In this case, there is also involvement of the posterior cerebral artery territory within the area of the infarct, which further increases the risk of herniation.

Case 6.4 Posterior circulation acute ischemic stroke

CASE DESCRIPTION

The patient presented to the ED with acute onset of headache, right arm and leg weakness, and tongue deviation to the left. Symptoms started 90 minutes prior to arrival to the ED, where neurologic evaluation demonstrated a fluctuating degree of weakness, with NIHSS score ranging from 3 to 9. Non-contrast CT head was unremarkable. MRI fast sequence was ordered and was interpreted as "normal" (Figure 6.5).

PRACTICAL POINTS

- This case represents several challenging topics relevant to evaluation of patients with acute ischemic stroke who present within the time window for IV alteplase. First, an alternative diagnose could be a complex migraine. Headaches frequently accompany patients with acute ischemic stroke. Patients with complex migraine will often describe multiple prior episodes with stereotypical symptoms. Second, patients with fluctuating symptoms should not be confused with patients with rapidly improving symptoms. If the severity of fluctuating deficits still reaches the lower threshold for IV alteplase, administration of alteplase should be considered. Finally, MRI brain can show no acute stroke when performed in a hyperacute state. If symptoms are suggestive of a stroke, IV alteplase should be considered.
- There is a lack of strong evidence regarding the role of EVT in this population of patients, if LVO is seen on angiography. The guidelines recommend EVT in patients with NIHSS ≥6. Reports of cases of endovascular therapy in patients with NIHSS score <6 exist, but more data are needed to compare the natural history of these patients with outcomes following EVT.[51,52]

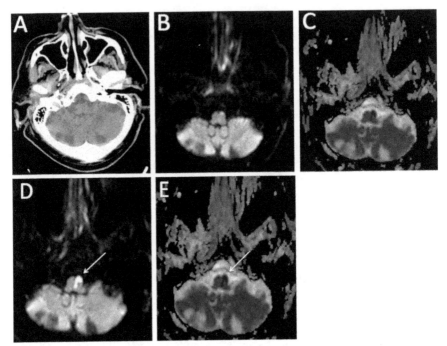

Figure 6.5 Posterior circulation acute ischemic stroke.
(A) Non contrast head computed tomography and (B) magnetic resonance imaging
(MRI) diffusion weighted image (DWI) and (C) apparent diffusion coefficient (ADC)
sequences show no findings suggestive of acute ischemia, which is commonly referred to
as "normal" or "negative" studies. Multiple areas of encephalomalacia suggestive of old
cerebellar strokes are present.
(D,E) Repeat MRI at 24 hours shows acute an area of restricted diffusion on DWI
with the corresponding signal changes on ADC, suggestive of acute ischemic stroke
of the left medial medulla. Together with the patient's clinical presentation, it
represents the medial medullary (Dejerine) syndrome. On careful examination of
the initial MRI DWI sequence (panel B), there is a subtle indication of hyperacute
stroke within this region; however, it was originally interpreted as an artifact by a
radiologist.

Case 6.5 Perfusion-based selection for revascularization therapy in acute ischemic stroke

CASE DESCRIPTION

The patient was found by the neighbor at 2 PM. The patient's deficits included confusion, left hemiplegia and neglect, and NIHSS score of 16. The patient's past medical history was unknown, and time of last known normal could not be established,
and non-contrast CT head was unremarkable. CT perfusion was processed with
automated RAPID software package (iSchemaView, Inc; Menlo Park, California)
(Figure 6.6).

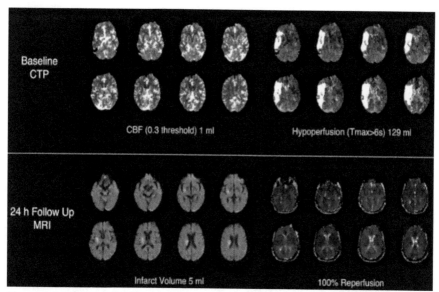

Figure 6.6 Perfusion-based selection for revascularization therapy in acute ischemic stroke. Computed tomography perfusion is processed with fully automated RAPID software package (iSchemaView, Inc; California). Top row shows the size and location of the ischemic core lesion (labeled "CBF," 1 ml volume) and ischemic penumbra (labeled "Hypoperfusion," 129 ml volume). Following successful recanalization with thrombectomy, a small final infarct is seen on magnetic resonance imaging at 24 hours (labeled "Infarct volume," 5 ml volume). Complete reperfusion was achieved in this case.

PRACTICAL POINTS

- This scenario is similar to the earlier case of wake-up stroke. Due to lack of history to determine contraindications to IV alteplase and no clear time of symptom onset, this patient would not be eligible for IV alteplase. Perfusion imaging showed a small ischemic core and a large area of potentially salvageable tissue, indicating a high chance for clinical recovery with endovascular therapy. Some clinicians also rely on "clinical penumbra," where the degree of clinical cortical deficits helps establish the extent of brain tissue at risk.
- In this case, perfusion imaging also helped differentiate between alternative causes of focal neurologic deficits, such as postictal state. Because the size of the ischemic core was so small, initial CT head was interpreted as "normal."

REFERENCES

1. Dubosh NM, Bellolio MF, Rabinstein AA, Edlow JA. Sensitivity of early brain computed tomography to exclude aneurysmal subarachnoid hemorrhage: a systematic review and meta-analysis. *Stroke.* 2016;47(3):750–755.

2. Chalela, JA, Kidwell CS, Nentwich LM, et al. Magnetic resonance imaging and computed tomography in emergency assessment of patients with suspected acute stroke: a prospective comparison. *Lancet*. 2007;369(9558):293–298.

3. Kothari RU, Brott T, Broderick JP, et al. The ABCs of measuring intracerebral hemorrhage volumes. *Stroke*. 1996;27(8):1304–1305.

4. Brazzelli M, Sandercock PA, Chappell FM, et al. Magnetic resonance imaging versus computed tomography for detection of acute vascular lesions in patients presenting with stroke symptoms. *Cochrane Db Syst Rev*. 2009;7(4):CD007424.

5. Lansberg MG, Albers GW, Beaulieu C, Marks MP. Comparison of diffusion-weighted MRI and CT in acute stroke. *Neurology*. (2000);54(8):1557–1561.

6. Demaerschalk BM, Kleindorfer DO, Adeoye OM, et al. Scientific rationale for the inclusion and exclusion criteria for intravenous alteplase in acute ischemic stroke: a statement for healthcare professionals from the American Heart Association/ American Stroke Association. *Stroke*. 2016;47(2):581–641.

7. Barber PA, Demchuk AM, Zhang J, Buchan AM. Validity and reliability of a quantitative computed tomography score in predicting outcome of hyperacute stroke before thrombolytic therapy. ASPECTS Study Group. Alberta Stroke Programme Early CT Score. *Lancet*. 2000;355(9216):1670–1674.

8. Herweh C, Ringleb PA, Rauch G. Performance of e-ASPECTS software in comparison to that of stroke physicians on assessing CT scans of acute ischemic stroke patients. *Int J Stroke*. 2016;11(4):438–445.

9. Song D, Lee K, Kim EH, et al. Gray-matter volume estimate score: a novel semi-automatic method measuring early ischemic change on CT. *J Stroke*. 2016;18(1):80–86.

10. Goyal M, Menon BK, van Zwam WH, et al. Endovascular thrombectomy after large-vessel ischaemic stroke: a meta-analysis of individual patient data from five randomised trials. *Lancet*. 2016;387(10029):1723–1731.

11. Noorian AR, Rangaraju S, Sun C-H, et al. Endovascular therapy in strokes with ASPECTS 5–7 may result in smaller infarcts and better outcomes as compared to medical treatment alone. *Interv Neurol*. 2015;4(1–2), 30–37.

12. Arboix A, García-Eroles L, Sellarés N, et al. Infarction in the territory of the anterior cerebral artery: clinical study of 51 patients. *BMC Neurol*. 2009;9:30.

13. Beslow LA, Vossough A, Dahmoush HM, et al. Modified pediatric ASPECTS correlates with infarct volume in childhood arterial ischemic stroke. *Front Neurol*. 2012;3:122.

14. Puetz V, Sylaja PN, Coutts SB, et al. Extent of hypoattenuation on CT angiography source images predicts functional outcome in patients with basilar artery occlusion. *Stroke*. 2008;39(9), 2485–2490.

15. Sun CH, Connelly K, Nogueira RG, et al. ASPECTS decay during inter-facility transfer predicts patient outcomes in endovascular reperfusion for ischemic stroke: a unique assessment of dynamic physiologic change over time. *J Neurointerv Surg*. 2015;7(1):22–26.

16. Liebeskind DS, Jahan R, Nogueira RG, et al. Serial Alberta Stroke Program early CT score from baseline to 24 hours in Solitaire Flow Restoration with the Intention for Thrombectomy study: a novel surrogate end point for revascularization in acute stroke. *Stroke*. 2014;45(3), 723–727.

17. Liebeskind DS, Jahan R, Nogueira, RG, et al. Impact of collaterals on successful revascularization in Solitaire FR with the intention for thrombectomy. *Stroke*. 2014;45(7):2036–2040.

18. Mokin M, Gupta R, Guerrero1 WR, et al. ASPECTS decay during inter-facility transfer in patients with large vessel occlusion strokes. *J Neurointerv Surg*. 2017;9:442–444.

19. Launes J, Ketonen L. Dense middle cerebral artery sign: an indicator of poor outcome in middle cerebral artery area infarction. *J Neurol Neurosurg Psychiatry*. 1987;50(11):1550–1552 (1987).

20. Goldmakher GV, Camargo EC, Furie KL, et al. Hyperdense basilar artery sign on unenhanced CT predicts thrombus and outcome in acute posterior circulation stroke. *Stroke*. 2009;40(1):134–139.

21. Paciaroni M, Agnelli G, Floridi P, et al. Hyperdense middle cerebral and/or internal carotid arteries in acute ischemic stroke: rate, predictive factors and influence on clinical outcome. *Cerebrovasc Dis*. 2011;32(3):239–245.

22. Leary MC, Kidwell CS, Villablanca JP, et al. Validation of computed tomographic middle cerebral artery "dot"sign: an angiographic correlation study. *Stroke*. 2003;34(11):2636–2640, doi:10.1161/01.STR.0000092123.00938.83 (2003).

23. Koo CK, Teasdale E, Muir KW. What constitutes a true hyperdense middle cerebral artery sign? *Cerebrovasc Dis*. 2000;10(6):419–423.

24. Manelfe C, Larrue V, von Kummer R, et al. Association of hyperdense middle cerebral artery sign with clinical outcome in patients treated with tissue plasminogen activator. *Stroke*. 1999;30(4):769–772.

25. Rauch RA, Bazan C, 3rd, Larsson EM, Jinkins JR. Hyperdense middle cerebral arteries identified on CT as a false sign of vascular occlusion. *Am J Neuroradiol*. 1993;14(3):669–673.

26. Mehta BP, Nogueira RG. Should clot composition affect choice of endovascular therapy? *Neurology*. 2012;79(13 Supp 1), S63–S67.

27. Brinjikji W, Duffy S, Burrows A, et al. Correlation of imaging and histopathology of thrombi in acute ischemic stroke with etiology and outcome: a systematic review. *J Neurointerv Surg*. 2017;9(6):529–534.

28. Charidimou A, Kakar P, Fox Z, Werring DJ. Cerebral microbleeds and the risk of intracerebral haemorrhage after thrombolysis for acute ischaemic stroke: systematic review and meta-analysis. *J Neurol Neurosurg Psychiatry*. 2013;84(3):277–280.

29. Charidimou A, Shoamanesh A, Wilson D, et al. Cerebral microbleeds and postthrombolysis intracerebral hemorrhage risk Updated meta-analysis. *Neurology*. 2015;85(11):927–934.

30. Erdur H, Scheitz JF, Tütüncü S, et al. Safety of thrombolysis in patients with acute ischemic stroke and cerebral cavernous malformations. *Stroke*. (2014);45(6):1846–1848.

31. Rosso C, Drier A, Lacroix D, et al. Diffusion-weighted MRI in acute stroke within the first 6 hours: 1.5 or 3.0 Tesla? *Neurology*. 2010:74(24):1946–1953.

32. Oppenheim C, Stanescu R, Dormont D, et al. False-negative diffusion-weighted MR findings in acute ischemic stroke. *Am J Neuroradiol*. 2000;21(8):1434–1440.

33. de Margerie-Mellon C, Turc G, Tisserand M, et al. Can DWI-ASPECTS substitute for lesion volume in acute stroke? *Stroke* 2013;44(12):3565–3567.

34. Olivot JM, Mosimann PJ, Labreuche J, et al. Impact of diffusion-weighted imaging lesion volume on the success of endovascular reperfusion therapy. *Stroke.* 2013;44(8):2205–2211.

35. Soize S, Tisserand M, Charron S, et al. How sustained is 24-hour diffusion-weighted imaging lesion reversal? Serial magnetic resonance imaging in a patient cohort thrombolyzed within 4.5 hours of stroke onset. *Stroke.* 2015;46(3):704–710.

36. Labeyrie MA, Turc G, Hess A, et al. Diffusion lesion reversal after thrombolysis: a MR correlate of early neurological improvement. *Stroke.* 2012;43(11):2986–2991.

37. Wada R, Aviv RI, Fox AJ, et al. CT angiography "spot sign" predicts hematoma expansion in acute intracerebral hemorrhage. *Stroke.* 2007;38(4):1257–1262.

38. Du FZ, Jiang R, Gu M, He C, Guan, J. The accuracy of spot sign in predicting hematoma expansion after intracerebral hemorrhage: a systematic review and meta-analysis. *PLoS ONE.* 2014;9(12):e115777.

39. Wartenberg KE, Mayer SA. Ultra-early hemostatic therapy for intracerebral hemorrhage: future directions. *Front Neurol Neurosci.* 2015;37:107–129.

40. Menon BK, Almekhlafi MA, Pereira VM, et al. Optimal workflow and process-based performance measures for endovascular therapy in acute ischemic stroke: analysis of the Solitaire FR thrombectomy for acute revascularization study. *Stroke.* 2014;45(7):2024–2029.

41. Frei D, McGraw C, McCarthy K, et al. A standardized neurointerventional thrombectomy protocol leads to faster recanalization times. *J Neurointerv Surg.* 2016;9(11):1035–1040.

42. Van Schaik SM, Van der Veen B, Van den Berg-Vos RM, Weinstein HC, Bosboom,WM. Achieving a door-to-needle time of 25 minutes in thrombolysis for acute ischemic stroke: a quality improvement project. *J Stroke Cerebrovasc Dis.* 2014;23(10):2900–2906.

43. Saqqur M, Uchino K, Demchuk AM, et al. Site of arterial occlusion identified by transcranial Doppler predicts the response to intravenous thrombolysis for stroke. *Stroke.* 2007;38(3):948–954.

44. Riedel CH, Zimmermann P, Jensen-Kondering U, et al. The importance of size: successful recanalization by intravenous thrombolysis in acute anterior stroke depends on thrombus length. *Stroke.* 2011;42(6):1775–1777.

45. Goyal M, Demchuk AM, Menon, BK, et al. Randomized assessment of rapid endovascular treatment of ischemic stroke. *N Engl J Med.* 2015;372(11):1019–1030.

46. Menon BK, d'Esterre CD, Qazi EM, et al. Multiphase CT angiography: a new tool for the imaging triage of patients with acute ischemic stroke. *Radiology.* 2015;275(2):510–520.

47. Yu AY, Zerna C, Assis Z, et al. Multiphase CT angiography increases detection of anterior circulation intracranial occlusion. *Neurology.* 2016;87(6):609–616.

48. Boned S, Padroni M, Rubiera M, et al. Admission CT perfusion may overestimate initial infarct core: the ghost infarct core concept. *J Neurointerv Surg.* 2017;9(1):66–69.

49. Fiorella D, Arthur A, Bain M, Mocco J. Minimally invasive surgery for intracerebral and intraventricular hemorrhage: rationale, review of existing data and emerging technologies. *Stroke.* 2016;47(5):1399–1406.

50. Wijdicks EF, Sheth KN, Carter BS, et al. Recommendations for the management of cerebral and cerebellar infarction with swelling: a statement for healthcare professionals from the American Heart Association/American Stroke Association. *Stroke.* 2014;45(4):1222–1238.

51. Haussen DC, Bouslama M, Grossberg JA, et al. Too good to intervene? Thrombectomy for large vessel occlusion strokes with minimal symptoms: an intention-to-treat analysis. *J Neurointerv Surg.* 2016;9(10):917–921.

52. Mokin M, Masud MW, Dumont TM, et al. Outcomes in patients with acute ischemic stroke from proximal intracranial vessel occlusion and NIHSS score below 8. *J Neurointerv Surg.* 2014;6(6):413–417.

7

Telemedicine for Evaluation of Stroke Patients

KAUSTUBH LIMAYE AND LAWRENCE R. WECHSLER ∎

CONTENTS

1 INTRODUCTION

The initial use of precursors to telemedicine consultations occurred the fields of psychiatry and radiology.[1,2] Unfortunately, these pilot projects did not succeed, in part due to poor organization, a lack of financial sustainability, and an absence of standards and laws in this area of healthcare.

More recently, evolving economic and healthcare policies fostered a slow but steady revival of telemedicine.

Telestroke was developed to apply telemedicine for the delivery of stroke expertise, including evaluation and treatment of acute stroke, secondary prevention, and patient follow-up and stroke rehabilitation. Recent developments in the field have increased the need for emergent evaluation by experienced stroke specialists. Such developments include the evidence supporting endovascular thrombectomy (EVT), either in combination with intravenous (IV) alteplase or alone, along with the rapidly changing and expanding criteria for patient selection for recanalization therapies, advances in minimally invasive treatment of intracerebral hemorrhage (ICH). Telestroke effectively provides such expertise and allows at least a partial shift of the burden of managing these complex patients from the Emergency Department (ED) physicians to a remotely located stroke specialist.

For example, in the Telemedicine in Stroke in Swabia (TESS) study, in which stroke patients presenting to several rural hospitals in Germany were evaluated via telestroke, consultations in a rural setting led to a modification in the diagnosis and/or management of nearly 75% of the consultations.[3] These consultations included patients with transient ischemic attacks, ischemic stroke, and ICH; they averaged 15 minutes in duration and included diagnostic workup, computed tomography (CT) assessment, and therapeutic recommendations.

The technology used as a part of the modern telestroke consultation comprises high quality two-way, interactive videoconferencing (Figure 7.1). This is typically accomplished using video codecs or Web-based interfaces and, more recently, with smartphones and tablet devices.

2 TELESTROKE MODELS

Telestroke networks most commonly consist of originating sites (spokes) where the patient is located and distant site (hub) where the provider is located. Telestroke offers stroke expertise to such remote sites and small hospitals with limited stroke neurology (and often even no general neurology) coverage. Telestroke is a growing model, with an increasing number of spoke hospitals per hub.[4] The two most commonly used telestroke models are a hub and spoke model and a distributed model.

Question 7.1: What types of hospitals most commonly rely on telestroke coverage?

Answer: More than 80% of spoke sites are rural or small hospitals.

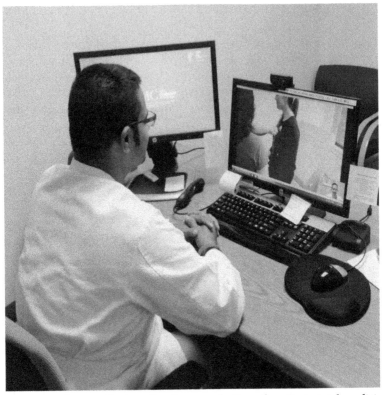

Figure 7.1 A stroke specialist is performing an evaluation of a patient via telemedicine using two-way videoconferencing.

2.1 Hub and spoke model

The hub and spoke is the most common model used in the United States.[4] In this model, a provider group, usually consisting of vascular neurologists or other stroke specialists residing in a tertiary stroke center (typically, a comprehensive stroke center [CSC]), serves as the acute stroke team for one or more community or rural hospitals, evaluating stroke patients with 24/7/365 availability. The vascular neurologists often join the medical staff of the spoke hospitals, which means the hospitals will grant them consultation or telemedicine privileges, allow them to enter orders, and document directly in the patient's record. Depending upon the specific arrangements, the stroke team or the ED physicians might obtain consent and order alteplase when appropriate. If the spoke hospital has adequate facilities to achieve primary stroke center certification, patients may be admitted there after treatment with alteplase. In other cases, patients are assessed and treated at the spoke hospital and then transferred for post alteplase care. The stroke team also assesses the eligibility for EVT and arranges transfer to the hub hospital for patients who are candidates for EVT.

2.2 Distributed model

The distributed telestroke model differs in that a group of providers consult at originating sites but without a clinical hub and spoke relationship. In this model, stroke specialists evaluate patients by telemedicine and give advice on eligibility for IV alteplase or EVT. Other than this interaction, the consulting physician has no ongoing relationship with the spoke hospital. Alteplase is given at the originating site after consultation with the telestroke provider, and each site needs to have a transfer relationship with a local CSC capable of providing post alteplase care as well as EVT. These transfer sites should be chosen to minimize transfer time and, in the case of mechanical thrombectomy, door-to-groin puncture time.

3 EVIDENCE FOR TELESTROKE

The majority of studies evaluating the impact of telestroke focus on acute stroke triage and treatment with IV alteplase. The role telestroke plays in accurately identifying and triaging patients eligible for EVT has not been well studied.

3.1 Telestroke and treatment with IV alteplase

In small community hospitals, before the availability of telestroke services, a "ship and drip" model was often used, where the patient first had to be transferred to the nearest hospital capable of administering alteplase before the treatment with IV alteplase could be initiated.[5] The ship and drip model caused considerable treatment delay, and not infrequently the patients reaching the stroke centers were outside the time window for the alteplase treatment. In a study of 4750 hospitals in the MEDPAR database, an alarming 64% of hospitals reported no administration of alteplase within a 2-year period.[6] These hospitals tended to be small, with fewer than 100 beds, and located in sparsely populated areas.

One of the earliest pilot studies of telestroke, the Telemedic Pilot Project for Integrative Stroke Care (TEMPiS) in Bavaria, examined telestroke consultations in community hospitals without pre-existing specialized stroke care using telemedical support from academic hospitals.[7] Stroke and TIA admissions to a stroke unit increased from 19% to 78% over a 10-year period. At the same time, the number of patients who were treated with alteplase increased from 3% to 16%.

The Stroke DOC Trial sought to compare the effect of video versus telephone consultation on establishing the correct diagnosis and decisions regarding thrombolysis.[8] Patients were randomly assigned to receive telestroke evaluation (real-time, two-way audio and video and digital imaging interpretation) or phone consultation from a single stroke center. An independent review committee retrospectively judged whether the correct decision was made regarding treatment with alteplase. Telemedicine consultations resulted in more accurate decision-making compared with telephone consultations. Specifically, the review committee agreed with the decision regarding treatment in 98% of patients in the telestroke group, and 82% of those assessed over the telephone. In those patients treated with alteplase A, the difference between the two groups was even greater.

3.1.1 SAFETY OF ALTEPLASE WITH TELESTROKE

Results from multiple studies reveal that the rates of post IV alteplase hemorrhages, mortality, and the length of hospital stay in patients treated using telestroke consultations are comparable to rates reported at the hub sites.[8–11] Based on these and other studies, the American Heart Association (AHA) now endorses the use of distant video-based examination to determine eligibility for IV alteplase in patients with suspected acute ischemic stroke.[12]

3.2 Telestroke and endovascular therapy

CT or magnetic resonance (MR) angiography is not always available at small community hospitals to determine which patients with acute stroke have emergent large vessel occlusion (LVO) requiring EVT. As we usher in a new era of endovascular management of acute ischemic stroke, telestroke is likely to play an important role in selection of patients for transfer to CSCs or acute stroke ready hospital for EVT using various stroke severity screens (discussed in Chapter 3 of this book). Telestroke also allows assessment of early infarct signs and the Alberta Stroke Program Early CT Score (ASPECTS) on initial CT, avoiding futile transfers, and facilitates discussion of risks and benefits, as well as goals of care with patients and families prior to transfer. Several studies have shown that patients transferred from community hospitals with telestroke coverage are more likely to be treated with EVT, have a faster door-to-groin time and better clinical outcomes than patients transferred from hospitals without telestroke.[13,14]

3.3 Telestroke for patients with intracerebral hemorrhage

The recommendations state that, once diagnosed, patients with ICH should be transferred to tertiary hospitals with neurology, neuroradiology, neurosurgery, and critical care physicians.[15] Alternatively, the guidelines state that a telestroke-based consultation can be utilized for hospitals without on-site presence of such consultants.[15]

A study from Italy included 733 patients with ICH whose radiological and clinical data were transmitted within a hub and spoke telestroke network and neurosurgical teleconsulting was provided by the hub hospital.[16] Using telestroke, a neurosurgical consultation was provided in 38 minutes, whereas a consultation without telestroke coverage took an average of 160 minutes. Twenty-four percent of patients with ICH were transferred to the hub, and 54% of these patients required surgical treatment. Only 1.4% of patients who remained and were treated at the spoke hospitals needed a subsequent transfer for surgical treatment because of a worsening clinical condition or imaging CT findings. This study illustrates the value of telestroke in optimizing utilization of resourses at smaller peripheral spoke hospitals and larger specialized hub hospitals.

Telestroke can also help in the initial management of acute ICH. A small study from southern California demonstrated that telestroke consultation of patients with ICH presenting urban primary stroke centers improved time to blood pressure control and anticoagulation reversal agent initiation.[17]

> **Question 7.2:** What are the common barriers to developing a telestroke program?
>
> **Answer:** Licensing restrictions, lack of reimbursement, and liability are cited as the most common barriers in the literature.

4 LEGAL AND LEGISLATIVE ISSUES AND TELESTROKE

Telemedicine presents unique challenges to existing rules and regulations regarding the practice of medicine. Most regulations were formulated before telemedicine was commonly used. State medical boards and new legislation are beginning to address some of these issues; however, much work remains to be done. The major areas of concern include training, licensing, credentialing, and professional liability.

4.1 Training

As telestroke consists of evaluating a patient present at a distant site, the physician, nursing staff, and other ancillary staff should be trained for these situations. At the originating site, all personnel involved in telestroke consultations should be familiar with the technology and basic troubleshooting processes if a connection cannot be established. Workflows regarding contacting the distant provider, activating equipment, performing consultations, entering orders, and treating with IV alteplase should be reviewed. The training may start preferably in a non-emergent basis in patients with acute ischemic stroke who are out of the time window for treatment. IT personnel, hospital administrators, and the legal team should be involved to make the telestroke program a success.[18]

4.2 Licensing

Licensing is a necessary step before physicians can care for patients in any setting. The physician should be licensed in the state in which the patient resides to perform consultations regardless of the provider site. Many large telestroke networks cover hospitals in several states and the physicians must be licensed in all states where service is provided.

Recognizing these limitations, the Federation of State Medical Boards proposed an Interstate Medical Licensure Compact (IMLC) that establishes an expedited licensure process for physicians in a participating state and requesting licensure in other participating states. The expedited processing would not override the individual states licensing authority, but streamlines the process for licensure. Despite the similarities in the state-to-state licensing, there is no interstate reciprocity or a single federal telestroke license.

As of June 2017, Maine became the 22nd state to join Alabama, Arizona, Colorado, Idaho, Illinois, Iowa, Kansas, Minnesota, Mississippi, Montana, Nebraska, Nevada, New Hampshire, Pennsylvania, South Dakota, Tennessee, Utah, Washington, West Virginia, and Wyoming to enact legislation that expedite multistate licensure as a part of IMLC. This initiative remains under consideration in Michigan, Rhode Island, Texas, the District of Columbia, and Guam. These changes certainly increase access to quality healthcare by expediting and streamlining the licensure process.

4.3 Credentialing

The Center for Medicaid and Medicare (CMS) in 2011 permitted "credentialing by proxy" in small community hospitals. This allows small community hospitals to rely on the credentialing process of larger stroke centers. However, at the state level, most states have yet to change the board requirements accordingly. Proxy credentialing reduces the administrative burden on the small community hospitals and thus increases the population that has access to expert care.

4.4 Medicolegal ramifications

Another concern for telestroke providers is liability and medicolegal responsibility. Whether or not treatment is initiated, the use of alteplase carries a known medicolegal risk. Liang et al. have studied the malpractice suits related to acute ischemic stroke. They conclude that, in most cases, medicolegal risks arise from the patient not getting alteplase in time rather than the complications of its use.[19,20] Similarly, with EVT now being the standard of treatment for patients with emergent LVO, failure to recognize and refer these patients in a timely fashion for endovascular therapy may have medicolegal consequences. Telestroke likely carries the same medicolegal risk as does the evaluation of acute stroke.

5 ECONOMICS OF TELESTROKE

At present, reimbursement for telestroke services remains limited, and this lack of reimbursement significantly impedes further growth. CMS reimburses for telemedicine services only in rural areas, and few other insurers cover telemedicine or telestroke.[18,21] The AHA has recommended new billing codes that would reflect the

---

Box 7.1

FUNDING FOR TELESTROKE

- Grants
- Institutional funding
- State and federal government incentives
- Health insurance reimbursements (public and private)
- Philanthropy

---

start-up as well as the long-term costs incurred by the insurers.[12] The AHA has also recommended that increased reimbursements for thrombolysis diagnosis-related group (DRG; MS-DRG 61–63) be available to the hospitals that supervise the delivery to stroke thrombolysis through telestroke.[12] Box 7.1 describes potential funding options for a telestroke program.

5.1 Defraying start-up cost of telestroke

The cost-effectiveness of telestroke has been previously examined. Nelson and colleagues reported that telestroke is more cost-effective over a life time with incremental cost-effective ratio of $2449 per quality-adjusted life years.[22] Another study from the same group showed that telestroke was most cost-effective for severe strokes.[23] Telestroke was least cost-effective for the spoke hospitals if spokes paid for more than half of implementation costs.[23]

Liang et al. developed a model to study costs and effectiveness with and without a telestroke network over a 5-year period.[20] They found that a network model with 1 hub and 7 spoke hospitals using telestroke would result in 45 more patients treated with alteplase and 20 more patients treated with EVT per year. Each year, such a network was associated with overall $358,435 in cost savings; each of the seven spokes had $109,080 in cost savings, whereas the hub had positive costs of $405,121, indicating the need for cost sharing.

6 CLINICAL CASE

Case 7.1 Evaluation of ischemic stroke via telemedicine

CASE DESCRIPTION

An 80-year-old man was talking to his wife when he suddenly slumped over and collapsed in the chair. The patient was taken to the nearest stroke-ready hospital. He was 1 hour from symptom onset upon arrival to the hospital's ED, and non-contrast CT head reveal no major hypodensity or hemorrhage. The hospital was a part of a hub and spoke network, and the telestroke team at the hub CSC was consulted. The patient's NIHSS was fluctuating between 9 and 27, there were no contraindications to alteplase, and after discussing the case with the local hospital ED attending physician, IV alteplase was started 92 minutes from symptom onset.

There was no rapid availability of CT or MR angiography at the facility. The consulting stroke specialist suspected high likelihood of LVO responsible for patient's stroke symptoms, and the patient was transferred to the hub CSC where CT angiogram demonstrated the top of the basilar occlusion. The patient was immediately taken to the angiography suite and had a successful mechanical thrombectomy.

PRACTICAL POINT

- Ischemic stroke cause by the top of the basilar occlusion is a challenging diagnosis and can often be missed in the emergency setting. A telestroke consultation allows rapid evaluation of such patients by a stroke specialist, resulting in timely decision to proceed with currently available treatments, namely, IV alteplase and EVT.

REFERENCES

1. Wittson CL, Affleck DC, Johnson V. Two-way television in group therapy. *Ment Hosp.* 1961;12:22–23.
2. Jutras A. Teleroentgen diagnosis by means of video-tape recording. *Am J Roentgenol Radium Ther Nucl Med.* 1959;82:1099–1102.
3. Wiborg A, Widder B. Teleneurology to improve stroke care in rural areas: The Telemedicine in Stroke in Swabia (TESS) Project. *Stroke.* 2003;34(12):2951–2956.
4. Silva GS, Farrell S, Shandra E, Viswanathan A, Schwamm LH. The status of telestroke in the United States: a survey of currently active stroke telemedicine programs. *Stroke.* 2012;43(8):2078–2085.
5. Hess DC, Audebert HJ. The history and future of telestroke. *Nat Rev Neurol.* 2013;9(6):340–350.
6. Kleindorfer D, Xu Y, Moomaw CJ, Khatri P, Adeoye O, Hornung R. US geographic distribution of rt-PA utilization by hospital for acute ischemic stroke. *Stroke.* 2009;40(11):3580–3584.
7. Audebert HJ, Schenkel J, Heuschmann PU, Bogdahn U, Haberl RL. Effects of the implementation of a telemedical stroke network: the Telemedic Pilot Project for Integrative Stroke Care (TEMPiS) in Bavaria, Germany. *Lancet Neurol.* 2006;5(9):742–748.
8. Meyer BC, Raman R, Hemmen T, et al. Efficacy of site-independent telemedicine in the STRokE DOC trial: a randomised, blinded, prospective study. *Lancet Neurol.* 2008;7(9):787–795.
9. Shafqat S, Kvedar JC, Guanci MM, Chang Y, Schwamm LH. Role for telemedicine in acute stroke: feasibility and reliability of remote administration of the NIH stroke scale. *Stroke.* 1999;30(10):2141–2145.

10. Demaerschalk BM, Vargas JE, Channer DD, et al. Smartphone teleradiology application is successfully incorporated into a telestroke network environment. *Stroke.* 2012;43(11):3098–3101.

11. Sairanen T, Soinila S, Nikkanen M, et al. Two years of Finnish telestroke: thrombolysis at spokes equal to that at the hub. *Neurology.* 2011;76(13):1145–1152.

12. Schwamm LH, Holloway RG, Amarenco P, et al. A review of the evidence for the use of telemedicine within stroke systems of care: a scientific statement from the American Heart Association/American Stroke Association. *Stroke.* 2009;40(7):2616–2634.

13. Pedragosa A, Alvarez-Sabin J, Rubiera M, et al. Impact of telemedicine on acute management of stroke patients undergoing endovascular procedures. *Cerebrovasc Dis.* 2012;34(5–6):436–442.

14. Kepplinger J, Dzialowski I, Barlinn K, et al. Emergency transfer of acute stroke patients within the East Saxony telemedicine stroke network: a descriptive analysis. *Int J Stroke.* 2014;9(2):160–165.

15. Hemphill JC, 3rd, Greenberg SM, Anderson CS, et al. Guidelines for the management of spontaneous intracerebral hemorrhage: A guideline for healthcare professionals from the American Heart Association/American Stroke Association. *Stroke.* 2015;46(7):2032–2060.

16. Angileri FF, Cardali S, Conti A, Raffa G, Tomasello F. Telemedicine-assisted treatment of patients with intracerebral hemorrhage. *Neurosurg Focus.* 2012;32(4):E6.

17. Sierra C, Ford ZAA, Chen Q, et al. Comparison of standard emergency room care with tele-stroke evaluation in acute intracerebral hemorrhage management. Neurology. 2016;86(16 Suppl):P6:030.

18. Wechsler LR, Demaerschalk BM, Schwamm LH, et al. Telemedicine quality and outcomes in stroke: a scientific statement for healthcare professionals from the American Heart Association/American Stroke Association. *Stroke.* 2017;48(1):e3–e25.

19. Liang BA, Zivin JA. Empirical characteristics of litigation involving tissue plasminogen activator and ischemic stroke. *Ann Emerg Med.* 2008;52(2):160–164.

20. Liang BA, Lew R, Zivin JA. Review of tissue plasminogen activator, ischemic stroke, and potential legal issues. *Arch Neurol.* 2008;65(11):1429–1433.

21. Katie Horton M-BM, Naomi Seiler. Medicare payment rules and telemedicine. *Public Health Rep.* 2014;129(2):196–199.

22. Nelson RE, Saltzman GM, Skalabrin EJ, Demaerschalk BM, Majersik JJ. The cost-effectiveness of telestroke in the treatment of acute ischemic stroke. *Neurology.* 2011;77(17):1590–1598.

23. Nelson RE, Okon N, Lesko AC, Majersik JJ, Bhatt A, Baraban E. The cost-effectiveness of telestroke in the Pacific Northwest region of the USA. *J Telemed Telecare.* 2016;22(7):413–421.

Intravenous Thrombolysis in Acute Ischemic Stroke

WALDO R. GUERRERO, EDGAR A. SAMANIEGO,
AND SANTIAGO ORTEGA-GUTIERREZ ■

CONTENTS

1 INTRODUCTION

Recombinant tissue-type plasminogen activate (rtPA, alteplase) underwent the Food and Drug Administration (FDA) approval in the Unites States in 1996 and is currently the only proven medication to affect outcomes when administered in the hyperacute time frame after ischemic stroke. Since the landmark National Institute of Neurological Disorders and Stroke (NINDS) trial of intravenous (IV) alteplase, there have been several other studies and stroke registries demonstrating the beneficial effect of alteplase on stroke disability.[2–6] Unfortunately, despite its proven benefit, only a minority of patients with acute ischemic stroke (AIS) receive treatment.

2 BARRIERS TO INTRAVENOUS ALTEPLASE

IV alteplase utilization currently ranges from 3–5% since 2004.[7,8] Several factors have been blamed for this dismal use including the lack of community public education about recognition and response to acute stroke symptoms and signs, the slow adjustment of the medical world to thrombolysis, and the complexity of the large system changes at the hospital level that are required for this medication to be provided safely and timely.[9]

However, one of the most likely reasons for the low rate of alteplase utilization is the low eligibility of stroke patients to receive this medication. The most common reason for exclusion is delayed presentation. It is estimated that that roughly 22–31% of patients present within 3 hours from symptom onset.

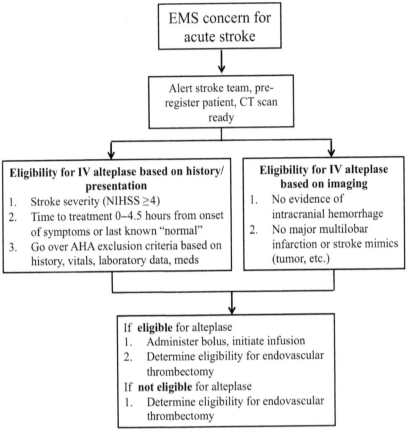

Figure 8.1 Basic algorithm for emergent evaluation of patients for intravenous alteplase.
ABBREVIATIONS: AHA, American Heart Association; CT, computed tomography;
IV, intravenous; NIHSS, National Institutes of Health Stroke Scale.

3 INDICATIONS AND CONTRAINDICATIONS FOR INTRAVENOUS ALTEPLASE

Given the consideration for benefit with the concern for hemorrhagic complications
with IV alteplase, there are various clinical, radiological, and laboratory considerations
that create an individual benefit versus risk determination for each patient. Figure 8.1
describes the basic emergent protocol when evaluating patients with suspected AIS
for IV thrombolysis.

The initial exclusion criteria for alteplase administration were developed for the
original alteplase pilot studies, and many were derived from the cardiac thrombolysis
and basic science literature, all with a focus on safety.[10-15] However, over the years
there have been some modifications to these exclusions. In fact, until recently the

Box 8.1

ORIGINAL EXCLUSION CRITERIA FOR INTRAVENOUS THROMBOLYSIS
BASED ON THE PIVOTAL NATIONAL INSTITUTE OF NEUROLOGICAL
DISORDERS AND STROKE (NINDS) ALTEPLASE TRIAL

- Onset of symptoms >3 hours
- Stroke or serious head trauma within 3 months
- Major surgery within 14 days
- History of intracranial hemorrhage
- Systolic blood pressure >185 mm Hg or diastolic blood pressure >110 mm Hg
- Rapidly improving or minor symptoms
- Symptoms suggestive of subarachnoid hemorrhage
- GI hemorrhage or urinary tract hemorrhage within 21 days
- Arterial puncture at a noncompressible site within 7 days
- Seizure at the onset of stroke
- Taking anticoagulants or received heparin within the 48 hours and an elevated partial-thromboplastin time
- Prothrombin time (PT) >15 seconds
- Platelet counts below 100,000
- Glucose concentrations <50 mg or >400 mg/dL

Adapted from the NINDS and Stroke rt-PA Stroke Study Group study.[1]

---

exclusion criteria listed by the American Heart Association/American Stroke Association (AHA/ASA) was mainly based on the original criteria listed in the pivotal NINDS alteplase trial from 1996 (Box 8.1).[1]

In 2016, the AHA critically reviewed and evaluated the science in terms of these inclusions and exclusions to publish a new set of inclusion/exclusion criteria (Box 8.2).[16] The goal was to help inform the decision-making process for clinicians in terms of the absolute and relative risks and benefits of alteplase treatment, to incorporate 2 decades of experience, to dispel uncertainty and myths about exclusion criteria, and to further quantify estimates of benefit and risk in zones of former uncertainty. In the next couple of paragraphs, we will address some of the more historically controversial inclusion/exclusion criteria.

Question 8.1: What is the recommended time window for IV alteplase?

Answer: Treatment with IV alteplase is recommended up to 4.5 hours from onset of symptoms. Any treatment with IV alteplase beyond this time window is currently considered experimental.

Box 8.2

INCLUSION AND EXCLUSION CRITERIA FOR THE TREATMENT OF ACUTE ISCHEMIC STROKE WITH IV ALTEPLASE

Inclusion criteria

- Diagnosis of ischemic stroke causing measurable neurological deficit
- AHA currently recommends administration of alteplase within 4.5 hours of onset of symptoms
- Age ≥18 years

Exclusion criteria

- Significant head trauma or prior stroke in the previous 3 months
- Symptoms suggest subarachnoid hemorrhage
- Arterial puncture at noncompressible site in previous 7 days
- History of previous intracranial hemorrhage
- Intracranial neoplasm, arteriovenous malformation, or aneurysm
- Recent intracranial or intraspinal surgery
- Elevated blood pressure (systolic >185 mm Hg or diastolic >110 mm Hg)
- Active internal bleeding
- Acute bleeding diathesis, including but not limited to
- Platelet count <100,000/mm^3
- Heparin received within 48 hours resulting in abnormally elevated aPTT above the upper limit of normal
- Current use of anticoagulant with INR >1.7 or PT >15 seconds
- Current use of direct thrombin inhibitors or direct factor Xa inhibitors with elevated sensitive laboratory tests (e.g., aPTT, INR, platelet count, ecarin clotting time, thrombin time, or appropriate factor Xa activity assays)
- Blood glucose concentration <50 mg/dL (2.7 mmol/L)
- CT demonstrates multilobar infarction (hypodensity >1/3 cerebral hemisphere)

Relative exclusion criteria

- Recent experience suggests that under some circumstances, with careful consideration and weighting of risk to benefit, patients may receive fibrinolytic therapy despite ≥1 relative contraindications. Consider risk to benefit of intravenous alteplase administration carefully if any of these relative contraindications is present
- Only minor or rapidly improving stroke symptoms (clearing spontaneously)
- Pregnancy
- Seizure at onset with postictal residual neurological impairments

- Major surgery or serious trauma within previous 14 days
- Recent GI or urinary tract hemorrhage (within previous 21 days)
- Recent acute MI (within previous 3 months)

Adapted from the 2016 AHA criteria for intravenous Alteplase in AIS.[16]

3.1 Time from symptom onset

Time from symptom onset is the most common reason patients are excluded from receiving IV alteplase. Treating physicians are expected to obtain corroborating history on onset time because families often confuse the time of symptom onset with the time the patient was found. The scientific rationale for choosing such a restrictive time window by the original NINDS studies started with ischemic stroke models in rodents and primates, which demonstrated that after 2 to 3 hours occlusion of the middle cerebral artery (MCA) led to permanent larger infarcts compared.[17] The importance of time with a 3-hour window has been shown in multiple studies.[18-20] Earlier thrombolytic treatment within the 3-hour window results in increased odds of a good outcome for the patient.

Recently the European Cooperative Acute Stroke Study III (ECASS III) trial, performed in Europe, included thrombolytic therapy from 3 to 4.5 hours, with the addition of 4 exclusion criteria: age >80 years, National Institutes of Health Stroke Scale (NIHSS) score >25, history of diabetes mellitus and prior stroke, and taking oral anticoagulants (OACs) demonstrate a favorable outcome in patients receiving IV alteplase within 3–4.5 hours.[2]

This pivotal trial led to a revision of the AHA/ASA acute stroke management guidelines, which now **recommended IV alteplase out to 4.5 hours from symptom onset**, provided that the additional exclusion criteria are followed (Case 8.1).

Question 8.2: Why is it critical to rapidly administer IV alteplase to those who are eligible for this treatment?

Answer: The effect of IV alteplase is time-dependent. For example, there is approximately a twofold decrease in the efficacy of alteplase when given within 3–4.5 hour versus treatment in the first 90 minutes of symptom onset.

3.2 Age

One of the most controversial issues in the decision to treat patients with alteplase is age. The FDA alteplase label states that for patients over 75 years of age the risks of alteplase may be increased and should be balanced against the anticipated benefits. Age is a critical factor in terms of the incident risk of stroke and the associated outcomes.[21,22] The risk of ischemic stroke doubles for each successive decade after 55 years of age.[23,24] Furthermore, death at discharge is two- and threefold higher among octogenarians and those >90 years of age, respectively, compared with younger individuals.[25]

The benefits of alteplase in stroke patients over 80 years of age has been assessed and demonstrated in both randomized and observational studies. A recent meta-analysis from 6 randomized trials demonstrated that among patients treated within 3 hours, for every 1000 patients >80 years of age, there would be 96 more patients alive and independent at follow-up.[26] In fact, results from the two largest observational studies evaluating the benefits of alteplase by age were the Safe Implementation of Treatments in Stroke–International Stroke Thrombolysis Registry (SITS-ISTR) and the Virtual International Stroke Trials Archive (VISTA). A study combining these registries and including 29,500 patients of which 3472 (11.8%) were over 80 years of age concluded that patients in this age group who received IV alteplase had a higher odds of excellent outcome as defined by a modified Rankin Score (mRS) score of 0–1 after receiving IV alteplase.[27,28] In addition, patients over 80 years of age who received IV alteplase had decreased mortality when compared to patients who did not receive it.[28]

The main concern and feared complication of treating patients over 80 years of age is symptomatic intracerebral hemorrhage (sICH). All studies consistently showed an increased risk of hemorrhagic conversion after alteplase compared with no alteplase in all age groups. However, a more relevant question is the risk of intracerebral hemorrhage after alteplase among those ≥80 years of age compared with younger patients. A meta-analysis including studies comparing the risk of sICH in patients receiving alteplase who were >80 and <80 years of age demonstrated no significant difference in risk of sICH between groups.[29] Therefore, age over 80 should not be a contraindication for alteplase administration in AIS.

3.3 Rapidly improving symptoms

Rapid improvement of neurologic deficits is one of the most commons reasons for excluding patients from IV alteplase.[30–32] Rapid improvement usually is incomplete, thus leaving patients with disabling deficits. Deterioration can also follow spontaneous improvement because of persistent occlusion or partial recanalization with subsequent re-occlusion and often results in deficits worsening. Many patients with stroke with initial rapid improvement are ultimately disabled.[30–32]

The AHA guidelines state that alteplase treatment is reasonable for patients who present with moderate to severe ischemic stroke and demonstrate early improvement but remain moderately impaired and potentially disabled in the judgment of the examiner (Case 8.2).

3.4 Use of novel oral anticoagulants

Increasing numbers of patients are anticoagulated with the oral factor Xa inhibitors such as apixaban and rivaroxaban and direct thrombin inhibitors such as dabigatran. These agents known as novel OACs (NOACs) are rapidly emerging, and the evidence demonstrates that they are as effective (if not more effective) as warfarin in preventing stroke in patients with atrial fibrillation.[29,32,33] However, the safety and efficacy of alteplase in patients who have been taking these agents is not been well elucidated. The literature on IV alteplase administration in stroke patients taking dabigatran is limited to only case reports.[34–39]

Currently the use of alteplase in patients taking NOACs is not recommended unless laboratory tests such as activated partial thromboplastin time (aPTT), international normalized ratio (INR), platelet count, ecarin clotting time, thrombin time, or appropriate direct factor Xa activity assays are normal or the patient has not received a dose of these agents for >48 hours[16] (Case 8.3).

3.5 Gastrointestinal bleeding

The current FDA product insert lists gastrointestinal (GI) bleeding without a time limit as a warning for treatment. In the clinical setting, stroke physicians often attempt to distinguish patients with a known source or structural lesion from those with an occult source of GI bleeding. Patients with defined sources of bleeding may have therapeutic options such as sclerotherapy or embolization in the event of hemorrhagic complications. However, in patients with an occult source of GI bleeding, the risk profile with systemic thrombolysis is likely more of an unknown.

Current guidelines suggest a low bleeding risk with IV alteplase administration in the setting of past GI bleeding. However, in patients with a structural GI malignancy or recent bleeding event within 21 days of their stroke event should be considered high risk and IV alteplase administration is potentially harmful.[16]

3.6 Myocardial infarction

Acute myocardial infarction (MI) is not a contraindication to IV alteplase (Case 8.4). IV alteplase as simultaneous treatment for acute cerebral and coronary occlusion is not possible as the two different vascular beds require different doses of IV alteplase.[1,2] The recommended treatment dose of alteplase for AIS is 0.9 mg/kg (not to exceed 90 mg total treatment dose) infused over 60 minutes. Ten percent of the total treatment dose should be administered as an initial bolus over 1 minute, and the remaining treatment dose should be infused intravenously over 60 minutes.

Alteplase is given at a higher dose to treat MI. Alteplase at doses higher than 0.9mg/kg in AIS may be associated with elevated risk of hemorrhagic complications. On the other hand, alteplase at lower stroke does for MI is of unknown efficacy, and primary angioplasty and stenting are preferred treatment options over IV alteplase for acute MI.[40] A potential option in these cases is to administer the stroke dose alteplase followed by percutaneous transluminal coronary angioplasty.

The major concerns with the administration of IV alteplase to patients with a recent MI are cardiac rupture caused by lysis of fibrin clot within necrotic myocardial wall, post-MI pericarditis that may be transformed to pericardial hemorrhage by lytics, and embolization of ventricular thrombi by lytics.

Current recommendations are that in these patients presenting with concurrent AIS and acute MI, treatment with IV alteplase at the dose appropriate for cerebral ischemia, followed by percutaneous coronary angioplasty and stenting if indicated, is reasonable.[16]

3.7 Seizure

Initially, seizure at stroke onset was considered a contraindication to IV alteplase. This was based on the thought that a focal neurological deficit in this scenario was most likely secondary to stroke mimic phenomenon of Todd's paralysis (postictal weakness) than to acute cerebral ischemia. These two occurrences are not mutually exclusive as seizures can occur at onset of AIS.[41] In fact, the risk of hemorrhagic complications after thrombolysis in the setting of a stroke mimic is extremely low.[42–44] Most of the evidence supporting that a seizure at symptoms onset should not be considered an absolute contraindication to IV alteplase administration is limited and derived from retrospective stroke registries.[42–50]

The AHA guidelines mention that alteplase is reasonable in patients with a seizure at the time of onset of acute stroke if evidence suggests that residual impairments are secondary to stroke and not a postictal phenomenon[16] (Case 8.5).

> **Question 8.3:** Is MRI better than non-contrast CT when selecting patients for IV thrombolysis?
>
> **Answer:** Presently, there is no scientific evidence that MRI-based selection of patients for IV alteplse is superior to that of non-contrast CT when considering risk/benefit in a large population of patients.

3.8 Imaging findings

Non-contrast head computed tomography (CT) is the main imaging modality utilized in the acute stroke setting and primarily used to exclude intracranial hemorrhage prior to the administration of IV alteplase. Non-contrast CT head is also used to evaluate for early ischemic changes (EICs) and frank hypodensity prior to IV alteplase administration and/or mechanical thrombolysis. If there is hypodensity involving more than one third of the MCA territory, IV alteplase is contraindicated and should be withheld.[16]

However, the issue of EICs is challenging even to the most seasoned vascular neurologist. EICs on cerebral non-contrast CT is defined as parenchymal hypoattenuation (gray–white indistinction or decreased density of brain tissue relative to attenuation of other parts of the same structure or of the contralateral hemisphere) or focal swelling of mass effect (any focal narrowing of the cerebrospinal fluid spaces as a result of compression of adjacent structures). EICs reflect primarily a decrease in x-ray attenuation, which is inversely correlated with tissue net water uptake and may be a marker of irreversibly damaged ischemic brain tissue.[51] There is still controversy on the degree of x-ray attenuation required for irreversible damage.

The Alberta Stroke Program Early CT Score (ASPECTS) was developed to systemically assess EICs on non-contrast CT. This scale divides the MCA territory into 10 regions of interest that are weighted on the basis of functional importance. The scale maximum is 10, and 1 point is substracted for each region that demonstrates hypoattenuation on non-contrast CT.[52] In a post hoc analysis of the NINDS stroke study, ASPECTS of >7 was associated with a trend toward decreased mortality and small final infarct volumes.[53] However, data are limited, and there remains insufficient evidence to identify a threshold of hypoattenuation severity or extent that affects treatment response to IV alteplase.

Administering IV alteplase to patients whose CT brain imaging exhibits extensive regions of clear hypoattenuation is not recommended.

Question 8.4: What are the symptoms of an intracranial hemorrhage from IV alteplase?

Answer: Nausea, vomiting, headache, and worsening neurological symptoms are the more common symptoms of a symptomatic ICH. The rate of symptomatic ICH for IV alteplase administration is 6.4%. The rate of asymptomatic ICH is 4.4%.

4 COMPLICATIONS OF INTRAVENOUS ALTEPLASE

The most dreaded complication of systemic thrombolysis is hemorrhage, of which ICH is the most serious. It typically presents with nausea, vomiting, headache, worsening neurologic deficit, and, in severe cases, altered level of alertness. In the original NINDS tPA trial, the rate of symptomatic ICH (sICH), defined as the presence of hemorrhage on CT of the head and a decline in neurologic status, was present in 6.4% of those receiving alteplase and 0.6% in those receiving placebo.[1] Of those patients who suffered sICH in the alteplase group, approximately 50% died at 3 months; 4.4% of patients had asymptomatic ICH. Major systemic hemorrhages were rare, while minor extracranial hemorrhage occurred in 23% of patients treated with IV alteplase (only 3% in placebo). Risk factors for developing sICH after systemic thrombolysis were hypoattenuation on head CT, elevated serum glucose and history of diabetes, hypertension, increased stroke severity, and protocol violations with treatment outside of the time window.[54-57]

Question 8.5: What are some reversal options for IV alteplase associated hemorrhagic complications?

Answer: Currently, there is no proven reversal agent for alteplase. However, agents that may be utilized include fresh-frozen plasma, platelet transfusion, or recombinant factor VII.

4.1 Management of alteplase-related intracranial hemorrhage

Management of sICH after IV alteplase usually starts with discontinuation of infusion followed by immediate non-contrast head CT. Furthermore, full coagulation panel including fibrinogen and complete blood count are usually ordered. Unfortunately, most patients usually have completed their IV alteplase infusion by the time a hemorrhage is detected on CT. There is no proven reversal agent for IV alteplase. However, reversal options include fresh-frozen plasma and platelet transfusion or even recombinant factor VII on a case by case basis.

4.2 Angioedema

Another uncommon complication of IV thrombolysis is angioedema which occurs 1–3% of patients. It typically occurs 30–120 minutes after IV alteplase infusion. It is thought to be caused by a similar pathway implicated in angiotensin-converting enzymes (ACEs) and tends to occur contralateral to the infarct. These patients are usually at a high risk of developing the same complication with ACE inhibitors.[58] Treatment involves the administration of diphenhydramine (50 mg IV) and H2 blockers, followed by 100 mg IV methylprednisolone or nebulized epinephrine. In very severe cases, IV alteplase should be stopped, and patients may require endotracheal intubation. An emergent tracheostomy may be necessary.

5 EMERGING RESEARCH ON EXPANDING THE TIME WINDOW FOR THROMBOLYSIS

As immediate and successful restoration of blood flow in the ischemic tissue has proven to be the paramount target in the treatment of acute cerebral ischemia,[59] clinical research has focused on the development of reperfusion therapies to aid/act as adjuncts to IV alteplase. Some of these strategies that have been tested in clinical trials include the use of systemic tenecteplase,[60,61] desmolteplase,[18,62] or the augmentation of systemic IV alteplase recanalization with ultrasound.[63,64] Next we will discuss some of these strategies.

5.1 Tenecteplase

The high rates of unsuccessful reperfusion observed with IV alteplase in patients with large thrombus burden (terminal internal carotid artery, tandem extracranial internal carotid artery/MCA occlusions) triggered the search for other thrombolytic agents in AIS.[1,65] Tenecteplase (TNK) is a genetically engineered variant of alteplase that has a longer half-life and is more fibrin specific than alteplase. TNK has properties that make it a faster and more complete thrombolytic agent and, at same time, with less bleeding complications and early re-occlusions.[66] Furthermore, TNK can be given as a one-time bolus without need for an infusion.[67] In the Tenecteplase versus Alteplase for Acute Ischemic Stroke (TAAIS) trial 75 patients, who arrived <6h after the onset of ischemic stroke were randomly assigned to receive either alteplase (0.9 mg/kg) or TNK (0.1 mg/kg or 0.25 mg/kg). Patient treated with TNK were found to have greater reperfusion rates and better clinical outcomes at 24 hours than the alteplase group, while no significant differences in intracranial bleeding or other serious adverse events were noted between the groups. Although TNK has been approved for the treatment of acute MI, its use instead of alteplase in the treatment of AIS has not been verified.[67,68]

5.2 Desmoteplase

Because of its high fibrin specificity, non-activation by β-amyloid, longer terminal half-life and absence of neurotoxicity, desmoteplase is an attractive alternative to alteplase for systemic thrombolytic treatment of AIS.[69,70] Recently DIAS (desmoteplase in acute stroke) assessed the safety and efficacy of desmoteplase given between 3 and 9 hours after symptom onset in patients with occlusion or high-grade stenosis in major cerebral arteries. Treatment with desmoteplase did not improve functional outcomes as measured by modified Rankin Scale of 0–2 at 90 days. Its use in the treatment of AIS remains investigational.

5.3 Ancrod

Ancrod is a serine protease, extracted from the venom of the Malayan pit viper that reduces blood fibrinogen levels when injected intravenously. This indirectly leads to anticoagulation, reduced blood viscosity, and increased circulation to affected areas of the brain.[71] It was initially shown to be beneficial in AIS if started within 3 hours of symptom onset.[72–74] The Stroke Treatment with Ancrod Trial (STAT) randomized 500 patients who presented within 3 hours of stroke onset to receive an infusion of ancrod or placebo over 72 hours and 1-hour infusions at 96 and 120 hours. Better functional outcome was observed in the ancrod group versus placebo. However, there was a trend of more symptomatic intracranial hemorrhage in the ancrod group versus placebo, 5.2% versus 2%.[73] Subsequent studies extending the treatment window to 6 hours from onset have not demonstrated any significant difference in clinical outcome.[72,74,75]

5.4 Glycoprotein IIb/IIIa antagonists

Glycoprotein IIb/IIIa antagonists prevent platelet aggregation thus preventing reocclusion and facilitate thrombus breakdown.[76] In the cardiac literature, they have demonstrated improved coronary revascularization in the acute MI in Phase IIb studies but no significant improvement in the Phase III studies.[74,77,78] Safety of Tirofiban in Acute Ischemic Stroke (SaTIS) was a Phase II placebo-controlled study on monotherapy with IV tirofiban in patients presenting up to 22 hours after onset. There was no neurological/functional benefit found compared with placebo at 5 months except for lower mortality shown in the treatment group.[74,79] The subsequent Abciximab in Emergency Treatment of Stroke Trial (AbESTT-II) trial was a Phase III study on GP IIb/IIIa inhibitor monotherapy which was terminated prematurely because of an unfavorable risk–benefit profile. There was no benefit in neurological recovery in any of the cohorts (within 5-hour onset, between 5–6 hours, and wake-up strokes) in the abciximab group compared to placebo. Furthermore, there was a significant increase in symptomatic intracranial hemorrhage.[74,80,81] Efficacy and safety of combined IV alteplase and eptifibatide compared with IV alteplase alone were investigated in the Phase II Combined Approach to Lysis Utilizing Eptifibatide and Recombinant Tissue Plasminogen Activator in Acute Ischemic Stroke-Enhanced Regimen stroke trial (CLEAR-ER) study. The combined treatment group had a lower rate of symptomatic intracranial hemorrhage (2%) and showed a trend toward better functional outcome, with 49.5% achieving mRS 0–1 versus 36% in the standard alteplase group.[82]

5.5 Argatroban

Argatroban is a direct thrombin inhibitor which has demonstrated safety in the Argatroban Anticoagulation in Patients with Acute Ischemic Stroke (ARGIS-I) trial.[83] The use of argatroban as an adjuvant to IV alteplase was investigated in the Argatroban TPA Stroke (ARTSS) study and demonstrated 63% complete recanalization rate at 24 hours.[74,83–89] In Phase II ARTSS-2 (Randomized Controlled Trial of Argatroban with tPA for Acute Stroke), Barreto et al. conducted a randomized exploratory study to assess safety and the probability of a favorable outcome with adjunctive argatroban and alteplase in AIS patients. Patients were treated with standard-dose alteplase versus full dose alteplase and argatroban (100 µg/kg bolus) followed by infusion of either 1 (low dose) or 3 µg/kg per minute (high dose) for 48 hours. They found that in patients treated with alteplase, adjunctive argatroban was not associated with increased risk of sICH. However, there was no difference in outcomes based on 90-day mRS.[90]

5.6 Sonothrombolysis

Sonothrombolysis is the ultrasound targeting of an arterial occlusive clot to accelerate the thrombolytic effect of systemic alteplase. Mechanical pressure waves, produced by 2 MHz frequency ultrasound energy, can improve the delivery and penetration of the thrombolytic drug inside the clot.[91,92] The first properly powered multicenter clinical trial that confirmed existence of ultrasound-enhanced thrombolysis in human subjects was the Combined Lysis of Thrombus in Brain ischemia using transcranial Ultrasound and Systemic TPA (CLOTBUST) trial. In this trial, patients with acute MCA occlusions that were randomized to the combination of IV alteplase with 2 hour continuous transcranial Doppler monitoring were found to achieve higher rates of recanalization within 2 hour of treatment (without having higher rates of sICH) when compared to patients treated only with IV alteplase.[63] Molina et al. pioneered the use of gaseous microspheres (that are able to cross the lung barrier due to their size and stability and undergo expansion in size followed by transient oscillation or complete break up, when intercepted intracranially by an ultrasound beam aimed at thrombus-residual flow interface) in combination with CLOTBUST monitoring methods and reported safety and recanalization rates of microsphere-potentiated sonothrombolysis in a pilot Phase IIb randomized controlled trial.[64] The main limitation of current sonothrombolysis technology (applied with or without microspheres) is that it is heavily operator-dependent. Skilled sonographers able to perform transcranial Doppler or duplex are usually unavailable 24/7 to treat strokes in the Emergency Department.[93-96] An operator-independent 2 MHz transcranial Doppler device, developed to provide therapeutic ultrasound regardless of sonography skills, was recently being tested in a pivotal, multicenter, Phase III randomized-controlled trial (CLOTBUST-ER) that was suspended secondary to futility.[97]

6 ONGOING TRIALS

6.1 Extending the time window for alteplase

To date, patients with wake-up ischemic stroke are excluded from IV alteplase in daily clinical practice even if they meet all other criteria for treatment. It is estimated that one of four ischemic strokes are identified upon awakening and are not candidates for IV alteplase because their symptoms are >4.5 hours from last known normal.[31] Nonetheless, emerging data suggest that IV alteplase in carefully selected wake-up stroke patients, showing no or EICs on brain imaging, might be safe and effective comparable to those patients with known time of symptom onset.[98,99] Barreto et al. published a prospective, open-label safety study of IV alteplase in wake-up strokes. 40 preplanned patients were enrolled (50% men) at five stroke centers. No symptomatic intraparenchymal hemorrhages or parenchymal hematomas occurred, and at 3 months, 52.6% patients achieved excellent recovery with mRS scores of 0 or 1.[90] WAKE-UP is another ongoing randomized controlled trial that is using diffusion weighted imaging–fluid-attenuated inversion recovery mismatch to identify patients for IV thrombolysis with alteplase among patients who wake up with stroke symptoms.[100]

6.2 Thrombolysis for patients with low NIHSS score

Over half of ischemic strokes in the United States are mild in severity (NIHSS ≤5).[101] Single-center, prospective cohorts suggest that 30% will have significant disability at 3 months after mild stroke.[102] However, the optimal acute treatment of patients with mild deficits, who are otherwise eligible for IV alteplase is still is not established. The initial randomized controlled trials of IV alteplase excluded mild strokes.[103] Recently PRISMS, a double-blind, multicenter, randomized, Phase IIIb study, was initiated to evaluate the efficacy and safety of IV alteplase in participants with mild AISs that do not appear to be clearly disabling. Participants were randomized to IV alteplase and 1 dose of oral aspirin placebo or 1 dose of IV placebo and 1 dose of oral aspirin 325 mg. However, study was terminated early due to poor enrollment. There is currently wide variation in the use of alteplase in patients with mild but judged nondisabling strokes, which further reflects this uncertainty.[4] The AHA states that for patients with mild but disabling stroke symptoms, IV alteplase is indicated within 3 hours from symptom onset of ischemic stroke. There should be no exclusion for patients with mild but nonetheless disabling stroke symptoms in the opinion of the treating physician from treatment with IV alteplase because there is proven clinical benefit for those patients.[16] However, for patients with milder ischemic stroke symptoms that are judged as nondisabling IV alteplase may be considered, and the risks should be weighed against possible benefits.[16]

6.3 Mobile stroke units

Despite two decades of substantial efforts to streamline systems of care, reported alteplase treatment rates extracted from hospital-derived databases range from 3.4–9.1% for patients with AIS,[7,104,105] and the rates of delivery of intra-arterial treatment are far lower. The leading reason for such under treatment is that patients do not reach the hospital quickly enough to be assessed and treated within the narrow therapeutic window. Only 15–60% of acute stroke patients arrive at the hospital within 3 hours after symptom onset.[106,107] The establishment of the first mobile stroke units in Germany and the United States has made earlier identification and treatment of ischemic stroke a reality and provides the potential to substantially improve outcomes and increase time and rates of IV alteplase administration.[108,109] However, crucial concerns regarding safety, clinical efficacy, best setting, and cost-effectiveness remain to be addressed in further studies.

7 CLINICAL CASES

Case 8.1 Left hemispheric syndrome within 0–4.5 hours of symptom onset

CASE DESCRIPTION
A 65-year-old patient arrives with right-sided weakness, global aphasia, and a right visual field cut. Admission blood pressure is 175/85 mmHg, and the NIHSS score is 18. Non-contrast head CT is read as "no acute findings" (Figure 8.2). History is obtained from patient's family who arrives in the Emergency Department and states symptoms started 4 hours ago. Is this patient eligible for IV alteplase?

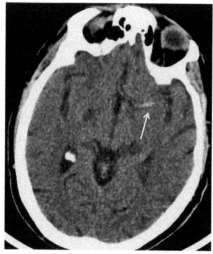

Figure 8.2 Acute ischemic stroke with large vessel occlusion. Hyperdense (bright) appearance of the proximal left middle cerebral artery (MCA) is shown (arrow). This suggests an acute thrombus within the left MCA.

PRACTICAL POINTS

- This patient is currently within the time window (0–4.5 hours) for IV alteplase. Based on the information provided, the patient is a candidate and should receive alteplase. However, additional information is needed to determine whether other major contraindications to systemic thrombolysis exist. In this case, only 30 minutes remain to gather additional information from patient's family and prepare and administer the alteplase.
- Given severity of NIHSS, there is high likelihood of large vessel occlusion. Based on the symptoms suggestive of left hemispheric syndromes (see Chapter 1 on stroke syndromes), proximal left MCA or left internal carotid artery occlusion is suspected. In fact, careful examination of admission CT shows the "hyperdense" MCA sign. Once alteplase drip is started, this patient should undergo emergent CT or magnetic resonance angiography to rule out large vessel occlusion. If proximal occlusion is confirmed, the patient will also be a candidate for intraarterial thrombectomy.

Case 8.2 Acute stroke with improvement of deficits

CASE DESCRIPTION

An 82-year-old patient presents with right hemiplegia and hemianesthesia, which started 2 hours ago. Non-contrast head CT is unrevealing. Admission blood pressure is 171/70 mmHg. Initial NIHSS score is 12 upon arrival to the Emergency

Department, however after CT head is completed, patient's exam has improved to a NIHSS of 7. Should IV alteplase still be administered?

PRACTICAL POINTS

- While there is spontaneous improvement of the NIHSS score by 5 points, this patient still continues to have significant neurologic deficits, indicated by repeat NIHSS score of 7. Partial improvement in stroke severity could be multifactorial, such as thrombus/embolus migration toward a more distal arterial segment, partial spontaneous thrombolysis, or changes in cerebral perfusion.
- As long as residual symptoms remain significant (typically, NIHSS of 4 or above), the patient should receive IV alteplase. Also, patient's age >80 years should not be considered a contraindication for IV alteplase.

Case 8.3 Thrombolysis and NOACs

CASE DESCRIPTION

69-year-old patient with a past medical history of atrial fibrillation on dabigatran presents with lethargy, dysarthria, dysconjugate gaze, diplopia, nystagmus, right-sided weakness, and right gaze preference, which started 3 hours prior to presentation to the emergency room. Patient's NIHSS score is above 20. Of note, patient had recently stopped (3 days prior to presentation) dabigatran for a routine screening colonoscopy. Does the history of dabigatran eliminate IV alteplase eligibility?

PRACTICAL POINTS

- Confirmation that this patient has been off dabigatran for more than 48 hours is critical in determining whether alteplase should be administered or withheld in this case.
- If the information regarding the timing of the last dose of NOAC administration is not available, the guidelines recommend testing aPTT, INR, platelet count, ecarin clotting time, thrombin time, or appropriate direct factor Xa activity assays.

Case 8.4 Simultaneous AIS and myocardial infarct

CASE DESCRIPTION

55-year-old patient with a past medical history of hypertension, hyperlipidemia, and diabetes presents with dysarthria, right arm, face, and leg weakness as well as right hemisensory loss. Patient also complains of chest pain, and electrocardiogram in the emergency room demonstrates ST elevations. Troponin is also elevated suggesting an acute MI. Patient's NIHSS score is 8. Can this patient receive IV alteplase safely in the setting of an acute MI? At what dose should the IV alteplase be administered?

Practical points

- Acute MI is not a contraindication to IV alteplase. The major concerns with the administration of IV alteplase to patients with a recent MI are cardiac rupture caused by lysis of fibrin clot within necrotic myocardial wall, post-MI pericarditis that may be transformed to pericardial hemorrhage by thrombolysis, and embolization of ventricular thrombi by alteplase. However, there are limited data supporting these as common events after IV alteplase administration.
- In fact, current recommendation for patients presenting with concurrent AIS and acute MI is the administration of IV alteplase at the dose appropriate for cerebral ischemia (0.9 mg/kg), followed by percutaneous coronary angioplasty and stenting if indicated.

Case 8.5 Seizure at the onset of stroke symptoms

Case description

45-year-old patient with no past medical history presents with right-sided weakness and expressive aphasia. Per emergency responders, patient was initially witnessed to have right upper and lower extremity shaking prior to onset of weakness and aphasia. Symptoms started approximately 2 hours ago. Upon Emergency Department arrival, blood pressure is 150/80 mmHg, and the NHSS score is 9 mainly for language components. Patient's right-sided strength has significantly improved over the last hour based on the report from the emergency responders. Non-contrast head computed tomography demonstrates a large frontal hypodensity with a calcified center (Figure 8.3). Should this patient receive IV alteplase?

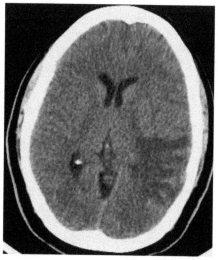

Figure 8.3 Brain tumor causing a seizure. Non-contrast computed tomography scan showing cytotoxic edema sparing cortex, suggestive of an underlyling brain tumor.

PRACTICAL POINTS

- This patient seems to have had a seizure based on the history previously described. Although seizures are not considered to be an absolute contraindication to IV alteplase, this patient's presentation of a seizure in the setting of a large frontal hypodensity with a calcified center suggest a stroke mimic, more specifically a central nervous system tumor/mass.
- Based on the information provided, the patient should not get IV alteplase. In fact, we would advise on obtaining further emergent imaging such as a magnetic resonance imaging (MRI) of the brain with gadolinium for further evaluation.

REFERENCES

1. National Institute of Neurological Disorders and Stroke rt-PA Stroke Study Group. Tissue plasminogen activator for acute ischemic stroke. *New Engl J Med.* 1995;333(24):1581–1587.
2. Hacke W, Kaste M, Bluhmki E, et al. Thrombolysis with alteplase 3 to 4.5 hours after acute ischemic stroke. *New Engl J Med.* 2008;359(13):1317–1329.
3. Hill MD, Buchan AM. Thrombolysis for acute ischemic stroke: results of the Canadian Alteplase for Stroke Effectiveness Study. *Can Med Assoc J.* 2005;172(10): 1307–1312.
4. Wahlgren N, Ahmed N, Davalos A, et al. Thrombolysis with alteplase for acute ischaemic stroke in the Safe Implementation of Thrombolysis in Stroke-Monitoring Study (SITS-MOST): an observational study. *Lancet.* 2007;369(9558):275–282.
5. Hacke W, Donnan G, Fieschi C, et al. Association of outcome with early stroke treatment: pooled analysis of ATLANTIS, ECASS, and NINDS rt-PA stroke trials. *Lancet.* 2004;363(9411):768–774.
6. Sandercock P, Wardlaw JM, Lindley RI, et al. The benefits and harms of intravenous thrombolysis with recombinant tissue plasminogen activator within 6 h of acute ischaemic stroke (the Third International Stroke Trial [IST-3]): a randomised controlled trial. *Lancet.* 2012;379(9834):2352–2363.
7. Adeoye O, Hornung R, Khatri P, Kleindorfer D. Recombinant tissue-type plasminogen activator use for ischemic stroke in the United States: a doubling of treatment rates over the course of 5 years. *Stroke.* 2011;42(7):1952–1955.
8. Nasr DM, Brinjikji W, Cloft HJ, Rabinstein AA. Utilization of intravenous thrombolysis is increasing in the United States. *Int J Stroke.* 2013;8(8):681–688.
9. Schwamm LH, Audebert HJ, Amarenco P, et al. Recommendations for the implementation of telemedicine within stroke systems of care: a policy statement from the American Heart Association. *Stroke.* 2009;40(7):2635–2660.
10. The Thrombolysis in Myocardial Infarction (TIMI) trial: Phase I findings. *New Engl J Med.* 1985;312(14):932–936.
11. Brott T, Haley EC, Levy DE, et al. The investigational use of tPA for stroke. *Ann Emerg Med.* 1988;17(11):1202–1205.

12. Haley EC, Jr., Brott TG, Sheppard GL, et al. Pilot randomized trial of tissue plasminogen activator in acute ischemic stroke: The TPA Bridging Study Group. *Stroke*. 1993;24(7):1000–1004.

13. Brott TG, Haley EC, Jr., Levy DE, et al. Urgent therapy for stroke: Part I. Pilot study of tissue plasminogen activator administered within 90 minutes. *Stroke*. 1992;23(5):632–640.

14. Sundt TM, Jr., Grant WC, Garcia JH. Restoration of middle cerebral artery flow in experimental infarction. *J Neurosurg*. 1969;31(3):311–321.

15. Crowell RM, Olsson Y, Klatzo I, Ommaya A. Temporary occlusion of the middle cerebral artery in the monkey: clinical and pathological observations. *Stroke*. 1970;1(6):439–448.

16. Demaerschalk BM, Kleindorfer DO, Adeoye OM, et al. Scientific rationale for the inclusion and exclusion criteria for intravenous alteplase in acute ischemic stroke: a statement for healthcare professionals from the American Heart Association/American Stroke Association. *Stroke*. 2016;47(2):581–641.

17. Jones TH, Morawetz RB, Crowell RM, et al. Thresholds of focal cerebral ischemia in awake monkeys. *J Neurosurg*. 1981;54(6):773–782.

18. Hacke W, Albers G, Al-Rawi Y, et al. The Desmoteplase in Acute Ischemic Stroke Trial (DIAS): a Phase II MRI-based 9-hour window acute stroke thrombolysis trial with intravenous desmoteplase. *Stroke*. 2005;36(1):66–73.

19. Lees KR, Bluhmki E, von Kummer R, et al. Time to treatment with intravenous alteplase and outcome in stroke: an updated pooled analysis of ECASS, ATLANTIS, NINDS, and EPITHET trials. *Lancet*. 2010;375(9727):1695–1703.

20. Fonarow GC, Zhao X, Smith EE, et al. Door-to-needle times for tissue plasminogen activator administration and clinical outcomes in acute ischemic stroke before and after a quality improvement initiative. *JAMA*. 2014;311(16):1632–1640.

21. Furie KL, Kasner SE, Adams RJ, et al. Guidelines for the prevention of stroke in patients with stroke or transient ischemic attack: a guideline for healthcare professionals from the american heart association/american stroke association. *Stroke*. 2011;42(1):227–276.

22. Goldstein LB, Bushnell CD, Adams RJ, et al. Guidelines for the primary prevention of stroke: a guideline for healthcare professionals from the American Heart Association/American Stroke Association. *Stroke*. 2011;42(2):517–584.

23. Carandang R, Seshadri S, Beiser A, et al. Trends in incidence, lifetime risk, severity, and 30-day mortality of stroke over the past 50 years. *JAMA*. 2006;296(24):2939–2946.

24. Wolf PA, D'Agostino RB, O'Neal MA, et al. Secular trends in stroke incidence and mortality. The Framingham Study. *Stroke*. 1992;23(11):1551–1555.

25. Fonarow GC, Reeves MJ, Zhao X, et al. Age-related differences in characteristics, performance measures, treatment trends, and outcomes in patients with ischemic stroke. *Circulation*. 2010;121(7):879–891.

26. Wardlaw JM, Murray V, Berge E, et al. Recombinant tissue plasminogen activator for acute ischaemic stroke: an updated systematic review and meta-analysis. *Lancet*. 2012;379(9834):2364–2372.

27. Ford GA, Ahmed N, Azevedo E, et al. Intravenous alteplase for stroke in those older than 80 years old. *Stroke*. 2010;41(11):2568–2574.

28. Mishra NK, Ahmed N, Andersen G, et al. Thrombolysis in very elderly people: controlled comparison of SITS International Stroke Thrombolysis Registry and Virtual International Stroke Trials Archive. *BMJ*. 2010;341:c6046.
29. Granger CB, Alexander JH, McMurray JJ, et al. Apixaban versus warfarin in patients with atrial fibrillation. *New Engl J Med*. 2011;365(11):981–992.
30. Smith EE, Fonarow GC, Reeves MJ, et al. Outcomes in mild or rapidly improving stroke not treated with intravenous recombinant tissue-type plasminogen activator: findings from Get with the Guidelines-Stroke. *Stroke*. 2011;42(11):3110–3115.
31. Barber PA, Zhang J, Demchuk AM, Hill MD, Buchan AM. Why are stroke patients excluded from TPA therapy? An analysis of patient eligibility. *Neurology*. 2001;56(8):1015–1020.
32. Balucani C, Levine SR. Mild stroke and rapidly improving symptoms: it's not always a happy ending. *Stroke*. 2011;42(11):3005–3007.
33. Connolly SJ, Ezekowitz MD, Yusuf S, et al. Dabigatran versus warfarin in patients with atrial fibrillation. *New Engl J Med*. 2009;361(12):1139–1151.
34. Matute MC, Masjuan J, Egido JA, et al. Safety and outcomes following thrombolytic treatment in stroke patients who had received prior treatment with anticoagulants. *Cerebrovasc Dis*. 2012;33(3):231–239.
35. De Smedt A, De Raedt S, Nieboer K, De Keyser J, Brouns R. Intravenous thrombolysis with recombinant tissue plasminogen activator in a stroke patient treated with dabigatran. *Cerebrovasc Dis*. 2010;30(5):533–534.
36. Casado Naranjo I, Portilla-Cuenca JC, Jimenez Caballero PE, Calle Escobar ML, Romero Sevilla RM. Fatal intracerebral hemorrhage associated with administration of recombinant tissue plasminogen activator in a stroke patient on treatment with dabigatran. *Cerebrovasc Dis*. 2011;32(6):614–615.
37. Lee VH, Conners JJ, Prabhakaran S. Intravenous thrombolysis in a stroke patient taking dabigatran. *J Stroke Cerebrovasc*. 2012;21(8):916.e911–912.
38. Marrone LC, Marrone AC. Thrombolysis in an ischemic stroke patient on dabigatran anticoagulation: a case report. *Cerebrovasc Dis*. 2012;34(3):246–247.
39. Sangha N, El Khoury R, Misra V, Lopez G. Acute ischemic stroke treated with intravenous tissue plasminogen activator in a patient taking dabigatran with radiographic evidence of recanalization. *J Stroke Cerebrovasc*. 2012;21(8):917.e5–e8.
40. O'Gara PT, Kushner FG, Ascheim DD, et al. 2013 ACCF/AHA guideline for the management of ST-elevation myocardial infarction: executive summary: a report of the American College of Cardiology Foundation/American Heart Association Task Force on Practice Guidelines. *Circulation*. 2013;127(4):529–555.
41. Shinton RA, Gill JS, Melnick SC, Gupta AK, Beevers DG. The frequency, characteristics and prognosis of epileptic seizures at the onset of stroke. *J Neurol Neurosur Ps*. 1988;51(2):273–276.
42. Winkler DT, Fluri F, Fuhr P, et al. Thrombolysis in stroke mimics: frequency, clinical characteristics, and outcome. *Stroke*. 2009;40(4):1522–1525.
43. Scott PA, Silbergleit R. Misdiagnosis of stroke in tissue plasminogen activator-treated patients: characteristics and outcomes. *Ann Emerg Med*. 2003;42(5):611–618.
44. Chernyshev OY, Martin-Schild S, Albright KC, et al. Safety of tPA in stroke mimics and neuroimaging-negative cerebral ischemia. *Neurology*. 2010;74(17):1340–1345.

45. Zinkstok SM, Engelter ST, Gensicke H, et al. Safety of thrombolysis in stroke mimics: results from a multicenter cohort study. *Stroke.* 2013;44(4):1080–1084.

46. Tsivgoulis G, Alexandrov AV, Chang J, et al. Safety and outcomes of intravenous thrombolysis in stroke mimics: a 6-year, single-care center study and a pooled analysis of reported series. *Stroke.* 2011;42(6):1771–1774.

47. Chang J, Teleb M, Yang JP, et al. A model to prevent fibrinolysis in patients with stroke mimics. *J Stroke Cerebrovasc.* 2012;21(8):839–843.

48. Forster A, Griebe M, Wolf ME, Szabo K, Hennerici MG, Kern R. How to identify stroke mimics in patients eligible for intravenous thrombolysis? *J Neurol.* 2012;259(7):1347–1353.

49. Giraldo EA, Khalid A, Zand R. Safety of intravenous thrombolysis within 4.5 h of symptom onset in patients with negative post-treatment stroke imaging for cerebral infarction. *Neurocrit Care.* 2011;15(1):76–79.

50. Selim M, Kumar S, Fink J, Schlaug G, Caplan LR, Linfante I. Seizure at stroke onset: should it be an absolute contraindication to thrombolysis? *Cerebrovasc Dis.* 2002;14(1):54–57.

51. Dzialowski I, Hill MD, Coutts SB, et al. Extent of early ischemic changes on computed tomography (CT) before thrombolysis: prognostic value of the Alberta Stroke Program Early CT Score in ECASS II. *Stroke.* 2006;37(4):973–978.

52. Barber PA, Demchuk AM, Zhang J, Buchan AM. Validity and reliability of a quantitative computed tomography score in predicting outcome of hyperacute stroke before thrombolytic therapy. ASPECTS Study Group. Alberta Stroke Programme Early CT Score. *Lancet.* 2000;355(9216):1670–1674.

53. Puetz V, Dzialowski I, Hill MD, Demchuk AM. The Alberta Stroke Program Early CT Score in clinical practice: what have we learned? *Int J Stroke.* 2009;4(5):354–364.

54. Butcher K, Christensen S, Parsons M, et al. Postthrombolysis blood pressure elevation is associated with hemorrhagic transformation. *Stroke.* 2010;41(1):72–77.

55. Amlie-Lefond C, deVeber G, Chan AK, et al. Use of alteplase in childhood arterial ischaemic stroke: a multicentre, observational, cohort study. *Lancet Neurol.* 2009;8(6):530–536.

56. Lansberg MG, Albers GW, Wijman CA. Symptomatic intracerebral hemorrhage following thrombolytic therapy for acute ischemic stroke: a review of the risk factors. *Cerebrovasc Dis.* 2007;24(1):1–10.

57. Marti-Fabregas J, Bravo Y, Cocho D, et al. Frequency and predictors of symptomatic intracerebral hemorrhage in patients with ischemic stroke treated with recombinant tissue plasminogen activator outside clinical trials. *Cerebrovasc Dis.* 2007;23(2–3):85–90.

58. Hill MD, Barber PA, Takahashi J, Demchuk AM, Feasby TE, Buchan AM. Anaphylactoid reactions and angioedema during alteplase treatment of acute ischemic stroke. *Can Med Assoc J.* 2000;162(9):1281–1284.

59. Hill MD, Hachinski V. Stroke treatment: time is brain. *Lancet.* 1998;352(Suppl 3):SIII10–SIII14.

60. Haley EC, Jr., Thompson JL, Grotta JC, et al. Phase IIB/III trial of tenecteplase in acute ischemic stroke: results of a prematurely terminated randomized clinical trial. *Stroke.* 2010;41(4):707–711.

61. Parsons M, Spratt N, Bivard A, et al. A randomized trial of tenecteplase versus alteplase for acute ischemic stroke. *New Engl J Med.* 2012;366(12):1099–1107.
62. Hacke W, Furlan AJ, Al-Rawi Y, et al. Intravenous desmoteplase in patients with acute ischaemic stroke selected by MRI perfusion-diffusion weighted imaging or perfusion CT (DIAS-2): a prospective, randomised, double-blind, placebo-controlled study. *Lancet Neurol.* 2009;8(2):141–150.
63. Alexandrov AV, Molina CA, Grotta JC, et al. Ultrasound-enhanced systemic thrombolysis for acute ischemic stroke. *New Engl J Med.* 2004;351(21):2170–2178.
64. Molina CA, Barreto AD, Tsivgoulis G, et al. Transcranial ultrasound in clinical sonothrombolysis (TUCSON) trial. *Ann Neurol.* 2009;66(1):28–38.
65. Rother J, Ford GA, Thijs VN. Thrombolytics in acute ischaemic stroke: historical perspective and future opportunities. *Cerebrovasc Dis.* 2013;35(4):313–319.
66. Martinez-Sanchez P, Diez-Tejedor E, Fuentes B, Ortega-Casarrubios MA, Hacke W. Systemic reperfusion therapy in acute ischemic stroke. *Cerebrovasc Dis.* 2007;24(Suppl 1):143–152.
67. Bivard A, Lin L, Parsonsb MW. Review of stroke thrombolytics. *J Stroke.* 2013;15(2):90–98.
68. Behrouz R. Intravenous tenecteplase in acute ischemic stroke: an updated review. *J Neurol.* 2014;261(6):1069–1072.
69. Liberatore GT, Samson A, Bladin C, Schleuning WD, Medcalf RL. Vampire bat salivary plasminogen activator (desmoteplase): a unique fibrinolytic enzyme that does not promote neurodegeneration. *Stroke.* 2003;34(2):537–543.
70. Reddrop C, Moldrich RX, Beart PM, et al. Vampire bat salivary plasminogen activator (desmoteplase) inhibits tissue-type plasminogen activator-induced potentiation of excitotoxic injury. *Stroke.* 2005;36(6):1241–1246.
71. Kirmani JF, Alkawi A, Panezai S, Gizzi M. Advances in thrombolytics for treatment of acute ischemic stroke. *Neurology.* 2012;79(13 Suppl 1):S119–125.
72. Levy DE, del Zoppo GJ, Demaerschalk BM, et al. Ancrod in acute ischemic stroke: results of 500 subjects beginning treatment within 6 hours of stroke onset in the ancrod stroke program. *Stroke.* 2009;40(12):3796–3803.
73. Sherman DG, Atkinson RP, Chippendale T, et al. Intravenous ancrod for treatment of acute ischemic stroke: the STAT study: a randomized controlled trial. Stroke Treatment with Ancrod Trial. *JAMA.* 2000;283(18):2395–2403.
74. Barreto AD, Alexandrov AV. Adjunctive and alternative approaches to current reperfusion therapy. *Stroke.* 2012;43(2):591–598.
75. Hennerici MG, Kay R, Bogousslavsky J, Lenzi GL, Verstraete M, Orgogozo JM. Intravenous ancrod for acute ischaemic stroke in the European Stroke Treatment with Ancrod Trial: a randomised controlled trial. *Lancet.* 2006;368(9550):1871–1878.
76. Eisenberg PR, Sobel BE, Jaffe AS. Activation of prothrombin accompanying thrombolysis with recombinant tissue-type plasminogen activator. *J Am Coll Cardiol.* 1992;19(5):1065–1069.
77. Ohman EM, Kleiman NS, Gacioch G, et al. Combined accelerated tissue-plasminogen activator and platelet glycoprotein IIb/IIIa integrin receptor blockade with Integrilin in acute myocardial infarction. Results of a randomized, placebo-controlled, dose-ranging trial. IMPACT-AMI Investigators. *Circulation.* 1997;95(4):846–854.

78. Pereira H. Reperfusion therapy for acute myocardial infarction with fibrinolytic therapy or combination reduced fibrinolytic therapy and platelet glycoprotein IIb/IIIa inhibition: the GUSTO V randomised trial. *Rev Port Cardiol.* 2001;20(6):687–688.

79. Siebler M, Hennerici MG, Schneider D, et al. Safety of Tirofiban in acute Ischemic Stroke: the SaTIS trial. *Stroke.* 2011;42(9):2388–2392.

80. Adams HP, Jr., Effron MB, Torner J, et al. Emergency administration of abciximab for treatment of patients with acute ischemic stroke: results of an international Phase III trial: Abciximab in Emergency Treatment of Stroke Trial (AbESTT-II). *Stroke.* 2008;39(1):87–99.

81. Torgano G, Zecca B, Monzani V, et al. Effect of intravenous tirofiban and aspirin in reducing short-term and long-term neurologic deficit in patients with ischemic stroke: a double-blind randomized trial. *Cerebrovasc Dis.* 2010;29(3):275–281.

82. Pancioli AM, Adeoye O, Schmit PA, et al. Combined approach to lysis utilizing eptifibatide and recombinant tissue plasminogen activator in acute ischemic stroke-enhanced regimen stroke trial. *Stroke.* 2013;44(9):2381–2387.

83. LaMonte MP, Nash ML, Wang DZ, et al. Argatroban anticoagulation in patients with acute ischemic stroke (ARGIS-1): a randomized, placebo-controlled safety study. *Stroke.* 2004;35(7):1677–1682.

84. Barreto AD, Alexandrov AV, Lyden P, et al. The argatroban and tissue-type plasminogen activator stroke study: final results of a pilot safety study. *Stroke.* 2012;43(3):770–775.

85. Barreto AD, Alexandrov AV, Shen L, et al. CLOTBUST-Hands Free: pilot safety study of a novel operator-independent ultrasound device in patients with acute ischemic stroke. *Stroke.* 2013;44(12):3376–3381.

86. Jang IK, Brown DF, Giugliano RP, et al. A multicenter, randomized study of argatroban versus heparin as adjunct to tissue plasminogen activator (TPA) in acute myocardial infarction: myocardial infarction with novastan and TPA (MINT) study. *J Am Coll Cardiol.* 1999;33(7):1879–1885.

87. Kawai H, Umemura K, Nakashima M. Effect of argatroban on microthrombi formation and brain damage in the rat middle cerebral artery thrombosis model. *Jpn J Pharmacol.* 1995;69(2):143–148.

88. Morris DC, Zhang L, Zhang ZG, et al. Extension of the therapeutic window for recombinant tissue plasminogen activator with argatroban in a rat model of embolic stroke. *Stroke.* 2001;32(11):2635–2640.

89. Sugg RM, Pary JK, Uchino K, et al. Argatroban tPA stroke study: study design and results in the first treated cohort. *Arch Neurol.* 2006;63(8):1057–1062.

90. Barreto AD, Fanale CV, Alexandrov AV, et al. Prospective, open-label safety study of intravenous recombinant tissue plasminogen activator in wake-up stroke. *Ann Neurol.* 2016;80(2):211–218.

91. Alexandrov AV, Barlinn K. Taboos and opportunities in sonothrombolysis for stroke. *Int J Hyperther.* 2012;28(4):397–404.

92. Rubiera M, Alexandrov AV. Sonothrombolysis in the management of acute ischemic stroke. *Am J Cardiovasc Drug.* 2010;10(1):5–10.

93. Barreto AD, Ford GA, Shen L, et al. Randomized, multicenter trial of ARTSS-2 (Argatroban with Recombinant Tissue Plasminogen Activator for Acute Stroke). *Stroke.* 2017;48(6):1608–1616.

94. Tsivgoulis G, Alexandrov A. Ultrasound-enhanced thrombolysis: from bedside to bench. *Stroke.* 2008;39(5):1404–1405.

95. Tsivgoulis G, Alexandrov AV, Sloan MA. Advances in transcranial Doppler ultrasonography. *Curr Neurol Neurosci.* 2009;9(1):46–54.

96. Tsivgoulis G, Culp WC, Alexandrov AV. Ultrasound enhanced thrombolysis in acute arterial ischemia. *Ultrasonics.* 2008;48(4):303–311.

97. Schellinger PD, Alexandrov AV, Barreto AD, et al. Combined lysis of thrombus with ultrasound and systemic tissue plasminogen activator for emergent revascularization in acute ischemic stroke (CLOTBUST-ER): design and methodology of a multinational Phase 3 trial. *Int J Stroke.* 2015;10(7):1141–1148.

98. Albers GW, Thijs VN, Wechsler L, et al. Magnetic resonance imaging profiles predict clinical response to early reperfusion: the diffusion and perfusion imaging evaluation for understanding stroke evolution (DEFUSE) study. *Ann Neurol.* 2006;60(5):508–517.

99. Davis SM, Donnan GA, Parsons MW, et al. Effects of alteplase beyond 3 h after stroke in the Echoplanar Imaging Thrombolytic Evaluation Trial (EPITHET): a placebo-controlled randomised trial. *Lancet Neurol.* 2008;7(4):299–309.

100. Thomalla G, Fiebach JB, Ostergaard L, et al. A multicenter, randomized, double-blind, placebo-controlled trial to test efficacy and safety of magnetic resonance imaging-based thrombolysis in wake-up stroke (WAKE-UP). *Int J Stroke.* 2014;9(6):829–836.

101. Reeves M, Khoury J, Alwell K, et al. Distribution of National Institutes of Health stroke scale in the Cincinnati/Northern Kentucky Stroke Study. *Stroke.* 2013;44(11):3211–3213.

102. Khatri P, Conaway MR, Johnston KC. Ninety-day outcome rates of a prospective cohort of consecutive patients with mild ischemic stroke. *Stroke.* 2012;43(2):560–562.

103. Khatri P, Kleindorfer DO, Yeatts SD, et al. Strokes with minor symptoms: an exploratory analysis of the National Institute of Neurological Disorders and Stroke recombinant tissue plasminogen activator trials. *Stroke.* 2010;41(11):2581–2586.

104. Schwamm LH, Ali SF, Reeves MJ, et al. Temporal trends in patient characteristics and treatment with intravenous thrombolysis among acute ischemic stroke patients at Get with rhe Guidelines-Stroke hospitals. *Circ-Cardiovasc Qual.* 2013;6(5):543–549.

105. Scholten N, Pfaff H, Lehmann HC, Fink GR, Karbach U. [Thrombolysis for acute stroke—a nationwide analysis of regional medical care]. *Fortschr Neurol Psyc.* 2013;81(10):579–585.

106. Agyeman O, Nedeltchev K, Arnold M, et al. Time to admission in acute ischemic stroke and transient ischemic attack. *Stroke.* 2006;37(4):963–966.

107. Evenson KR, Foraker RE, Morris DL, Rosamond WD. A comprehensive review of prehospital and in-hospital delay times in acute stroke care. *Int J Stroke.* 2009;4(3):187–199.

108. Ebinger M, Winter B, Wendt M, et al. Effect of the use of ambulance-based thrombolysis on time to thrombolysis in acute ischemic stroke: a randomized clinical trial. *JAMA.* 2014;311(16):1622–1631.

109. Walter S, Kostopoulos P, Haass A, et al. Diagnosis and treatment of patients with stroke in a mobile stroke unit versus in hospital: a randomised controlled trial. *Lancet Neurol.* 2012;11(5):397–404.

9

Endovascular Treatment of Stroke

MANDY J. BINNING AND DANIEL R. FELBAUM ■

CONTENTS

1 INTRODUCTION

Thrombolysis with intravenous (IV) alteplase has traditionally been the first line of treatment in patients presenting within 4.5 hours of the onset of stroke symptoms. However, recent multicenter, randomized controlled trials have demonstrated that select patients with large vessel arterial occlusions are found to have higher recanalization rates and better outcomes when IV alteplase is used in conjunction with endovascular thrombectomy (EVT).[1-5] Thrombectomy is the physical removal of intra-arterial thrombus from cervical or intracranial arteries with endovascular devices. HERMES, a meta-analysis of the 5 randomized EVT trials, found that the number of patients needed to treat (NNT) to positively impact 1 patient was 2.6.[6] Contrast this to the NNT for IV alteplase of 5, 9, and 14 for the <90-minute, 90-minute to 3-hour, and 3 to 4.5-hour windows, respectively.[7]

This chapter will explain the presentation, workup (diagnostic imaging modalities) and indications for EVT for acute ischemic stroke as well as explain the devices and procedure with some illustrative cases. Figure 9.1 summarizes an algorithm in stroke triage with clinical decision-making for diagnostic imaging workup and subsequent involvement of the neurointerventionalist for potential EVT.

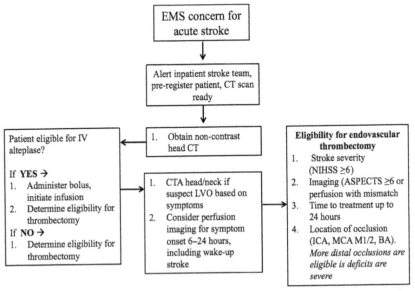

Figure 9.1 Basic algorithm for the initial pathway for managing patients being worked up and considered for potential endovascular thrombectomy.
ABBREVIATIONS: ASPECTS, Alberta stroke program early CT score; BA, basilar artery; CT, computed tomography, CTA, computed tomography angiography; EMS, emergency medical services; ICA, internal carotid artery; MCA, middle cerebral artery; NIHSS, National Institutes of Health Stroke Scale.

Question 9.1: Can you treat a patient with EVT who has had symptoms more than 6 hours?

Answer: The clinical exam in combination with radiographic studies become more important than a strict time limit. Patients with symptoms onset up to 24 hours are eligible for thrombectomy using currently available imaging and treatment technology.

2 PRESENTATION

All patients who present with the acute onset of focal neurological symptoms should be evaluated and worked up for the possibility of a large vessel occlusion (LVO). In practice, LVO is an acute, symptomatic occlusion of the internal carotid artery (ICA), middle cerebral artery (MCA), vertebral artery (VA), or basilar artery (BA). Anterior and posterior cerebral artery (ACA/PCA) occlusions can be treated as well, though these are encountered less frequently. For the purposes of the randomized trials, only ICA and MCA occlusions were treated.

The patient's presentation is determined by the location and laterality (side) of the LVO. Refer to Chapter 1 for a more detailed description of stroke syndromes associated with LVO. First order LVO (such as proximal M1 segment of MCA) tend to cause greater deficits and patients will typically present with the National Institutes of Health Stroke Scale (NIHSS) score of >6. For example, a left MCA occlusion (Case 9.1) will present with right hemiparesis/plegia, aphasia in most patients, and a left gaze preference. A right MCA occlusion is more commonly associated with left-sided neglect and hemiparesis/plegia and right gaze preference. BA occlusions early on can be mistaken for and mimic many other conditions but should be considered in any patient with the acute onset of dizziness, vertigo, nausea, vomiting, cranial nerve findings, paresthesia, paresis, visual field cut, altered mental status, and lethargy.

Second order vessel occlusion, such as MCA occlusion after the bifurcation (M2) tend to present with a lower NIHSS, but deficits are often still disabling. An example would be a left M2 occlusion causing aphasia without significant weakness. Patients with very low NIHSS scores and pure sensory or pure motor symptoms are unlikely to have an LVO but still warrant investigation if their deficits are disabling.

3 DIAGNOSTIC STUDIES

3.1 Computed tomography

When patients arrive to the emergency department (ED) with acute stroke symptoms, non-contrast computed tomography (CT) should be performed immediately to evaluate for intracranial hemorrhage (ICH), early signs of ischemic infarct (Case 9.2) or hyperdensity (acute thrombus) within the vasculature (e.g., hyperdense MCA sign). In most instances of acute ischemic stroke, the CT will appear normal if the patient arrives early.

Question 9.2: The patient has unknown kidney function; can he or she still receive contrast for CT angiography/perfusion?

Answer: Yes. In emergency situations such as stroke from LVO, the diagnosis and potential treatment is much more important and time-dependent. The risks must be counseled with the patient or family if possible, but this should not delay a diagnosis and life-saving therapy.

3.2 Computed tomography angiography and perfusion

CT angiography (CTA) utilizes a contrast bolus to opacify the cervical and intracranial arteries to evaluate for LVO. This study diagnostically is as useful as catheter angiography to diagnose LVO.

CT perfusion (CTP) is a physiologic study that utilizes an IV contrast bolus to measure components of cerebral perfusion. Cerebral blood flow (CBF) is decreased in the territory of an LVO. In potentially reversible strokes, the cerebral blood volume (CBV) will be maintained in areas of potentially reversible ischemia or penumbra.[8,9] This creates a "mismatch" between CBF and CBV maps when the studies are compared side by side. In completed, or irreversible strokes, the CBV will be diminished to match the CBF (Case 9.2).

3.3 Magnetic resonance imaging

Magnetic resonance imaging (MRI) and magnetic resonance angiography (MRA) are utilized in some centers instead of CTA/CTP to determine areas of reversible ischemia. An LVO seen on MRA coupled with a diffusion weighted image (DWI) sequence on MRI showing no acute stroke suggests reversible ischemia. A large area of DWI restriction or change suggests that the stroke is completed, although reversible DWI changes have been well described.[10,11]

In most stroke centers, CTA/CTP is a more readily available and quicker test, as 24/7 MRI availability can vary and requires screening sheets that aphasic patients or disabled patients cannot fill out and family members may not know the answers to. Not all community hospitals have the software to perform CTP, but most have the capability to perform CTA. In these cases, it is common to reserve performing the CTA/CTP until the patient arrives at the comprehensive stroke center so as one to minimize contrast and radiation exposure.

3.4 Digital subtraction angiography

Formal catheter-based cerebral angiography is typically reserved for those patients undergoing stroke intervention. Angiography is both diagnostic and potentially therapeutic and is described in detail in the following discussion.

Question 9.3: Should I wait for IV alteplase to "fail" prior to considering endovascular therapy?

Answer: Appropriate imaging such as CTA and perfusion can be performed in real time as alteplase drip is being administered. The neuroendovascular team should be alerted, and thrombectomy should be initiated as soon as possible. Remember that trials show that EVT thrombectomy plus alteplase is more effective than alteplase alone.

4 INDICATIONS FOR ENDOVASCULAR TREATMENT

4.1 Patient selection

In brief, any patient with acute stroke symptoms referable to an LVO and imaging showing reversible ischemia in that territory is a candidate for EVT. The previously mentioned randomized trials mainly treated patients within 6 hours of symptom onset and with ICA or MCA occlusions. From a practical standpoint, a much broader group of patients might be candidates for treatment (Table 9.1). This will be discussed in detail.

Table 9.1 2015 AMERICAN HEART ASSOCIATION GUIDELINE CRITERIA VERSUS REAL WORLD CRITERIA REGARDING ENDOVASCULAR TREATMENT OF STROKE

	2015 AHA Guidelines Criteria[12]	Real-world Criteria
Age	≥18	No limit
Neurological exam	NIHSS≥6	Any potentially reversible disabling deficit
Imaging findings	ASPECTS ≥6	Salvageable penumbra on CT, CTP, or MRI
Time to treatment	0–6 hours	Dependent on the extent salvageable tissue versus size of core (irreversible injury), often up to 24 hours
Location	ICA or proximal MCA	Any symptomatic vessel with salvageable tissue

ABBREVIATIONS: ASPECTS, Alberta stroke program early CT score; CT, computed tomography, CTP, computed tomography perfusion; ICA, internal carotid artery; MCA, middle cerebral artery; MRI, magnetic resonance imaging; NIHSS, National Institutes of Health Stroke Scale.

SOURCE: Powers WJ, Derdeyn CP, Biller J et al. 2015 American Heart Association/ American Stroke Association Focused Update of the 2013 Guidelines for the Early Management of Patients With Acute Ischemic Stroke Regarding Endovascular Treatment Stroke. 2015; 46(10):3020–3035.

From an imaging standpoint, non-contrast head CT can be used as a guide to appropriateness for intervention. Deficits resulting from hemorrhagic stroke (intracerebral hemorrhage, subarachnoid hemorrhage, etc.) will be seen immediately on CT and excluded. Patients with a large territory of acute ischemic changes (loss of gray–white differentiation) would not be candidates for intervention as this area represents completed or irreversible infarct (Case 9.2).

However, most non-contrast CT studies are initially "negative" if the patient presents acutely. Therefore, CTA and CTP are very helpful in this situation in determining the patients who are candidates for intervention. It is common, for example, for a patient with an internal capsule lacunar infarct to present with hemiplegia. In most instances, this patient will not have a LVO as these strokes are caused by small vessel disease. The CTA can prove that all of the arteries are patent in these cases in which the stroke may not be visible on plain CT and prevent an unnecessary catheter angiogram.

CTA is also helpful in identifying the exact location of a LVO. In practice, a patient with LVO of the ICA, MCA, VA, BA, or, less commonly, ACA/PCA with a correlating area of reversible ischemia/penumbra and a deficit would be a candidate for intervention. While the aforementioned randomized trials only treated patients within 6 hours of symptom onset, that window is often extended beyond that arbitrary cut-off if the CTP shows that the area of ischemia is still reversible. For this reason, many centers will call stroke alerts even for symptoms that have been present for 24 hours to hasten evaluation with CTA/CTP.

Question 9.4: How old is too old? How sick is too sick?

Answer: Every patient should be considered individually on a case-by-case basis. There is no definite age limit to the therapy, but careful discussion with the family is important in cases of extremely elderly or infirm patients.

4.2 2015 American Heart Association guidelines

The guidelines for the management of patients with acute ischemic stroke were updated in 2015 to include EVT.[12] The following outlines the most current recommendations.

- Eligible patients should still receive IV alteplase therapy as first-line treatment.
- Endovascular therapy with a stent retriever should be considered if the patient had a good preoperative baseline, age >18 years, NIHSS >6, ASPECT of >6, the ICA or proximal M1 is affected, and groin puncture is performed within 6 hours of symptom onset.
- A technically successful EVT is if a near-complete or complete recanalization is obtained (i.e., the thrombolysis in cerebral infarction grading score 2b/3).

- If treatment with EVT is to be performed beyond 6 hours, the benefit is less certain. If IV alteplase is contraindicated, EVT is an option if performed within 6 hours of stroke onset.
- If groin puncture is performed within 6 hours, stent retriever EVT may be considered, and there is an occlusion of the distal MCA, ACA, or vessels of the posterior circulation.
- In the pediatric population with a LVO, EVT within 6 hours of onset does not have established benefit.
- Waiting for an effect after initiating IV alteplase therapy before proceeding with mechanical thrombectomy (MT) is not recommended.
- A non-contrasted CT head is the preferred initial emergency imaging in suspected stroke cases.
- A non-invasive vascular test should be considered if EVT is contemplated, although IV alteplase should not be delayed.
- Patients should be transported to the closest available primary stroke center. The center must meet specific facility standards, including capability of performing emergency non-invasive vascular imaging, administration of IV alteplase, and be able to provide access to experienced neuro-interventionalists.

4.3 Controversies

In real-world situations, adhering to rigid guidelines is difficult, as most patients do not fit neatly into categories established by randomized trials.[13,14] In general, regardless of location of occlusion or time of onset, the goal is brain preservation. Establishing a means of identifying patients with salvageable brain is paramount and the use of advanced imaging such as a CT perfusion can more rapidly identify patients with penumbra.

4.3.1 WAKE-UP STOKE AND INTERVENTION BEYOND 6 HOURS

For example, patients who woke up with their symptoms were not included in the thrombectomy trials. Despite this fact, we routinely intervene on these patients if imaging suggests salvageable tissue. Until recently, smaller retrospective reviews suggested a benefit in treating carefully selected patients with wake-up strokes.[15,16] However, we now have the benefit of a randomized trial looking at MT in carefully selected patients versus medical therapy in patients presenting after 6 hours of symptom onset. The DAWN trial, demonstrated a 2-point difference in the 90-day modified Rankin Scale (mRS) score in favor of the thrombectomy group.[17,18] A 73% relative reduction of dependency in activities of daily living was found with an NNT for any lower disability of 2.0.

As a result, a 24-hour window to treatment in select cases is an established paradigm, and any age limits are much less important. Furthermore, patients that are not eligible for IV alteplase are potential candidates for EVT.

4.3.2 POSTERIOR CIRCULATION STROKES AND DISTAL OCCLUSIONS

Patients with posterior circulation strokes do not fit into any randomized trial. However, it is widely recognized that a BA occlusion is a fatal condition, and we recommend treatment unless the patient has an exam consistent with brain death or massive infarction or hemorrhage on imaging (Case 9.3). A retrospective review by Mokin et al. found that posterior circulation thrombectomy was safe and most effective if performed within 6 hours of symptom onset.[19]

Other less common strokes such as M2/3 occlusion, ACA strokes can be treated if they are also acutely symptomatic and demonstrate salvageable brain on perfusion imaging.[20,21]

Question 9.5: The patient cannot receive IV alteplase. Is the patient still a candidate for EVT?

Answer: IV alteplase and EVT are not exclusive therapies. Thrombectomy can be performed alone if the patient is not eligible for IV alteplase. In fact, some studies have challenged whether alteplase has any added benefit when combined with EVT.

4.3.3 QUESTIONING THE BENEFIT OF IV ALTEPLASE IN THROMBECTOMY

In addition, there is doubt that "bridging" with alteplase in patients with LVO has any added benefit. IV alteplase alone was used as the control arm in the randomized trials given that it was the standard of care at the time. However, some studies suggest that there may be no advantage to using alteplase in patients who are candidates for EVT.[22] A retrospective review of patients receiving alteplase plus EVT versus EVT alone suggested that in patients with anterior circulation LVO, EVT alone was equally effective to alteplase plus EVT.[23,24]

5 ENDOVASCULAR TREATMENT

5.1 Systems of care

It is important to remember that the NNT for EVT is 2.6–4 in comparison to other well-established therapies such with less efficacy such as ST-elevation myocardial infarction (STEMI) with IV lysis (NNT = 45–91), aspirin for STEMI (NNT = 42), IV alteplase within 0–3 hours for ischemic stroke (NNT = 8), and IV alteplase for stroke within 3–4.5 hours (NNT = 14). Performing EVT can provide a robust and lasting improved outcomes effect in a majority of appropriately selected stroke patients.

With every 30 minutes elapsed, there is a 10% decrease in probability of independent function. Hence, time barriers to treatment—be it IV alteplase or IV alteplase plus EVT—are important to overcome. The lag between groin puncture time and time to arrival begins with the prearrival emergency medical services (EMS) activation system and stream lining access to designated stroke centers. In a review by Saver et al., in 1000 patients with technically successful EVT, for every 15-minute more rapid door-to-reperfusion time, 39 patients would have a higher likelihood of a less-disabled outcome at 3 months.[25] Furthermore, 25 more patients would likely obtain functional independence.

Stroke centers should have a prehospital stroke alert system in combination with the local EMS services. Part of this is overcoming that stroke is a true emergency on the same level of magnitude as a heart attack or trauma. Local EMS can be trained in early recognition of stroke and potentially determining a LVO. They can then alert the stroke center to activate all relevant services, such as the ED, CT scan and technician, laboratory, pharmacy, and so on. The patient can be preregistered and delivered to the imaging suite immediately rather than a delay within the ED. Upon arrival to CT, the patient can be rapidly assessed by the stroke trained clinical team.

IV alteplase in eligible patients can be delivered while the CT is being read by the radiologist in real time. In appropriately selected patients, a CTA/CTP can be performed immediately or once the alteplase bolus is given, without leaving the CT suite to further streamline the process. The imaging can be reconstructed and read in real time. The neurointerventionalist can then be called immediately if the patient is a candidate for MT. The entirety of the neuroendovascular team, potentially including the anesthesiology team, can be notified and prepare for MT.

Most community hospitals will have the capability to administer IV alteplase, but fewer have the infrastructure and staff available to perform neurointerventions 24 hours a day. Therefore, it is crucial for stroke-ready or primary stroke centers to have an affiliation with a comprehensive stroke center who can accept the patient in transfer and can provide endovascular treatment for stroke 24/7. This relationship makes it possible for a neurointerventional team to be ready to take the patient to the neurointerventional suite as soon as they arrive for rapid thrombectomy.

5.2 Endovascular procedure

Most interventions are carried out via femoral artery access. A guide catheter is advanced over a wire through femoral sheath, through the descending aorta, over the aortic arch and the cervical vessel of interest is selected. Once the guide catheter is in place, the guidewire is removed, and a small catheter (microcatheter) is placed in the guide and advanced over a microwire into the intracranial vessel of interest, either proximal or distal to the thrombus depending on the type of stroke device that is utilized. All of this is performed using direct fluoroscopic guidance, typically with biplane anteroposterior and lateral fluoroscopy. Radiopaque contrast is injected under fluoroscopy to visualize the arteries, diagnose the vessel occlusion, make roadmaps for navigation, and assess flow before and after thrombectomy.

While many devices for EVT exist, in general, there are two basic types: stent retrievers and suction thrombectomy.[24] All the randomized studies cited earlier utilized stent retrievers. Stent retrievers are stents that expand across the thrombus when pushed with a wire that it is attached to. The stent then incorporates the arterial thrombus after deployment while simultaneously restoring blood flow to the ischemic territory. Upon retrieval (pulling the stent back) it is designed to remove the incorporated thrombus through the guide catheter as a unit (stent retriever and thrombus).

Table 9.2 COMPLICATION RATES BETWEEN ENDOVASCULAR THROMBECTOMY AND MEDICAL THERAPY

	Endovascular thrombectomy	Control (medical therapy)	Risk Difference (95% CI)	Adjusted ratio (95% CI)	Adjusted odds (95% CI)
Symptomatic ICH	4.4% (28/634)	4.3% (28/653)	0.1	1.07, p = 0.81	1.07, p = 0.81
Parenchymal hematoma type-2	5.1% (32/629)	5.3% (34/641)	−0.2	1.04, p = 0.88	1.04, p = 0.88
Mortality	15.3% (97/633)	18.9% (122/646)	−3.6	0.82, p = 0.15	0.73, p = 0.16

NOTE: Data are based on pulled analysis of five randomized trials of endovascular therarpy.[6]

ABBREVIATIONS: CI, confidence interval; ICH, intracranial hemorrhage.

Suction thrombectomy devices work by placing suction on a larger bore catheter that is positioned on the proximal end of the thrombus. When suction is applied to the catheter, the clot will become attached to the catheter by suction and can often be removed in its entirety.

Both devices are approved by the Food and Drug Administration for EVT for stroke and are readily available and commonly used at most stroke centers. For the most part, the decision which device to use is individualized to the patient and the specifics of the clot locations, size, and etiology as well as surgeon's preference.

There are associated risks with performing EVT. Direct complications from EVT include groin hematoma (1.8–10.7%), retroperitoneal hematoma (0.15–6%), symptomatic ICH (0–7.7%), perforation (0.9–4.9%), and mortality 7–18.4%).[6] These are listed in Table 9.2.

6 CLINICAL CASES

Case 9.1 Acute ischemic stroke with LVO

CASE DESCRIPTION

A patient developed the inability to speak (aphasia) and right-sided weakness (hemiplegia). After a 911 call, the patient was taken to her local ED. Her local primary stroke center ED was alerted that she was coming by paramedics via a prehospital stroke alert system, and the ED was prepared to receive her as a stroke alert upon arrival. The patient was immediately taken for a non-contrast head CT, which was "negative." The recommendation was made to give IV alteplase and then transfer the patient to a comprehensive stroke center for possible EVT while the alteplase drip was running (drip and ship). Upon arrival to the comprehensive stroke center, the patient went directly for CT angiography and perfusion, which revealed a left MCA

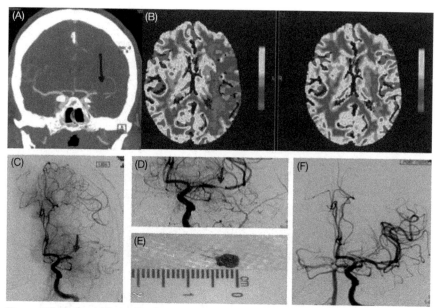

Figure 9.2 Left middle cerebral artery occlusion treatment with endovascular thrombectomy.

(A) Computed tomography angiography shows a left middle cerebral artery (MCA) occlusion (arrow).

(B) Computed tomography perfusion shows a mismatch between cerebral blood flow (CBF, left) and cerebral blood volume (CBV, right), indicating ischemic penumbra.

(C) Digital subtraction angiography again demonstrates the left MCA occlusion (arrow).

(D) The stent retriever is in place and has incorporated the thrombus while restoring blood flow (arrow).

(E) After retrieval of the stent retriever, a clot has been removed and (F) normal blood flow has been restored.

occlusion with a large area of ischemic penumbra or potentially salvageable brain tissue (Figure 9.2).

PRACTICAL POINTS

- This case represents a common scenario when a patient with suspected LVO first receives IV alteplase at a small local hospital, followed by transfer to a comprehensive stroke center capable of providing 24/7 neuroendovascular coverage.
- EMS alerting primary stroke responder team allows an expedited clinical evaluation, triage, and immediate diagnostic testing
- Advanced imaging such as CT or MR angiography with perfusion and rapid involvement of a neurointerventionalist are key to technical successful and expedient clot retrieval, increasing the odds for a good clinical outcome.

Case 9.2 Non-candidate for endovascular intervention

CASE DESCRIPTION

A man was found down at home next to his bed. He was found not moving his right side; he was not speaking and had a left gaze preference. He was last seen well the day before. The patient came to the ED by ambulance and underwent a non-contrast head CT (Figure 9.3).

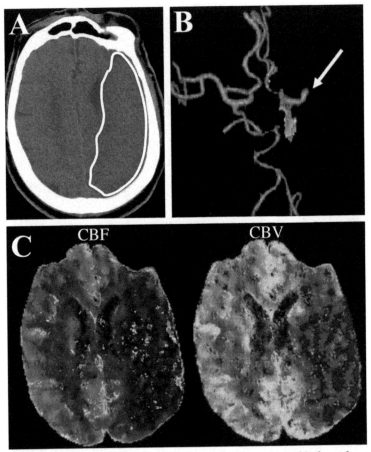

Figure 9.3 A completed left middle cerebral artery occlusion, ineligible for endovascular thrombectomy.

(A) Non-contrast head computed tomography shows early signs of ischemia with loss of gray-white differentiation in the left middle cerebral artery (MCA) territory (indicated by the white border).

(B) Computed tomography angiography shows a proximal left MCA occlusion (arrow).

(C) Computed tomography perfusion maps show further evidence that the stroke is not reversible with depression in the cerebral blood flow (CBF) and cerebral blood volume (CBV) maps without signs of mismatch between the two.

PRACTICAL POINTS

- The non-contrast CT showed early evidence of a large left MCA infarct. Perfusion imaging demonstrated decreased CBV and CBF without mismatch and CTA revealed a left MCA occlusion.
- Although the patient had a LVO, the ischemic changes on the CT alone would be enough to conclude that the stroke was not reversible.
- The CTP is a nice example of what it means to have no mismatch between CBF and CBV in contrast to Case 9.1. Despite the presence of LVO and severe deficits, EVT is not indicated in this situation.

Case 9.3 Posterior circulation acute ischemic stroke

CASE DESCRIPTION

A woman presented with a 2-day history of headaches, neck pain, and nausea and vomiting. On the day that she presented to the hospital, her symptoms progressed to left hemiplegia and obtundation. She required intubation in the ED for airway protection. A non-contrast head CT showed some questionable patchy hypodensities in the posterior fossa (cerebellum and brainstem). CTA revealed a BA occlusion and bilateral VA dissections (Figure 9.4).

PRACTICAL POINTS

- The patient was taken emergently to the angiography suite for neurointervention. The neurointerventional team proceeded with EVT using a stent retriever (see panel C of Figure 9.4). Following retrieval of the stent retriever and clot, a very large thrombus was removed, and angiography following thrombectomy demonstrated recanalization of the BA.
- Inclusion criteria of recent Class I trials involved LVO of the anterior circulation (i.e., ICA, proximal MCA), but that should not exclude EVT for patients with posterior circulation strokes (i.e., VA, BA).
- LVO of the posterior circulation is uniformly disabling. Time to intervention is less well-defined in this patient population. Because of such a poor natural history, EVT should always be considered even in a delayed presentation, such as >24 hours in this case if the patient has any neurological function.
- General anesthesia should be considered to protect the airway, but with specific instructions to avoid hypotension with induction. Normotension should be maintained throughout the procedure.

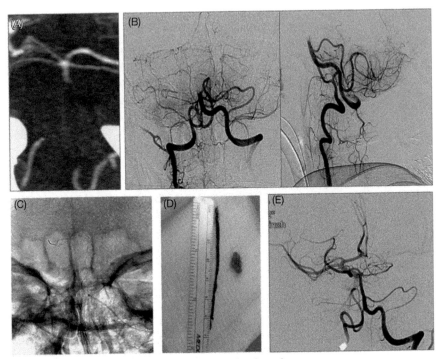

Figure 9.4 Basilar artery stroke with endovascular thrombectomy.
(A) Computed tomography angiography shows occlusion of the midbasilar artery. The top of the basilar artery (BA) is filling retrograde from the posterior communicating arteries.
(B) Digital subtraction angiograhy, AP and lateral views confirm occlusion of the BA.
(C) A still xray of a stent retriever in the right posterior cerebral artery and basilar artery BA.
(D) The thrombus was retrieved.
(E) AP angiography after thrombectomy shows recanalization of the BA.

REFERENCES

1. Berkhemer OA, Fransen PS, Beumer D, et al. A randomized trial of intraarterial treatment for acute ischemic stroke. *N Engl J Med.* 2015;372(1):11–20.
2. Campbell BC, Mitchell PJ, Kleinig TJ, et al. Endovascular therapy for ischemic stroke with perfusion-imaging selection. *N Engl J Med.* 2015;372(11):1009–1018.
3. Goyal M, Demchuk AM, Menon BK, et al. Randomized assessment of rapid endovascular treatment of ischemic stroke. *N Engl J Med.* 2015;372(11):1019–1030.
4. Jovin TG, Chamorro A, Cobo E, et al. Thrombectomy within 8 hours after symptom onset in ischemic stroke. *N Engl J Med.* 2015;372(24):2296–2306.
5. Saver JL, Goyal M, Bonafe A, et al. Stent-retriever thrombectomy after intravenous t-PA vs. t-PA alone in stroke. *N Engl J Med.* 2015;372(24):2285–2295.
6. Goyal M, Menon BK, van Zwam WH, et al. Endovascular thrombectomy after large-vessel ischaemic stroke: a meta-analysis of individual patient data from five randomised trials. *Lancet.* 2016;387(10029):1723–1731.

7. Lees KR, Bluhmki E, von Kummer R, et al. Time to treatment with intravenous alteplase and outcome in stroke: an updated pooled analysis of ECASS, ATLANTIS, NINDS, and EPITHET trials. *Lancet*. 2010;375(9727):1695–1703.

8. Amenta PS, Ali MS, Dumont AS, et al. Computed tomography perfusion-based selection of patients for endovascular recanalization. *Neurosurg Focus*. 2011;30(6):E6.

9. Wintermark M, Sincic R, Sridhar D, Chien JD. Cerebral perfusion CT: technique and clinical applications. *J Neuroradiol*. 2008;35(5):253–260.

10. Labeyrie MA, Turc G, Hess A, et al. Diffusion lesion reversal after thrombolysis: a MR correlate of early neurological improvement. *Stroke*. 2012;43(11):2986–2991.

11. Soize S, Tisserand M, Charron S, et al. How sustained is 24-hour diffusion-weighted imaging lesion reversal? Serial magnetic resonance imaging in a patient cohort thrombolyzed within 4.5 hours of stroke onset. *Stroke*. 2015;46(3):704–710.

12. Powers WJ, Derdeyn CP, Biller J, et al. 2015 American Heart Association/American Stroke Association focused update of the 2013 guidelines for the early management of patients with acute ischemic stroke regarding endovascular treatment: a guideline for healthcare professionals from the American Heart Association/American Stroke Association. *Stroke*. 2015;46(10):3020–3035.

13. Goyal N, Tsivgoulis G, Frei D, et al. A multicenter study of the safety and effectiveness of mechanical thrombectomy for patients with acute ischemic stroke not meeting top-tier evidence criteria. *J Neurointerv Surg*. 2017. doi:10.1136/neurintsurg-2016-012905

14. Bhole R, Goyal N, Nearing K, et al. Implications of limiting mechanical thrombectomy to patients with emergent large vessel occlusion meeting top tier evidence criteria. *J Neurointerv Surg*. 2017;9(3):225–228.

15. Mokin M, Kan P, Sivakanthan S, et al. Endovascular therapy of wake-up strokes in the modern era of stent retriever thrombectomy. *J Neurointerv Surg*. 2016;8(3):240–243.

16. Aghaebrahim A, Leiva-Salinas C, Jadhav AP, et al. Outcomes after endovascular treatment for anterior circulation stroke presenting as wake-up strokes are not different than those with witnessed onset beyond 8 hours. *J Neurointerv Surg*. 2015;7(12):875–880.

17. Nogueira RG, Jadhav AP, Haussen DC, et al. Thrombectomy 6 to 24 hours after stroke with a mismatch between deficit and infarct. *N Engl J Med*. 2018;378(1):11–21.

18. Jovin TG, Saver JL, Ribo M, et al. Diffusion-weighted imaging or computerized tomography perfusion assessment with clinical mismatch in the triage of wake up and late presenting strokes undergoing neurointervention with Trevo (DAWN) trial methods. *Int J Stroke*. 2017;2(6):641–652.

19. Mokin M, Sonig A, Sivakanthan S, et al. Clinical and procedural predictors of outcomes from the endovascular treatment of posterior circulation strokes. *Stroke*. 2016;47(3):782–788.

20. Mokin M, Primiani CT, Ren Z, et al. Endovascular treatment of middle cerebral artery M2 occlusion strokes: clinical and procedural predictors of outcomes. *Neurosurgery*. 2017;81(5):795–802.

21. Sarraj A, Sangha N, Hussain MS, et al. Endovascular therapy for acute ischemic stroke with occlusion of the middle cerebral artery M2 segment. *JAMA Neurol*. 2016;73(11):1291–1296.

22. Levy EI, Mokin M. Stroke: Stroke thrombolysis and thrombectomy—not stronger together? *Nat Rev Neurol.* 2017;13(4):198–200.
23. Abilleira S, Ribera A, Cardona P, et al. Outcomes after direct thrombectomy or combined intravenous and endovascular treatment are not different. *Stroke.* 2017;48(2):375–378.
24. Coutinho JM, Liebeskind DS, Slater LA, et al. Combined intravenous thrombolysis and thrombectomy vs thrombectomy alone for acute ischemic stroke: a pooled analysis of the SWIFT and STAR studies. *JAMA Neurol.* 2017;74(3):268–274.
25. Saver JL, Goyal M, van der Lugt A, et al. Time to treatment with endovascular thrombectomy and outcomes from ischemic stroke: a meta-analysis. *JAMA.* 2016;316(12):1279–1288.

10

Care of Stroke Patients Post Intravenous Alteplase and Endovascular Thrombectomy

VIOLIZA INOA AND LUCAS ELIJOVICH ■

CONTENTS

1 INTRODUCTION

There is a large amount of high quality data on post intravenous (IV) thrombolysis care for acute ischemic stroke (AIS) patients who are treated with IV alteplase. Less in known on the basic principles of managing patients treated with endovascular thrombectomy (EVT), such as the use of antithrombotic agents, optimal blood pressure (BP) parameters, and optimal imaging protocols. This chapter will review the latest literature and describe basic postinterventional algorithms applicable to the neurocritical intensive care unit settings, as well as recognition and management of complications, which are summarized in Figure 10.1.

2 STROKE AND INTENSIVE CARE UNIT MANAGEMENT

Current practice in the management of AIS patients that are candidates for IV alteplase or EVT is that they be treated at high-volume stroke centers that provide rapid access to neurointerventionalists and posttreatment care in advanced stroke and neurocritical care units (NICU). The care of patients with AIS in a stroke unit improves clinical outcome compared with treatment in a non-stroke unit or general medical ward.[1]

AIS patients that have been treated with IV alteplase and/or EVT require continuous monitoring after these interventions. Certain institutions have designated step-down beds for the care of patients after IV alteplase. This should only be considered appropriate when these units can offer continuous and standardized

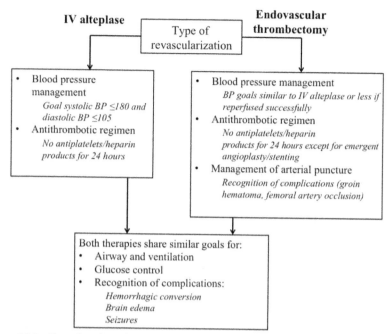

Figure 10.1 Algorithm describing care of the stroke patients post intravenous thrombolysis and endovascular intervention.
ABBREVIATIONS: BP, blood pressure; IV, intravenous.

post-IV alteplase care, as provided by experienced personnel. However, when EVT is performed, more intense neurological monitoring is routinely required, and these patients should be admitted to an intensive care unit (ICU). Endovascular patients may differ in their level of revascularization and require individually tailored BP goals for optimal cerebral perfusion. They may be treated with antithrombotic medications, which increases their bleeding risk. They also have the added complexity and additional potential complications related to arterial vascular access.

For these and other reasons, patients undergoing EVT often require more intensive neurologic monitoring and should be admitted to the ICU. Ideally, transfer to a NICU is preferred since frequent postthrombolytic and postprocedural standardized assessments are recommended. Such assessments are most adequately provided by medical and nursing personnel trained in neurocritical care. When NICU beds are not available, transfer to a non-neurological ICU is acceptable. The role of the clinician and the ICU staff is to provide continuous observation of vital signs, vascular access site checks, and cardiac monitoring and to administer uniform neurological evaluations to identify potential clinical fluctuations and/ or complications. The duration of this intensive surveillance should last at least

24 hours after the endovascular procedure or until the patient is deemed clinically stable to leave the ICU.

3 COMPLICATIONS ASSOCIATED WITH ACUTE STROKE

Early recognition and appropriate management of neurological and non-neurological complications in the ICU can be a significant factor in reducing mortality during the acute hospitalization of these patients.[2] Standardized care implemented by a neurointensivist and a critical care team can not only decrease the length of admission but can also offer a greater chance of being discharged home. There is a positive correlation between the care provided by a specialized neurovascular care team and favorable stroke outcomes. This could be in part related to continual improvements in the quality of care and utilization of neuroprotective measures, in conjunction with the therapeutic approaches that are currently available for the prevention and management of some of the common complications after AIS.[3]

The potential neurological complications related to brain ischemia and revascularization strategies are well described. These include increased intracranial pressure (due to malignant cerebral edema or hemorrhagic transformation of the infarct), seizures, impaired level of consciousness, infarct growth, arterial re-occlusion, and recurrent strokes. There are also typical non-neurological complications, which can be related to cardiac disease, hemodynamic instability, infections, deep venous thrombosis, pulmonary embolus, and many others that are outside of the scope of this chapter. The focus of this text relates to the acute management after IV alteplase administration and EVT; therefore, special consideration will be given to complications related to these revascularization techniques including arterial puncture, dissections, and other problems associated with revascularization therapies.

4 ARTERIAL PUNCTURE: POST THROMBECTOMY CARE AND MANAGEMENT

Percutaneous vascular access through the common femoral artery is the most commonly used approach for neuroendovascular procedures. The arteriotomy should be performed below the inguinal ligament. This technique has been considered easy and relatively safe, and a major advantage involves the ability to obtain hemostasis with compression against the femoral head after the sheath removal.[4]

Alternative approaches, such as direct carotid or brachial artery access, are also used when difficult femoral access or unfavorable anatomic situations are encountered. Although these techniques have been described for endovascular treatment of AIS, these are not commonly used and are reserved for distinct cases where catheter navigation into the vertebral, common, or internal carotid arteries is not possible.[5,6]

The angiography sheath size will depend on the catheters utilized for the procedure. Commonly, a large-bore introducer sheath (6–9 French size) will provide the path for a standard guide catheter, a distal access catheter or a relatively larger balloon guide catheter. At the completion of the procedure, a vascular closure device is often used due to the arteriotomy size and the attendant bleeding risks during, particularly after IV alteplase administration. Occasionally, the introducer sheath is left in place to be removed in the ICU under a more controlled environment. The decision to leave the sheath in place may be due to a variety of factors including vascular access complications, concomitant atherosclerosis precluding vascular closure device, or the need for arterial pressure monitoring. These and other pertinent details including the access site, sheath size and length, anatomical variations, and presence or absence of pedal pulses should be communicated with the accepting team post procedure.

Variations in protocol exist among different institutions regarding postprocedural clinical monitoring. Frequent access site checks should be documented every 15 minutes for at least 1 hour, followed by periodic assessments every 30–60 minutes for up to 5–6 hours. Additional or more frequent monitoring might be warranted if access site complications occur.

Question 10.1: What are the common signs of arterial access complications after stroke thrombectomy?

Answer: Pain at groin access site or abdomen pain, groin hematoma, and hypotension.

4.1 Complications associated with arterial access

Some of the arterial puncture site complications that are more often encountered during angiographic procedures include hematoma (most commonly), dissection, pseudoaneurysm formation, and arterial occlusion. Rarely, arteriovenous fistulas, femoral nerve damage, or focal and/or systemic infections can occur as a result of these procedures.[7,8] The rate of clinical significant groin complications utilizing large-bore sheaths in EVT has been recently reported to be as low as 0.4–0.8%,[9] but when present these conditions can result in hemodynamic compromise in cases of retroperitoneal bleeding with severe anemia and shock and may require surgery resulting in prolonged hospitalizations. Severe ischemic complications may also require surgical intervention; therefore, prompt recognition and management of these complications by the neurointerventional team or the NICU staff can lessen the likelihood of poor outcomes related to these circumstances.

A painful hematoma that continues to grow throughout the observation period should raise suspicion for a pseudoaneurysm, and rapid ultrasound evaluation is recommended. In fact, doppler ultrasound may also be a therapeutic option when a pseudoaneurysm develops, since manual compression of the puncture site with the doppler probe has proven adequate to thrombose the vascular abnormality.[10,11] This technique will occasionally avoid the need for surgical repair, although surgery is sometimes inevitable with large hematoma development and/or when focal compression of the adjacent structures take place.

Severe pain accompanied by focal tenderness and progressive discomfort should raise concern for retroperitoneal or pelvic bleeding. It is important to recognize that an obvious hematoma is generally not present on physical examination since the blood is accumulated within the abdominal cavity. Therefore, when suspected, emergent computed tomography (CT) of the pelvis should be obtained to establish the diagnosis.[12]

When identified, these vascular complications need prompt evaluation by the neurointervenionalist and a vascular surgery consultation should be immediate. The critical care staff should continue to coordinate care, provide clinical and laboratory monitoring, arrange for expedited blood transfusions when necessary, and offer hemodynamic support.

5 SUPPORTIVE CARE

5.1 Blood pressure, cardiac monitoring, and hemodynamics

Rapidly fluctuating arterial BP is common in the setting of AIS. Although it is more common to encounter elevation in the BP, arterial hypotension can also occur, and, theoretically, both, extreme hyper- and hypotension can be detrimental given the risk of cerebral and systemic complications from these situations.[13,14] Guidelines and recommendations for BP management after IV alteplase exist (Box 10.1), but less

---

Box 10.1

MANAGEMENT OF BLOOD PRESSURE DURING AND AFTER IV ALTEPLASE ADMINISTRATION

- Close monitoring of BP for the first 24 hours from the start of alteplase infusion:
  - Every 15 minutes for 2 hours
  - Every 30 minutes for 6 hours
  - Every hour for 16 hours
- BP goal is 180 mm Hg or less systolic and 105 mm Hg or less diastolic.
- Labetalol, hydralazine, or nicardipine can be used to control elevated BP if needed.

---

is known about optimal BP parameters after EVT. Prospective studies are needed to determine the ideal BP parameters during and immediately after EVT for acute stroke. Current clinical practice regarding BP management post endovascular intervention varies widely among institutions.

Question 10.2: What are the BP parameters after IV alteplase?

Answer: Following the administration of alteplase, BP should be maintained at or below 180/105 mm Hg.

5.1.1 INTRAVENOUS ALTEPLASE

Higher BP parameters within the first 24 hours after thrombolysis are associated with adverse events, with best outcomes correlated with systolic BP of 141 to 150 mm Hg.[15] Immediately after the administration of IV alteplase, BP should be maintained below 180/105 mm Hg.[16] During the EVT, before adequate reperfusion is achieved, it is reasonable to maintain a systolic BP of no less than 140 mm Hg with close intraprocedural BP monitoring to avoid extreme BP fluctuations. Hypotension has been known to be harmful in the setting of a large vessel occlusion, given the risk of cerebral hypoperfusion with resulting expansion of the core infarct and penumbral loss.

For patients undergoing general anesthesia, prolonged episodes of lower mean arterial pressures may have adverse effects,[17] and when necessary, fluids and vasopressors should be promptly administered by the anesthesia team in order to maintain a systolic BP of at least 140 mm Hg prior to revascularization.[18,19] As a rule of thumb, a mean arterial pressure drop >10% from baseline should be avoided, irrespective of the mode of sedation.[20]

The challenge in AIS is that patients often present with a pressor response and baseline BP is unknown. Acute cardiac conditions, volume depletion, and procedural complications can contribute to acute hypotension. When present, these conditions should be rapidly identified and treated. If fluid administration is needed, isotonic solutions are preferred over hypotonic solutions. The duration, volume, and route of fluid administration will vary according to the clinical scenario.[21]

Question 10.3: What are the BP parameters after EVT?

Answer: There is no agreement among stroke neurologists and neurointerventionalists. Some use the same parameters as with IV alteplase therapy (equal or less than 180/105 mm Hg). Others advocate for more aggressive BP control, once successful recanalization has been achieved.

5.1.2 ENDOVASCULAR THROMBECTOMY

A more complex dilemma still exits surrounding optimal BP parameters immediately after EVT. The premorbid characteristics of each patient can vary significantly, as well as their stroke mechanism, ultimate angiographic level of revascularization, grade of pial collateralization, infarct size, and risk for hemorrhagic complication. Important consideration should be given to each of these variables to individualize patient care accordingly. After thrombectomy, concern exists regarding the lack of cerebral autoregulation that may lead hyperperfusion of the revascularized tissue bed and hemorrhagic conversion of the infarct or conversely tissue hypoperfusion in the setting of incomplete revascularization. Therefore, increased variability and extreme BP fluctuations immediately after the procedure are considered detrimental and should be avoided.

Recommendations regarding specific BP parameters post thrombectomy are not available. Current practice adheres to treatment targets similar to those after IV alteplase, with BP goals of 180/105 mmHg or less.[16] Permissive hypertension is not recommended after successful recanalization has been achieved and goal BP <160/90 mmHg has been suggested when successful angiographic revascularization has resulted. Continuous BP monitoring for at least 24 hours after thrombectomy, with all attempts made to maintain BP parameters without major variations should be the objective until specific guidelines become available. The frequency of the surveillance should be similar to that after treatment with IV alteplase, with BP monitoring every 15 minutes for at least 2 hours, followed by repeated assessments every 30 minutes for 6 hours, and then hourly checks for at least 16 hours after treatment.[16]

Pre-morbid cardiac disease and acute serious cardiac events are highly prevalent in the stroke population, and cardiac mortality accounts for second most common cause of death after stroke.[22,23] On acute presentation, stroke patients are often found with new onset electrocardiography (ECG) abnormalities, which manifest frequently as cardiac arrhythmias.[24,25] Although this relationship is not fully understood, some cortical structures have been implicated in the control of cardiac rate and rhythm, and lesions to these regions may be considered arrhythmogenic. For example, cardiac chronotropic organization has been identified in the rostral posterior insula, with sympathetic predominance on the right side.[26] Hemispheric lesions affecting the right insular cortex can generate lethal cardiac arrhythmias and severe hemodynamic instability. Therefore, early recognition and assessments with a baseline ECG, ongoing cardiac telemetry and serial troponin checks should be included in the monitoring of all AIS patients. No special recommendations exist for the management of cardiac issues in the postthrombectomy stroke population, since these should be addressed similarly in all patients undergoing care for AIS.

5.2 Airway and ventilation

In the recent past, general anesthesia was the preferred mode of sedation of neurointerventionalists during EVT.[27] This practice is no longer the standard of care due to potential harm from both the inherent time delays and hypotension encountered with general anesthesia. Conscious sedation is now common practice for most EVT procedures. The choice of anesthetic technique, level of sedation, and pharmacological agent should be individualized based on clinical characteristics of each patient.

A novel agent that has been investigated for this purpose is dexmedetomidine (Precedex®), which has been reported safe and can be used for the induction and maintenance of sedation without causing respiratory depression nor obscuration of the neurological exam during mechanical thrombectomy.[28] This agent has been proven superior to benzodiazepines in reducing agitation and delirium in the ICU and represents an attractive alternative for postprocedural sedation when required. Endotracheal intubation is not required when adequate periprocedural oxygenation and ventilation can be maintained. Supplemental oxygen should be used during and after the procedure, especially in the setting of decreased consciousness. Continuous pulse oximetry, capnography, and monitoring of PaO_2 and $PaCO_2$ should be monitored intra-procedure, with the objective of maintaining SpO_2 >92% and PaO_2>60% by titrating the FiO_2. When clinically indicated, endotracheal intubation before, during or after the procedure should be performed. The goal is to maintain normocapnia with a $PaCO_2$ of 35–45 mm Hg.

5.3 Temperature

Temperature monitoring and management in patients undergoing EVT should follow usual stroke care parameters. Hyperthermia (>38C) is commonly encountered after stroke and is associated with poor outcome.[16] The fever etiology should be promptly investigated, and the use of antipyretics and cooling devices is recommended. A target body temperature of 35–37C should be maintained, and if shivering occurs, administration of meperidine is acceptable.

5.4 Glucose control

High glucose in the setting of non-lacunar acute stroke is an independent predictor of larger infarct size, poor outcome, and higher mortality.[29,30] The positive effects of recanalization after thrombolysis can be masked if hyperglycemia is not treated acutely.[31] There is a higher risk for clinical deterioration and intracranial hemorrhage in post-IV alteplase patients without strict hyperglycemic control, and theoretical benefits of good glucose management during and after endovascular stroke procedures are inferred.[32,33]

Inpatient hyperglycemia is defined as blood glucose >140 mg/dL. Insulin therapy is recommended when glucose levels are persistently >180 mg/dL, with target blood sugars between 110–140 mg/dL. A validated insulin infusion protocol should be administered when necessary, but the exclusive use of an insulin sliding scale is not supported.[34] Close glucose motoring every 4–6 hours should be implemented, and infusions with dextrose are permitted when glucose levels drop below 60 mg/dL. Dextrose therapy should be immediately discontinued once normoglycemia has been achieved. It is important to highlight that hypoglycemia is an equivalent if not more deleterious complication than hyperglycemia in stroke patients. Aggressive insulin infusion protocols, targeting strict normoglycemia (targets <120), have been demonstrated to result in frequent hypoglycemia and worse outcomes in the ICU and should be avoided.[35]

6 USE OF ANTITHROMBOTIC AGENTS

The use of antiplatelet agents and anticoagulants within the first 24 hours after IV alteplase and/or EVT is not recommended and can almost always be avoided.[16] The latest generation EVT devices (stent-retrievers and large bore aspiration catheters) have proven efficacy as stand-alone treatments for emergent large vessel occlusion, without the use of adjunctive intra-arterial thrombolytics or antiplatelet infusions.[36,37]

> **Question 10.4:** When is the optimal time to start antiplatelet agents after IV alteplase or EVT?
>
> **Answer:** It is typically advised to start antiplatelet therapy after the first 24 hours. Patients in whom emergent stenting was performed require immediate administration of antiplatelet agents to prevent in-stent thrombosis.

6.1 Acute stenting and antithrombotic agents

Acute stenting of the extracranial carotid artery in combination with intracranial thrombectomy is the most frequent indication for the use of antiplatelet medications with or without systemic anticoagulation (Case 10.1). The goal of this therapy is to prevent stent related thromboembolic complications. However, there is a legitimate risk of symptomatic intracranial hemorrhage (sICH) with periprocedural anticoagulation or with the use of an aggressive antiplatelet regimen.[38,39] Another scenario that may warrant immediate administration of antiplatelet agents is intracranial angioplasty and stenting.

6.1.1 GLYCOPROTEIN IIB/IIIA INHIBITORS
Certain medications may carry higher risks than others: abciximab (ReoPro®), for example, has been associated with increased risk of sICH when used during acute stroke treatments and other neuroendovascular procedures.[40] Its use is generally not recommended after thrombolysis given the theoretical risk of increased bleeding associated with this drug after IV alteplase has been given. Therefore, if abciximab is administered, caution and conservative dosage (bolus <0.25 mg/kg, without continuous infusion) are recommended. Although abciximab bolus followed by continued infusion is routinely used in percutaneous coronary interventions, clinical and safety data for abciximab or other platelet glycoprotein

IIb/IIIA inhibitors, such as eptifibatide or tirofiban, is scarce in emergent stenting during acute stroke; therefore, their routine use is not recommended in this setting.[41]

6.1.2 INTRAVENOUS HEPARIN

Treatment approaches for acute stenting during EVT vary widely among institutions and a protocol supporting standardized periprocedural antithrombotic recommendations are currently lacking. Intravenous heparin has been routinely used as an adjunctive therapy prior to the administration of antiplatelet agents. A common approach involves the use of IV heparin (1000–2500 units) immediately after arterial access has been obtained.[42,43] A more aggressive regimen consists of an IV bolus of 5000 units of heparin with additional boluses to achieve an activated clotting time of 230–250 seconds.[44] This second regimen with 5000 units of heparin has not been reported in patients who received thrombolysis with IV alteplase; therefore, its safety and efficacy is unclear.

6.1.3 ORAL ANTIPLATELET MEDICATIONS

Antiplatelet medications are often administered alone or in combination with a second antithrombotic agent. Loading doses of aspirin (300–600 mg) and/or clopidogrel (300–600 mg) are often used safely and are among the preferred agents during these procedures. A more conservative approach, with a single agent or a smaller dosage, is reasonable for patients who had been taking an antiplatelet agent in the preoperative period. These medications can be administered immediately prior, during, or at the completion of the procedure. The route of administration can be enteral or intravenous, and this decision is made based upon availability and preference of the treating physician. Table 10.1 summarizes some of the commonly used antiplatelet drugs that are currently available in the United States, along with details regarding their mechanism and action, administration route, and pharmacological properties.

6.2 Antithrombotic agents and intracranial hemorrhage

Assessment for hemorrhagic transformation and infarct size within the first 24 hours with a repeat head CT or magnetic resonance imaging (MRI) is common practice before adjustment or continuation of the antiplatelet regimen. This is routine imaging is often obtained even when the patient remains neurologically stable. The goal is to identify hemorrhagic conversion and/or large volumes of infarcted tissue prior to clinical deterioration.

Table 10.1 Summary table of commonly used antiplatelet drugs currently available in the United States

Agent	Brand name	Mechanism	Dosage	Onset of action	Half-life	Duration of effect
Oral use						
Aspirin	Aspir 81, Ecotrin, Bayer Aspirin, Bufferin, Aspir-Low, etc.	Cyclooxygenase-1 and 2 enzyme inhibitor	load 160–325 mg, 81–350 mg qd	20 minutes; peak 1–2 hours (nonenteric-coated); 3–4 hours (enteric- coated); rectal onset is slower, chewing nonenteric-coated is fastest	Dose dependent: 2–3 hours low dose, 5–6 hours after 1 g, 10 hours larger dose	Lifetime of a platelet (~10 days)
Clopidrogrel	Plavix	Inhibition of P2Y12 ADP receptor	300 or 600 mg load, 75 mg qd	2 hours after loading dose; within 48 hours after 50–100 mg	6–8 hours	~ 5 days
Prasugrel	Effient	Inhibition of P2Y12 ADP receptor	60 mg load, 10 mg qd	within 30 minutes after loading dose, peak effect 4 hours	7 hours (range 2–15)	~ 5–9 days
Ticagrelor	Brilinta	Inhibition of P2Y12 ADP receptor	180 mg load, 90 mg bid	within 30 minutes after loading dose, peak effect 2 hours	7 hours parent drug, 9 hours active metabolite	~ 3 days

Drug	Brand	Class	Dosage	Onset/peak	Half-life	Duration/discontinuation
Dipyridamole	Persantine	Adenosine reuptake inhibitor	75–100 mg qid	1–2 hours; peaks 2–2.5 hours	10–12 hours	
Cilostazol	Pletal	Phosphodiesterase (PDE) III inhibitor	100 mg bid	2–4 weeks, peaks up to 12 weeks	~ 11–13 hours	
Anagrelide	Agrylin	PDE inhibitor	0.5 mg aid–1 mg bid	7–14 days, complete response 4–12 weeks	1.5 hours	~ 4 days
Intravenous use						
Eptifibatide	Integrilin	Glycoprotein IIb/IIIa antagonist	Bolus: 180 mcg/kg Infusion: 2 mcg/kg/min	5 minutes, peaks 1 hour	2.5 hours	~ 4–8 hours after discontinuation
Abciximab	ReoPro	Glycoprotein IIb/IIIa antagonist	Bolus: 0.25 mg/kg bolus over 10–60 min Infusion: 0.125 mg/kg/min	10 minutes	30 min from plasma, remains bound to some receptors up to 15 days	72 hours (platelet function may remain abnormal for up to 7 days)
Tirofiban	Aggrastat	Glycoprotein IIb/IIIa antagonist	0.4 mcg/kg.min over 30 min + 0.1 mcg/kg/min	10 min	2 hours	4–8 hours after discontinuation

7 RECOGNITION AND MANAGEMENT OF ACUTE NEUROLOGICAL COMPLICATIONS

7.1 Periprocedural assessments during endovascular thrombectomy

Clinical and radiological monitoring are the cornerstones of identifying deterioration after acute stroke. Accurate clinical assessments are often difficult during and immediately after the endovascular therapy, mainly due to the use of procedural IV sedation or general anesthesia. Brain imaging during or postprocedure remains an indirect but effective mode for prompt and reliable evaluation (Case 10.2). Valuable information such as infarct volume, hemorrhagic transformation, and real-time estimates of tissue perfusion postthrombectomy may be promptly obtained to allow rapid recognition and management of potentially fatal complications.[45,46]

7.1.1 IMAGING TECHNOLOGY IN THE ANGIOGRAPHY SUITE

When available in the angiographic suite, biplane flat-panel detectors can generate three-dimensional (3D) volumes from data acquired during C-arm rotation using CT-like reconstruction algorithms. The reconstructed 3D volumes can be postprocessed for visualization and analysis, similar to multisection CT. Currently, available C-arm flat detectors allow for a contrast resolution that is comparable with conventional CT, making this system sufficient to diagnose suspected neurological complications in a timely manner.[47,48] Parenchymal blood volume (PBV) mapping with flat panel detectors remains a useful tool to estimate tissue perfusion prior and/or post intervention. This can be particularly useful in recognizing hypoperfused tissue after therapy. Determining lack of normalization of PBV can help clinicians distinguish between successful or failed reperfusion (despite recanalization). Hence, PBV mapping may have important implications in the periprocedural management of these patients.[49] When these techniques are not available in the angiographic suite, acquisition of a conventional CT or a brain MRI are recommended when neurological complications are suspected.

7.1.2 BRAIN HEMATOMA VERSUS CONTRAST ON IMAGING

When hyperdense lesions are present in flat-panel or conventional CT, differentiating hematoma from contrast is of extreme importance for decision-making and postprocedural management of these patients. Theoretically, contrast-related hyperdensities can be present due to endothelial permeability and ischemic injury and does represent bleeding. Therefore, if contrast-related hyperdensity is suspected, repeat imaging to demonstrate resolution of the hyperdense findings is recommended without reversal of the antithrombotic regimen. Lesions with lower densities (Hounsfield unit [HU] values below 50), are often suggestive of iodinated contrast. On the contrary, lesions with higher attenuation (HU values >58) have been reported to predict subsequent hemorrhage.[50–52]

7.2 Management of neurological complications

Neurological complications after endovascular procedures may be related to the procedure itself or to acute brain injury resulting from the stroke. Catheter perforation with hemorrhage, embolus to other circulations, and failed recanalization are all well described causes of periprocedural complications.[53] Antithrombotic reversal, tight BP control, and prompt neurosurgical evaluation are often necessary when hemorrhagic complications occur (Case 10.3). Hemorrhagic conversion of the infarcted tissue, malignant cerebral edema, and seizures are also well-known complications of AIS. Specific guidelines for the management of acute neurological complications after EVT do not exist, and it is reasonable to apply similar therapeutic strategies to those after IV alteplase. Although no standardized treatment approach exists, expert consensus guidance exists for the management of these adverse events.[16,54,55]

7.2.1 HEMORRHAGIC CONVERSION POST ALTEPLASE AND ENDOVASCULAR THROMBECTOMY

sICH represents the most feared complication after IV alteplase[54] and is associated with worse outcome.[55] Hematoma expansion can be seen in 40% of the cases in follow up CT scan, which suggests a therapeutic window and potential benefit from thrombolytic reversal.[56]

According to the neurocritical care guidelines for reversal of antithrombotics in intracranial hemorrhage (ICH),[56] reversal after IV alteplase is indicated in patients with symptomatic deterioration attributable to ICH and/or large ICH with associated mass effect. If an acute clinical deterioration is identified, the infusion should be stopped immediately, and a non-contrast head CT should be obtained. If the infusion has been completed, reversal is suggested when a thrombolytic agent has been administered in the previous 24 hours. Reversal agents that have been used include cryoprecipitate (10 units will raise fibrinogen levels by 70 mg/dL in a 70 kg patient), fresh-frozen plasma, vitamin K (when abnormal international normalized ratio), antifibrinolytics (aminocaproic acid and tranexamic acid) and platelets.[57] The goal is to raise fibrinogen levels to >150 mg/dL. Unfortunately, bleeding progression can still occur despite the prompt administration of these agents, and there are few data to support their efficacy. The use of antifibrinolytics remains as a conditional recommendation with very low-quality evidence, and the usefulness of platelet transfusions remain unclear in this setting.[58]

7.2.2 BRAIN EDEMA POST STROKE

Cerebral edema after AIS starts to develop within hours of stroke onset, peaks at 2 to 5 days, and then gradually resolves.[59] Acute brain swelling within the first 24 hours after AIS occurs when the infarct involves a large portion of the vascular distribution of the internal carotid or the middle cerebral artery (MCA).[58] "Malignant MCA infarction" is the term used to describe rapid neurological decline due to the effects of cerebral edema following MCA territory stroke. This is considered potentially fatal, since focal brain edema may result in brain herniation.

Some predictors of malignant stroke evolution include large infarct size (more than 50% of the MCA territory), presence of a "dense MCA sign," multiple vascular territories, high National Institutes of Health Stroke Scale (NIHSS) score, coma on admission, prior hypertension or congestive heart failure, and elevated white cell count. Intense clinical surveillance is recommended to identify potential neurological worsening. A non-contrast head CT is a useful imaging modality for monitoring the progression of the brain swelling, increasing midline shift and/ or development of hydrocephalus. Routine intracranial pressure monitoring or placement of a ventriculostomy is not indicated in hemispheric strokes, since the mechanism of herniation is due to focal mass effect, without an increase in intracranial pressure.[60]

Similarly, in patients with cerebellar stroke with early swelling, acute hydrocephalus may occur. Placement of a ventriculostomy for the treatment of acute hydrocephalus in this setting should be accompanied or followed by decompressive craniectomy.[61] The initial management focuses on reducing the brain edema. Although there is not robust evidence to support its use, osmotic therapy is considered a reasonable approach for patients with clinical deterioration from brain swelling associated with cerebral infarction. Agents that are currently used for this purpose, include mannitol (as a single loading dose and/or in scheduled doses every 4–6 hours) and hypertonic saline at concentrations of 3%, 7.5%, or 23%.[60,62]

Suboccipital craniectomy may be necessary in patients with cerebellar infarction and deteriorating mental status despite best medical therapy. Although patient's selection and timing for surgery have been controversial, surgical decompression after massive posterior fossa infarct can be associated with meaningful recovery, and its use is often recommended.[63] In patients with malignant MCA stroke, decompressive surgery, usually within 48 hours, reduces mortality and may increase favorable outcome in patients between 18 and 60 years.[64] It is important to recognize that randomized clinical trials that have studied patients with supratentorial infarctions treated with hemicraniectomy have shown a reproducible large reduction in mortality, but near all survivors remained with residual permanent disabilities.[63,65,66] Persistent moderate to severe disability can be more prevalent in patients older than 60 years, which could make treatment decisions more challenging for this population.[63] Nevertheless, surgical decompression remains as an effective life-saving procedure for malignant stroke, and it is generally agreed that the surgery should be performed in this setting before clinical signs of brainstem compression ensue.[67]

7.2.3 SEIZURES POST STROKE

Seizures after stroke are more often associated with large infarcts involving cortical regions and/or hemorrhagic conversion.[68,69] New onset seizures after AIS occur in less than 10% of the patients, and there is no role for the use prophylactic anticonvulsants in this setting.[67] When convulsive seizures present after AIS, aggressive management with antiepileptic drugs is recommended, similar to other acute neurological injuries.

Non-convulsive seizures are of special concern in the ICU setting, since these can be associated with poor outcome secondary to refractory status epilepticus and increased mortality. Hence, continued electroencephalogram monitoring is of high value in the ICU setting, and it is indicated in all AIS patients with unexplained and/ or persistently altered level of consciousness. Once identified, seizures should be treated aggressively, and a long-acting anticonvulsant agent should be considered. Phenytoin and levetiracetam are often used as first-line agents in this setting; however, the choice of an anticonvulsant drug should be made depending on the clinical setting and characteristics of each patient.[70]

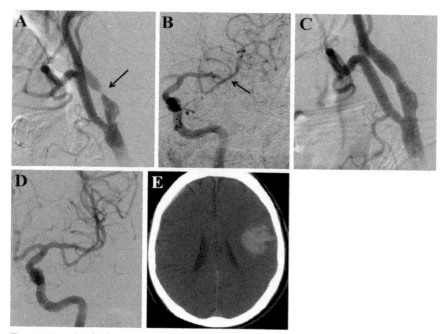

Figure 10.2 Stroke from tandem intracranial occlusion and cervical stenosis.
(A) Digital subtraction angiography (DSA), lateral cervical view and (B) antero-posterior view demonstrating high-grade stenosis of the left carotid artery (internal carotid artery [ICA], arrow) and occlusion of the proximal left middle cerebral artery (MCA).
(C) DSA, lateral cervical view after successful stent placement and revascularization of the left ICA.
(D) Complete flow restoration is achieved intracranially (arrow).
(E) Post-procedural non-contrast head computed tomography performed due to acute neurological deterioration, which evidenced a left frontal hematoma.

8 CLINICAL CASES

Case 10.1 Stroke from tandem intracranial occlusion and cervical stenosis

CASE DESCRIPTION

A 65-year-old man presents with sudden right-sided weakness and dysarthria. IV alteplase was administered at an outside hospital, and the patient was transferred for potential endovascular intervention. His initial NIHSS score was 4, but rapid neurological deterioration was noted after arrival, with a repeat NIHSS score of 20 with worsening right-sided weakness, aphasia, and right-sided neglect. The patient underwent EVT of the left MCA occlusion combined with emergent left carotid stenting of flow-limiting internal carotid artery stenosis (Figure 10.2). His exam improved immediately upon revascularization; however, several hours later he was noted to be aphasic and flaccid on the right arm. Repeated CT evidenced a left frontal hematoma (Figure 10.2).

PRACTICAL POINTS

- This represents a commonly encountered case of symptomatic carotid stenosis presenting with tandem intracranial occlusion. The rupture of the cervical internal carotid plaque results in thrombus formation and embolism. A rapid decision regarding the need for immediate versus delayed cervical carotid revascularization make these cases challenging. The potential benefits of early and complete revascularization must be balanced with the required use of antithrombotic agents post IV alteplase and the attendant risks for subsequent hemorrhagic complications. These patients are closely monitored in the ICU postoperatively. Tight BP parameters (such as systolic BP below 140 mm Hg) and frequent neurological evaluations are recommended.
- There is a potential augmented risk of increased hemorrhagic transformation when antithrombotic agents are administered after IV alteplase.[71] This case illustrates that this is possible even when the initial CT does not show significant ischemic changes. A postprocedural CT is not always performed, especially when there is clinical improvement after the thrombectomy. When clinical worsening is identified, brain imaging should be promptly obtained to rule out hemorrhagic conversion, progression of the ischemia, new stroke, or mass effect. In this case, rapid diagnosis of the intraparenchymal hematoma shifted management to a more aggressive BP control, neurosurgical surveillance, and a delayed antithrombotic regimen.
- Occasionally, temporary carotid revascularization is achieved during the EVT without the use of a stent. Techniques that have been used by interventionalists include angioplasty without stent and proximal thrombus suction with guiding or balloon guide catheter-assist. It is also possible that spontaneous revascularization occurs upon "crossing the lesion" during the EVT. Ultimately, the decision to proceed with acute stenting will be

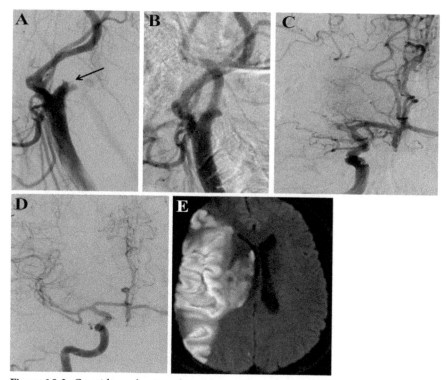

Figure 10.3 Carotid re-oclussion after endovascular revascularization.
(A) Digital subtraction angiography (DSA), common carotid artery injection demonstrating occlusion of the right internal carotid artery (ICA) at its bulb (arrow).
(B) This was treated with balloon angioplasty with good flow restoration immediately post-treatment.
(C) DSA, intracranial view showing the right middle cerebral artery occlusion.
(D) Post thrombectomy, successful recanalization is achieved.
(E) Magnetic resonance diffusion weighted imaging showing a complete right MCA territory infarct with mass effect despite adequate angiographic revascularization.

made by the interventionalist, depending on the angiographic appearance of the carotid lesion and the suspicion for reocclusion. If emergent stenting is not performed during the EVT, early revascularization during the same hospital stay may be safe and beneficial; therefore, this should be strongly considered.

Case 10.2 Carotid reoclussion after endovascular revascularization

CASE DESCRIPTION
A 59-year-old man presents with left-sided weakness and slurred speech. CT angiography showed right cervical internal carotid and proximal MCA occlusions. The

patient was treated with IV alteplase and EVT with balloon angioplasty of the cervical carotid stenosis (Figure 10.3). No clinical improvement was seen after the procedure. He was started on aspirin 325 mg 24 hours after the administration of IV alteplase. Brain MRI demonstrated a complete right MCA stroke with mass effect (Figure 10.3). Hypertonic saline was started, and neurosurgery was consulted. Follow-up imaging showed worsening edema, and the patient underwent a hemicraniectomy. A follow-up CT angiography demonstrated reocclusion of the cervical ICA.

PRACTICAL POINTS

- Despite successful recanalization, this patient developed a large stroke with malignant edema that required surgical decompression. It is presumed that he reoccluded his proximal ICA postoperatively, which resulted in cerebral hypoperfusion and further ischemia.
- Given that clinical evaluations are often difficult immediately after the endovascular therapy (due to the use of procedural IV sedation or general anesthesia), radiologic assessments can be effective in this setting and should be rapidly considered when there is clinical worsening or with lack of neurological improvement. Routinely, brain imaging will be performed within the first 24 hours after the treatment; however, in some cases with symptomatic carotid disease, it is reasonable to also reassess the affected carotid artery after treatment. This can be done noninvasively with ultrasound or with cross-sectional imaging (CT or MR angiography).

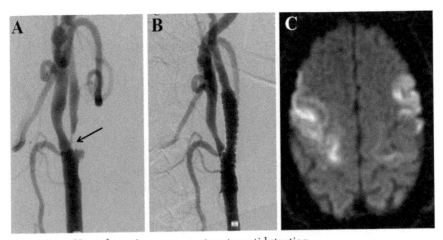

Figure 10.4 Hemodynamic management post carotid stenting.
(A) Digital subtraction angiography, left common carotid artery injection demonstrating critical stenosis of the left internal carotid artery (ICA) origin (arrow).
(B) Resolution of these near-occlusive findings is evident after placement of a carotid sent.
(C) Magnetic resonance diffusion weighted image performed one day after procedure showing bilateral strokes in both middle cerebral artery distributions.

Case 10.3 Hemodynamic management after carotid stenting

CASE DESCRIPTION

A 51-year-old hypertensive man presents with new onset speech difficulty for 6 hours. CT angiography demonstrated signs of left hemispheric ischemia, a severe (99%) left ICA stenosis, and a known chronic right ICA occlusion. He was outside of the window for IV alteplase. After appropriate antithrombotic loading and maintenance, he underwent successful left carotid stenting on the sixth day of his hospital stay (Figure 10.4). He remained in the NICU for monitoring postprocedure with target systolic BP parameters of less than 140 mmHg for 24 hours. The following day, the patient was noted with sudden right gaze preference, left-sided weakness, and left hemineglect in the setting of hypotension. His BP overnight was at times in the 90s systolic range, and the patient was intermittently bradycardic. MRI demonstrated a new right hemispheric infarct (Figure 10.4). After fluid administration and norepinephrine infusion for 48 hours, his symptoms resolved with augmented BP and heart rate.

PRACTICAL POINTS

- In patients with transient ischemic attacks or minor strokes, the benefit from carotid endarterectomy is greatest if it is done within 2 weeks after the event.[54] Patients with bilateral carotid disease carry a higher risk of periprocedural complications, which is encountered intra and postoperatively.[55] Strict BP parameters are recommended after carotid stenting with systolic BP maintained below 140 mm Hg in order to avoid hyperperfusion syndrome.[72] In patients with contralateral high grade stenosis or occlusion, avoidance of hypotension is equally important to avoid hypoperfusion.
- The hemodynamic depression that occurs commonly with the baroreceptor stimuli of angioplasty and stenting or carotid endarterectomy is generally transient but may be prolonged. In rare cases, such as this one it may result in clinically significant bradycardia and hypotension. This case illustrates the importance of not only setting an upper but also lower BP goal. Patients who experience significant or prolonged hypotension and bradycardia during carotid angioplasty and stenting should not be administered nodal agents (beta blockers or non-dihydropyridimine calcium channel blockers) until the heart rate recovers.

REFERENCES

1. Indredavik B, Bakke F, Solberg R, Rokseth R, Haaheim LL, Holme I. Benefit of a stroke unit: a randomized controlled trial. *Stroke.* 1991;22(8):1026–1031.

2. Zimmerman JE, Kramer AA, Knaus WA. Changes in hospital mortality for United States intensive care unit admissions from 1988 to 2012. *Crit Care.* 2013;17(2):R81.

3. Bershad EM, Feen ES, Hernandez OH, Suri MF, Suarez JI. Impact of a specialized neurointensive care team on outcomes of critically ill acute ischemic stroke patients. *Neurocrit Care.* 2008;9(3):287–292.

4. Spijkerboer AM, Scholten FG, Mali WP, van Schaik JP. Antegrade puncture of the femoral artery: morphologic study. *Radiology.* 1990;176(1):57–60.

5. Okawa M, Tateshima S, Liebeskind D, et al. Successful recanalization for acute ischemic stroke via the transbrachial approach. *J Neurointerv Surg.* 2016;8(2): 122–125.

6. Mokin M, Snyder KV, Levy EI, Hopkins LN, Siddiqui AH. Direct carotid artery puncture access for endovascular treatment of acute ischemic stroke: technical aspects, advantages, and limitations. *J Neurointerv Surg.* 2015;7(2):108–113.

7. Altin RS, Flicker S, Naidech HJ. Pseudoaneurysm and arteriovenous fistula after femoral artery catheterization: association with low femoral punctures. *Am J Roentgenol.* 1989;152(3):629–631.

8. Waugh JR, Sacharias N. Arteriographic complications in the DSA era. *Radiology.* 1992;182(1):243–246.

9. Shah VA, Martin CO, Hawkins AM, Holloway WE, Junna S, Akhtar N. Groin complications in endovascular mechanical thrombectomy for acute ischemic stroke: a 10-year single center experience. *J Neurointerv Surg.* 2016;8(6):568–570.

10. Feld R, Patton GM, Carabasi RA, Alexander A, Merton D, Needleman L. Treatment of iatrogenic femoral artery injuries with ultrasound-guided compression. *J Vasc Surg.* 1992;16(6):832–840.

11. Cox GS, Young JR, Gray BR, Grubb MW, Hertzer NR. Ultrasound-guided compression repair of postcatheterization pseudoaneurysms: results of treatment in one hundred cases. *J Vasc Surg.* 1994;19(4):683–686.

12. Spies JB, Berlin L. Complications of femoral artery puncture. *Am J Roentgenol.* 1998;170(1):9–11.

13. Leonardi-Bee J, Bath PM, Phillips SJ, Sandercock PA, Group ISTC. Blood pressure and clinical outcomes in the International Stroke Trial. *Stroke.* 2002;33(5):1315–1320.

14. Vemmos KN, Tsivgoulis G, Spengos K, et al. U-shaped relationship between mortality and admission blood pressure in patients with acute stroke. *J Intern Med.* 2004;255(2):257–265.

15. Ahmed N, Wahlgren N, Brainin M, et al. Relationship of blood pressure, antihypertensive therapy, and outcome in ischemic stroke treated with intravenous thrombolysis: retrospective analysis from Safe Implementation of Thrombolysis in Stroke-International Stroke Thrombolysis Register (SITS-ISTR). *Stroke.* 2009;40(7):2442–2449.

16. Jauch EC, Saver JL, Adams HP, Jr., et al. Guidelines for the early management of patients with acute ischemic stroke: a guideline for healthcare professionals from the American Heart Association/American Stroke Association. *Stroke.* 2013;44(3):870–947.

17. Treurniet KM, Berkhemer OA, Immink RV, et al. A decrease in blood pressure is associated with unfavorable outcome in patients undergoing thrombectomy under general anesthesia. *J Neurointerv Surg.* 2017. doi:10.1136/neurintsurg-2017-012988

18. Talke PO, Sharma D, Heyer EJ, Bergese SD, Blackham KA, Stevens RD. Republished: Society for Neuroscience in Anesthesiology and Critical Care expert consensus statement: Anesthetic management of endovascular treatment for acute ischemic stroke. *Stroke.* 2014;45(8):e138–e150.

19. Lowhagen Henden P, Rentzos A, Karlsson JE, et al. Hypotension during endovascular treatment of ischemic stroke is a risk factor for poor neurological outcome. *Stroke.* 2015;46(9):2678–2680.

20. Whalin MK, Halenda KM, Haussen DC, et al. Even small decreases in blood pressure during conscious sedation affect clinical outcome after stroke thrombectomy: an analysis of hemodynamic thresholds. *Am J Neuroradiol.* 2017;38(2):294–298.

21. Visvanathan A, Dennis M, Whiteley W. Parenteral fluid regimens for improving functional outcome in people with acute stroke. *Cochrane Db Syst Rev.* 2015(9):CD011138.

22. Adams RJ, Chimowitz MI, Alpert JS, et al. Coronary risk evaluation in patients with transient ischemic attack and ischemic stroke: a scientific statement for healthcare professionals from the Stroke Council and the Council on Clinical Cardiology of the American Heart Association/American Stroke Association. *Stroke.* 2003;34(9):2310–2322.

23. Prosser J, MacGregor L, Lees KR, et al. Predictors of early cardiac morbidity and mortality after ischemic stroke. *Stroke.* 2007;38(8):2295–2302.

24. Lavy S, Yaar I, Melamed E, Stern S. The effect of acute stroke on cardiac functions as observed in an intensive stroke care unit. *Stroke.* 1974;5(6):775–780.

25. Daniele O, Caravaglios G, Fierro B, Natale E. Stroke and cardiac arrhythmias. *J Stroke Cerebrovasc Dis.* 2002;11(1):28–33.

26. Oppenheimer SM, Cechetto DF. Cardiac chronotropic organization of the rat insular cortex. *Brain Res.* 1990;533(1):66–72.

27. McDonagh DL, Olson DM, Kalia JS, Gupta R, Abou-Chebl A, Zaidat OO. Anesthesia and sedation practices among neurointerventionalists during acute ischemic stroke endovascular therapy. *Front Neurol.* 2010;1:118.

28. Whalin MK, Lopian S, Wyatt K, et al. Dexmedetomidine: a safe alternative to general anesthesia for endovascular stroke treatment. *J Neurointerv Surg.* 2014;6(4):270–275.

29. Els T, Klisch J, Orszagh M, et al. Hyperglycemia in patients with focal cerebral ischemia after intravenous thrombolysis: influence on clinical outcome and infarct size. *Cerebrovasc Dis.* 2002;13(2):89–94.

30. Parsons MW, Barber PA, Desmond PM, et al. Acute hyperglycemia adversely affects stroke outcome: a magnetic resonance imaging and spectroscopy study. *Ann Neurol.* 2002;52(1):20–28.

31. Leigh R, Zaidat OO, Suri MF, et al. Predictors of hyperacute clinical worsening in ischemic stroke patients receiving thrombolytic therapy. *Stroke.* 2004;35(8):1903–1907.

32. Kase CS, Furlan AJ, Wechsler LR, et al. Cerebral hemorrhage after intra-arterial thrombolysis for ischemic stroke: the PROACT II trial. *Neurology.* 2001;57(9):1603–1610.

33. Won SJ, Tang XN, Suh SW, Yenari MA, Swanson RA. Hyperglycemia promotes tissue plasminogen activator-induced hemorrhage by Increasing superoxide production. *Ann Neurol.* 2011;70(4):583–590.

34. American Diabetes A. Standards of medical care in diabetes: 2016 abridged for primary care providers. *Clin Diabetes.* 2016;34(1):3–21.

35. Investigators N-SS, Finfer S, Chittock DR, et al. Intensive versus conventional glucose control in critically ill patients. *N Engl J Med.* 2009;360(13):1283–1297.

36. Powers WJ, Derdeyn CP, Biller J, et al. 2015 American Heart Association/American Stroke Association focused update of the 2013 guidelines for the early management of patients with acute ischemic stroke regarding endovascular treatment: a guideline for healthcare professionals from the American Heart Association/American Stroke Association. *Stroke.* 2015;46(10):3020–3035.

37. Goyal M, Menon BK, van Zwam WH, et al. Endovascular thrombectomy after large-vessel ischaemic stroke: a meta-analysis of individual patient data from five randomised trials. *Lancet.* 2016;387(10029):1723–1731.

38. Qureshi AI, Saad M, Zaidat OO, et al. Intracerebral hemorrhages associated with neurointerventional procedures using a combination of antithrombotic agents including abciximab. *Stroke.* 2002;33(7):1916–1919.

39. Heck DV, Brown MD. Carotid stenting and intracranial thrombectomy for treatment of acute stroke due to tandem occlusions with aggressive antiplatelet therapy may be associated with a high incidence of intracranial hemorrhage. *J Neurointerv Surg.* 2015;7(3):170–175.

40. Walsh RD, Barrett KM, Aguilar MI, et al. Intracranial hemorrhage following neuroendovascular procedures with abciximab is associated with high mortality: a multicenter series. *Neurocrit Care.* 2011;15(1):85–95.

41. Stampfl S, Ringleb PA, Mohlenbruch M, et al. Emergency cervical internal carotid artery stenting in combination with intracranial thrombectomy in acute stroke. *Am J Neuroradiol.* 2014;35(4):741–746.

42. Cohen JE, Gomori JM, Rajz G, Itshayek E, Eichel R, Leker RR. Extracranial carotid artery stenting followed by intracranial stent-based thrombectomy for acute tandem occlusive disease. *J Neurointerv Surg.* 2015;7(6):412–417.

43. Spiotta AM, Lena J, Vargas J, et al. Proximal to distal approach in the treatment of tandem occlusions causing an acute stroke. *J Neurointerv Surg.* 2015;7(3): 164–169.

44. Cohen JE, Gomori M, Rajz G, et al. Emergent stent-assisted angioplasty of extracranial internal carotid artery and intracranial stent-based thrombectomy in acute tandem occlusive disease: technical considerations. *J Neurointerv Surg.* 2013;5(5):440–446.

45. Heran NS, Song JK, Namba K, Smith W, Niimi Y, Berenstein A. The utility of DynaCT in neuroendovascular procedures. *Am J Neuroradiol.* 2006;27(2): 330–332.

46. Elijovich L, Doss VT, Theessen H, Khan M, Arthur AS. Intraprocedural parenchymal blood volume as a marker of reperfusion status in acute ischemic stroke intervention. *J Neurointerv Surg.* 2014;6(6):e36.

47. Kamran M, Nagaraja S, Byrne JV. C-arm flat detector computed tomography: the technique and its applications in interventional neuro-radiology. *Neuroradiology*. 2010;52(4):319–327.

48. Struffert T, Deuerling-Zheng Y, Kloska S, et al. Flat detector CT in the evaluation of brain parenchyma, intracranial vasculature, and cerebral blood volume: a pilot study in patients with acute symptoms of cerebral ischemia. *Am J Neuroradiol*. 2010;31(8):1462–1469.

49. Soares BP, Tong E, Hom J, et al. Reperfusion is a more accurate predictor of follow-up infarct volume than recanalization: a proof of concept using CT in acute ischemic stroke patients. *Stroke*. 2010;41(1):e34–e40.

50. Yoon W, Seo JJ, Kim JK, Cho KH, Park JG, Kang HK. Contrast enhancement and contrast extravasation on computed tomography after intra-arterial thrombolysis in patients with acute ischemic stroke. *Stroke*. 2004;35(4):876–881.

51. Jang YM, Lee DH, Kim HS, et al. The fate of high-density lesions on the non-contrast CT obtained immediately after intra-arterial thrombolysis in ischemic stroke patients. *Korean J Radiol*. 2006;7(4):221–228.

52. Payabvash S, Qureshi MH, Khan SM, et al. Differentiating intraparenchymal hemorrhage from contrast extravasation on post-procedural noncontrast CT scan in acute ischemic stroke patients undergoing endovascular treatment. *Neuroradiology*. 2014;56(9):737–744.

53. Gill HL, Siracuse JJ, Parrack IK, Huang ZS, Meltzer AJ. Complications of the endovascular management of acute ischemic stroke. *Vasc Health Risk Manag*. 2014;10:675–681.

54. National Collaborating Centre for Chronic Conditions. *Stroke: national clinical guideline for diagnosis and initial management of acute stroke and transient ischaemic attack: a quick reference guide*. London: NICE, 2008.

55. Schellinger PD, Ringleb P, Hacke W. [European Stroke Organisation 2008 guidelines for managing acute cerebral infarction or transient ischemic attack : part 2]. *Nervenarzt*. 2008;79(10):1180–1184, 1186–1188, 1190–1201.

56. Frontera JA, Lewin JJ, 3rd, Rabinstein AA, et al. Guideline for reversal of antithrombotics in intracranial hemorrhage: executive summary. a statement for healthcare professionals from the Neurocritical Care Society and the Society of Critical Care Medicine. *Crit Care Med*. 2016;44(12):2251–2257.

57. Goldstein JN, Marrero M, Masrur S, et al. Management of thrombolysis-associated symptomatic intracerebral hemorrhage. *Arch Neurol*. 2010;67(8):965–969.

58. Alderazi YJ, Barot NV, Peng H, et al. Clotting factors to treat thrombolysis-related symptomatic intracranial hemorrhage in acute ischemic stroke. *J Stroke Cerebrovasc Dis*. 2014;23(3):e207–214.

59. Yaghi S, Boehme AK, Dibu J, et al. Treatment and outcome of thrombolysis-related hemorrhage: a multicenter retrospective study. *JAMA Neurol*. 2015; 72(12):1451–1457.

60. Kasner SE, Demchuk AM, Berrouschot J, et al. Predictors of fatal brain edema in massive hemispheric ischemic stroke. *Stroke*. 2001;32(9):2117–2123.

61. Pullicino PM, Alexandrov AV, Shelton JA, Alexandrova NA, Smurawska LT, Norris JW. Mass effect and death from severe acute stroke. *Neurology*. 1997;49(4):1090–1095.

62. Oppenheim C, Samson Y, Manai R, et al. Prediction of malignant middle cerebral artery infarction by diffusion-weighted imaging. *Stroke.* 2000;31(9):2175–2181.

63. Wijdicks EF, Sheth KN, Carter BS, et al. Recommendations for the management of cerebral and cerebellar infarction with swelling: a statement for healthcare professionals from the American Heart Association/American Stroke Association. *Stroke.* 2014;45(4):1222–1238.

64. Berger C, Sakowitz OW, Kiening KL, Schwab S. Neurochemical monitoring of glycerol therapy in patients with ischemic brain edema. *Stroke.* 2005;36(2):e4–6.

65. Diringer MN, Scalfani MT, Zazulia AR, Videen TO, Dhar R. Cerebral hemodynamic and metabolic effects of equi-osmolar doses mannitol and 23.4% saline in patients with edema following large ischemic stroke. *Neurocrit Care.* 2011;14(1):11–17.

66. Jauss M, Krieger D, Hornig C, Schramm J, Busse O. Surgical and medical management of patients with massive cerebellar infarctions: results of the German-Austrian Cerebellar Infarction Study. *J Neurol.* 1999;246(4):257–264.

67. Vahedi K, Hofmeijer J, Juettler E, et al. Early decompressive surgery in malignant infarction of the middle cerebral artery: a pooled analysis of three randomised controlled trials. *Lancet Neurol.* 2007;6(3):215–222.

68. Hofmeijer J, Amelink GJ, Algra A, et al. Hemicraniectomy after middle cerebral artery infarction with life-threatening Edema trial (HAMLET): protocol for a randomised controlled trial of decompressive surgery in space-occupying hemispheric infarction. *Trials.* 2006;7:29.

69. Juttler E, Schwab S, Schmiedek P, et al. Decompressive Surgery for the Treatment of Malignant Infarction of the Middle Cerebral Artery (DESTINY): a randomized, controlled trial. *Stroke.* 2007;38(9):2518–2525.

70. Burn J, Dennis M, Bamford J, Sandercock P, Wade D, Warlow C. Epileptic seizures after a first stroke: the Oxfordshire Community Stroke Project. *BMJ.* 1997;315(7122):1582–1587.

71. Beghi E, D'Alessandro R, Beretta S, et al. Incidence and predictors of acute symptomatic seizures after stroke. *Neurology.* 2011;77(20):1785–1793.

72. Kirkman MA, Citerio G, Smith M. The intensive care management of acute ischemic stroke: an overview. *Intensive Care Med.* 2014;40(5):640–653.

11

In-Hospital Stroke

NOELLA J. CYPRESS WEST AND MAXIM MOKIN ■

CONTENTS

1 INTRODUCTION

The term "in-hospital stroke" (also referred to as "inpatient stroke") describes acute stroke occurring while a patient is already in the hospital for another diagnosis. A variable range of in-hospital stroke is reported in the literature, from 4–17% of all strokes.[1,2] Yet, the research on in-hospital strokes is limited in comparison to community-onset strokes presenting through the Emergency Department. Studies on in-hospital stroke mainly focus on barriers and delays to the recognition of

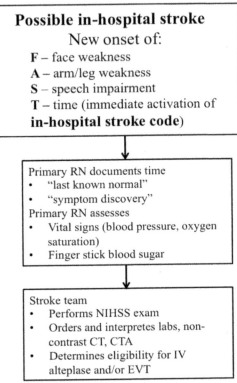

Figure 11.1 Basic algorithm for the in-hospital stroke code.
ABBREVIATIONS: CT, computed tomography; CTA, computed tomography angiography; EVT, endovascular thrombectomy; IV, intravenous; NIHSS, National Institutes of Health stroke scale; RN, registered nurse.

acute ischemic stroke and utilization of intravenous (IV) alteplase. The utilization of endovascular thrombectomy (EVT) for in-hospital ischemic stroke is largely unknown. Studies describing the occurrence and outcomes of in-patient hemorrhagic stroke are also lacking.

In-hospital stroke represents an area of quality improvement for better outcomes and shorter hospitalizations. In this chapter, we discuss the development of education for staff in the recognition of stroke symptoms, rapid assessment, and notification of key personnel for efficient treatment of inpatient stroke based on the previously published literature. An in-hospital acute stroke protocols is shown in Figure 11.1.

Question 11.1: When do most procedure-related in-hospital strokes occur?

Answer: Half of periprocedural strokes occur within first 24 hours of surgery or invasive procedure.

2 CHARACTERISTICS AND OUTCOMES OF IN-HOSPITAL STROKE

A large study comparing characteristics and outcomes for 21,349 patients with in-hospital strokes and 928,885 patients with community-onset strokes from the Get with the Guidelines (GWTG)-Stroke database demonstrated more comorbid conditions in patients with in-hospital strokes.[3] Specifically, these patients were more likely to have embolic risk factors, including atrial fibrillation, prosthetic heart valves, carotid stenosis, and heart failure.[4] Sixty to sixty-eight percent of in-patient strokes are associated with surgical or diagnostic invasive procedures prior to their reported event.[4,5] In-hospital strokes are more severe, with the median National Institutes of Health stroke scale score twice as high when compared to community-based strokes, and have higher mortality rates.[3-5]

Question 11.2: How many in-hospital strokes receive IV alteplase?

Answer: Get with the Guidelines-Stroke database shows that from 2006 to 2012 only 1 out of every 9 in-hospital strokes were treated with IV alteplase.

2.1 Intravenous alteplase for in-hospital strokes

Despite being in a monitored environment, in-hospital strokes are less likely to be treated with IV alteplase and have more significant delays to treatment than community strokes admitted through the ED.[3,6] This paradoxical effect is likely a combination of several factors including failure by the nursing staff and physicians to correctly identify stroke symptoms in a timely manner, the lack of established protocols for rapid diagnostic evaluation and treatment of acute stroke patients, and higher rates of contraindications to IV alteplase.

In a study of in-hospital strokes from 35 hospitals in the Colorado Stroke Alliance, 68% had contraindications to IV alteplase versus 37% for community strokes.[7] Recent surgery or trauma was the most common reported contraindication for IV alteplase (Case 11.1).

2.2 Endovascular thrombectomy for in-hospital strokes

Patients with in-hospital strokes were excluded from the recent randomized trials of EVT. Studies comparing technical and clinical outcomes of EVT between community and in-hospital strokes demonstrated similar rates of successful recanalization and intracranial hemorrhage.[8,9] Similar to the treatment effect observed with IV alteplase, in-hospital strokes treated with EVT had higher mortality than community strokes.

Because EVT can be safely performed in many cases where IV alteplase is contraindicated, in-patient strokes should be promptly evaluated for the presence of large vessel occlusion to determine eligibility for EVT (Case 11.1).

3 IN-HOSPITAL STROKE ALERT PROTOCOL

A dedicated in-hospital stroke response team can assist in improving recognition, evaluation, and treatment for patients with in-hospital stroke. Studies show that implementation of a code stroke team and quality improvement educational strategies reduces all major time outcome measures, such as the time from last seen normal to initial assessment, time to brain imaging, and time to treatment.[10–13]

The FAST (Face Arm Speech Time) stroke screening tool is commonly used for in-hospital stroke protocols.[10,14] Unilateral arm weakness is the most frequent identifying symptoms, present in 86% of in-hospital strokes, followed by speech deficits (46%) and facial droop (29%).[10] Stroke mimics are common for in-hospital strokes, corresponding to nearly half of all in-patient code stroke alerts (Case 11.2).[15] The most common stroke mimics are seizures, hypotension, delirium, and metabolic encephalopthy.[13,15]

3.1 National Stroke Association in-hospital stroke recourse center

Education is the key to change. The National Stroke Association provides valuable a series of tools educating hospital staff about the recognition and management of in-hospital stroke. These include protocols describing criteria for in-hospital stroke alerts, stroke alert protocol cards, practice trials, and alert records. This Web-based resource center also includes presentations describing individual hospital experiences and evidence-based publications.

The in-hospital stroke alert protocol provided by the National Stroke Association includes activating a special response to in-house stroke alerts, quick assessment of vitals and neurological status, emergent non-contrast computed tomography (CT) and defers the decision to initiate IV alteplase or EVT to a neurology team. The protocol does not incorporate any specific stroke screening tools or scales to evaluate for large vessel occlusion.

It should be noted that hospitals without a 24/7 EVT coverage should describe steps for rapid transfer of patients eligible for EVT to neuroendovascular-capable hospitals in their in-hospital stroke alert protocols.

4 CLINICAL CASES

Case 11.1 Acute stroke during percutaneous coronary intervention

CASE DESCRIPTION

A 74-year-old male with history of smoking and hypertension was admitted to the Emergency Department with acute onset of chest pain. The patient was admitted by the cardiology team with the diagnosis of acute coronary syndrome and was emergently taken to a cardiac catheterization lab for percutaneous coronary intervention (PCI). After the catheterization procedure was completed, the patient was immediately examined by the angiography team. The patient as noted to have new right-sided weakness, disconjugated gaze, and severe dysarthria, which were not present prior to PCI.

In-hospital stroke code was activated by the PCI lab personnel. The in-house stroke team arrived at 12:15 PM and gathered the following information: the patient was last known normal at 11:30 AM, discovery of stroke symptoms at 12:10 PM, National Institutes of Health stroke scale score of 12. Non-contrast CT of the head was ordered.

PRACTICAL POINTS

- Accurate recognition of acute stroke symptoms and immediate activation of in-patient stroke code team rather than requesting a neurology consultation or re-evaluating the patient in a delayed fashion anticipating spontaneous resolution of stroke symptoms are the correct steps in this clinical scenario.
- The patient developed stroke symptoms within the time window for IV alteplase, and cardiac catheterization procedure by itself is not considered a contraindication for IV alteplase. Either radial or femoral artery access is not considered a non-compressible site and should not preclude the administration of IV alteplase. Studies have shown safety and efficacy of IV alteplase in patients with strokes after catheterization procedures.
- However, in this case obtaining further history with a focus on recently administered medications revealed that the patient had received IV heparin and IIb/IIIa inhibitors during PCI. Most experts consider administration of these agents a contraindication for IV alteplase, which is summarized in the scientific statement for the inclusion and exclusion criteria for IV alteplase by the American Heart Association.[16]
- CT angiography was performed in this case confirming an occlusion of the distal basilar artery (Figure 11.2). A neurointerventionalist performed EVT resulting in successful recanalization of the occluded basilar artery (Figure 11.2). The likely etiology of this stroke was procedure-related (iatrogenic) embolic event, possibly from catheter manipulation in the aortic arch.

Case 11.2 Acute stroke mimic

CASE DESCRIPTION

An 84-year-old female with a history of arthritis, congestive heart failure, diabetes, and dementia was hospitalized for pneumonia. She was noted to be more sleepy by the nursing staff and "code stroke" was activated. Upon arrival of the in-patient stroke code team, the patient was noted to be diaphoretic and lethargic. She had generalized weakness of arms and legs. Her blood pressure was 86/52 mm Hg, and glucose finger stick was 22 mg/dL. The patient's exam improved after administration of IV dextrose.

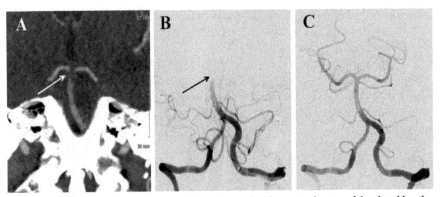

Figure 11.2 (A) Computed tomography angiography shows occlusion of the distal basilar artery (BA, arrow).
(B) Digital subtraction angiograhy (DSA), antero-posterior view confirms occlusion of the BA (arrow).
(C) DSA after thrombectomy shows successful recanalization of the BA.

PRACTICAL POINT

- This case represents a scenario where a change in mental status secondary to hypoglycemia was mistaken for an acute stroke. Even before laboratory and imaging data are available, non-focal neurological deficits (lethargy, generalized weakness) suggested that the change in patient's exam was unlikely to be an acute stroke. However, hypoglycemia can occasionally present with focal neurologic deficits; thus, it is critical that in-hospital stroke protocol includes a rapid blood sugar level test.[17]

REFERENCES

1. Kelley RE, Kovacs AG. Mechanism of in-hospital cerebral ischemia. *Stroke.* 1986;17(3):430–433.
2. Dulli D, Samaniego EA. Inpatient and community ischemic strokes in a university hospital. *Neuroepidemiology.* 2007;28(2):86–92.
3. Cumbler E, Wald H, Bhatt DL, et al. Quality of care and outcomes for in-hospital ischemic stroke: findings from the National Get with the Guidelines-Stroke. *Stroke.* 2014;45(1):231–238.
4. Park HJ, Cho HJ, Kim YD, et al. Comparison of the characteristics for in-hospital and out-of-hospital ischaemic strokes. *Eur J Neurol.* 2009;16(5):582–588.
5. Farooq MU, Reeves MJ, Gargano J, et al. In-hospital stroke in a statewide stroke registry. *Cerebrovasc Dis.* 2008;25(1–2):12–20.
6. Saltman AP, Silver FL, Fang J, Stamplecoski M, Kapral MK. Care and outcomes of patients with in-hospital stroke. *JAMA Neurol.* 2015;72(7):749–755.

7. Cumbler E, Murphy P, Jones WJ, Wald HL, Kutner JS, Smith DB. Quality of care for in-hospital stroke: analysis of a statewide registry. *Stroke.* 2011;42(1):207–210.

8. Yoo J, Song D, Lee K, Kim YD, Nam HS, Heo JH. Comparison of outcomes after reperfusion therapy between in-hospital and out-of-hospital stroke patients. *Cerebrovasc Dis.* 2015;40(1–2):28–34.

9. Moradiya Y, Levine SR. Comparison of short-term outcomes of thrombolysis for in-hospital stroke and out-of-hospital stroke in United States. *Stroke.* 2013;44(7):1903–1908.

10. Kassardjian CD, Willems JD, Skrabka K, et al. In-patient code stroke: a quality improvement strategy to overcome knowledge-to-action gaps in response time. *Stroke.* 2017;48(8):2176–2183.

11. Cumbler E, Zaemisch R, Graves A, Brega K, Jones W. Improving stroke alert response time: applying quality improvement methodology to the inpatient neurologic emergency. *J Hosp Med.* 2012;7(2):137–141.

12. Rucho M. Inpatient code stroke team improves IV-tPA treatment rates and decreases time to IV-tPA. International Stroke Conference; 2013.

13. Cumbler E, Anderson T, Neumann R, Jones WJ, Brega K. Stroke alert program improves recognition and evaluation time of in-hospital ischemic stroke. *J Stroke Cerebrovasc Dis.* 2010;19(6):494–496.

14. Cumbler E. In-hospital ischemic stroke. *Neurohospitalist.* 2015;5(3):173–181.

15. Cumbler E, Simpson J. Code stroke: multicenter experience with in-hospital stroke alerts. *J Hosp Med.* 2015;10(3):179–183.

16. Demaerschalk BM, Kleindorfer DO, Adeoye OM, et al. Scientific rationale for the inclusion and exclusion criteria for intravenous alteplase in acute ischemic stroke: a statement for healthcare professionals from the American Heart Association/American Stroke Association. *Stroke.* 2016;47(2):581–641.

17. Ohshita T, Imamura E, Nomura E, Wakabayashi S, Kajikawa H, Matsumoto M. Hypoglycemia with focal neurological signs as stroke mimic: clinical and neuroradiological characteristics. *J Neurol Sci.* 2015;353(1-2):98–101.

12

Medical Management
of Ischemic Stroke

MAXIM MOKIN AND JUAN RAMOS-CANSECO ■

CONTENTS

1 INTRODUCTION

The main principles of the initial medical management of ischemic stroke that can be applied to patients being evaluated in the Emergency Department or recently admitted to the hospital include general supportive care, blood pressure (BP) and glucose management, and the use of antiplatelet, anticoagulation, and lipid lowering agents. The discussion on these topics is based on the most recent American Heart Association (AHA) guidelines for the early management of patients with acute ischemic stroke.[1] Updates on the use of newer anticoagulation agents and management of specific conditions such as treatment of patients with intracranial stenosis or dissection based on the outcomes of the recent trials are also included. Figure 12.1 summarizes the basic algorithm for the initial medical management discussed throughout this chapter. The subject of treatment of acute ischemic stroke with intravenous (IV) alteplase is discussed in Chapter 8.

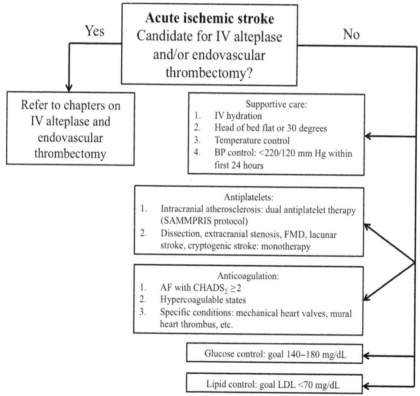

Figure 12.1 Basic algorithm for the initial medical management of ischemic stroke.
ABBREVIATIONS: AF, atrial fibrillation; BP, blood pressure; FMD, fibromuscular dysplasia; IV, intravenous; LDL, low-density lipoprotein; SAMMPRIS, Stenting Versus Aggressive Medical Therapy for Intracranial Arterial Stenosis trial.

2 GENERAL SUPPORTIVE CARE

The goals of initial care are to provide adequate cerebral perfusion pressure, oxygen saturation, and brain metabolic demands by avoiding hypoxia, hypotension, hyperthermia, and hyperglycemia.

2.1 Patient positioning

Lying flat is believed to facilitate cerebral perfusion pressure within the first 24 hours of stroke onset.[2] Some patients may not tolerate this position due to underlying pulmonary conditions, or when the risk of aspiration is high. However, a recently completed randomized trial of positioning patients lying flat or sitting up at ≥30° showed no difference in safety or disability outcomes.[3,4] Further investigations need to focus on specific populations of patients, such as those with large vessel occlusion, for whom differences in positioning may have a greater effect of cerebral perfusion and clinical outcomes.

2.2 Control of temperature

Elevated temperature (hyperthermia) is frequently observed in patients with acute stroke, and it negatively affects neurologic recovery. Acetaminophen is a typical first line agent of choice.[5] There is little evidence to support the use of other antipyretics in stroke. Physical cooling such as cooling blankets can induce shivering and requires a conjunct administration of antipyretics.[5]

Therapeutically induced hypothermia is believed to provide a neuroprotective effect against brain injury in patients with cardiac arrest, but its use in the treatment of stroke remains investigational. Some studies suggest association with an increased risk of pneumonia[6] in patients treated with therapeutic hypothermia.

2.3 Blood pressure

Hypertension is commonly seen in patients during the acute phase of ischemic stroke. Despite a large number of studies conducted, the mechanisms and effects of elevated BP on clinical outcomes remain unclear. The goal of BP parameters depends on whether treatment with systemic thrombolysis is being planned or performed. Prior to the administration of IV alteplase, BP should be below 185/100 mm Hg. Once IV tPA is started, BP should remain less than 180/105 mm Hg throughout the infusion and for the next 24 hours.[1]

Target BP parameters in patients treated with endovascular therapy are unknown. Some clinicians adopt guidelines for BP after IV alteplase to patients undergoing endovascular thrombectomy (EVT), whereas others advocate stricter control of BP once reperfusion is achieved.

In patients ineligible for IV alteplases, antihypertensive agents are usually not recommended unless the BP exceeds 220/120 mm Hg ("permissive" hypertension).[1] In patients previously treated for hypertension, it is advised to resume oral antihypertensive agents several days after the stroke.[7] If immediate correction of BP is needed, a gentle reduction of BP is advised. IV β-blocker such as labetalol or the smooth muscle vasodilator hydralazine are common first agents of choice. Continuous infusion of calcium channel blockers such as nicardipine can be used if the desired BP parameters cannot be achieved with a repeated use of "as needed" agents.

Hypotension in the setting of acute ischemic stroke is less common. It is typically initially managed by administration of IV fluids. Severe hypotension should warrant diagnostic workup for sepsis, myocardial infarction, blood loss, and other severe conditions that can result in low BP.

3 ANTIPLATELET AGENTS

In most of cases of acute ischemic stroke, aspirin is recommended to be given within 24 hours of stroke onset. Once a hemorrhagic stroke is ruled out and the decision is made not to proceed with the IV alteplase, a single dose of aspirin is often given by mouth in the emergency room. A true allergy to aspirin is rare. Usually, when patients are asked to describe their symptoms, dyspepsia or easy bruisability are the symptoms described. Daily aspirin dosed from 81 to 325 mg a day remains the mainstay therapy for patients with ischemic stroke or transient ischemic attack (TIA).

The early use of alternative antiplatelet agents such as clopidogrel and ticagrelor, or the use of a combination of antiplatelet agents (often referred to as dual antiplatelet therapy), has not been translated into the official guidelines despite the evidence from multiple randomized trials showing potential benefit.[8,9] Should treatment with dual antiplatelet therapy be pursued, the final decision on its duration is more complex because patients with acute stroke often have other comorbidities. A common clinical scenario is the determination of the most appropriate antiplatelet regimen in a patient with concurrent ischemic stroke and acute coronary syndrome, where dual antiplatelet therapy could be of benefit. However, the risk of using the two agents simultaneously should be weighed against the risk of hemorrhagic transformation, which can occur in patients with large ischemic strokes.

The following discussion provides specific clinical scenarios where specific modifications of the standard therapy with antiplatelet agents may be needed.

Question 12.1: Does the SAMMPRIS protocol apply to intracranial stenosis discovered incidentally?

Answer: No, there is no evidence to suggest dual antiplatelet therapy in patients with intracranial stenosis who are asymptomatic.

3.1 Intracranial stenosis

Stenosis of the intracranial arteries due to underlying atherosclerosis is present in approximately 8–12% of strokes in the United States.[10] This condition is more common in Asia, where it is estimated to be the primary cause of stroke in 50% of the adult population.[11] Initially treated with oral anticoagulation, antiplatelet therapy was subsequently demonstrated to provide a much safer and equally effective alternative to warfarin.[12] Intracranial stenting was also utilized in these patients with the expectations that stenting would be more a more effective strategy in preventing recurrent strokes than antiplatelets. However, a randomized trial of antiplatelet therapy for severe intracranial stenosis (SAMMPRIS) showed that use of dual antiplatelet therapy was beneficial in patients with severe intracranial stenosis.[13]

A combination of aspirin and clopidogrel in patients with severe intracranial stenosis is believed be effective if the treatment is started within 30 days of stroke onset. Some clinicians advocate for the earliest possible initiation of dual antiplatelet therapy. This may include prescribing a large initial dose of such agents, an "aspirin and clopidogrel load," such as 650 mg of aspirin and 300–600 mg of clopidogrel as a single dose. This practice has not been clinically validated; thus, it remains unknown if a large initial dose of these agents is generally recommended. The purportedly named "SAMMPRIS protocol" for the treatment of intracranial stenosis also includes aggressive life style modifications (smoking cessation, healthy diet) together with BP and glucose control (Case 12.1).

Question 12.2: How to interpret antiplatelet responses?

Answer: These are often referred to as ARU (Aspirin Reaction Units) and PRU (R2Y12 Reaction Units) for clopidogrel, ticlopidine, or prasugrel. ARU <550 and PRU <200 typically indicate adequate antiplatelet inhibition.

3.2 Testing antiplatelet inhibition

The use of high loading doses of antiplatelets is common in patients who are expecting to undergo interventional procedures, such as carotid or intracranial stenting, especially when such procedures are needed urgently. Therapeutic antiplatelet effect can be observed as early as 2–6 hours after the initial load is given.[14,15] However, unlike aspirin, which provides a very reliable antiplatelet response, the initial antiplatelet effect of clopidogrel can be inadequate in as many as 40% of patients.[16] In such cases additional administration of clopidogrel or the use of alternative antiplatelet agents such as ticagrelor may be required. Several commercial point-of-care devices are currently available, with variable design techniques for testing the rate of antiplatelet inhibition and diagnostic accuracy.[17]

3.3 Extracranial carotid stenosis

When a carotid artery lesion is believed to be the cause of patient's stroke or TIA, it is termed as symptomatic and requires medical treatment. Medical management includes monotherapy with an antiplatelet agent (typically, aspirin), a lipid lowering agent such as a statin, and control of vascular risk factors. Patients with stenosis of 50% or above should be evaluated for surgical revascularization, either endarterectomy or carotid artery stenting. Proceeding with either procedure depends on lesion's morphology and patient's characteristics such as age, cardiac, and pulmonary status. Carotid revascularization is rarely needed within with first 24–48 hours after a stroke unless fluctuating neurological symptoms are present. Patients treated with carotid stenting are typically managed with dual antiplatelet therapy for 30–90 days.

Question 12.3: Is Warfarin better than aspirin for dissection?

Answer: Latest data show similar efficacy of an antiplatelet and anticoagulation agents in preventing recurrent strokes in patients with dissection.

3.4 Dissection

One of the common causes of stroke in patients in the younger population is dissection of the carotid or vertebral artery. Carotid artery dissection most commonly occurs extracranially and involves the cervical segment of the internal carotid artery. An intraluminal hematoma or intimal tear can create a dissection, which, in turn, can cause a stroke. An extensive dissection flap or freshly formed clot can lead to a complete cutoff of arterial blood supply to the brain. Computed tomographic angiography (CTA) and magnetic resonance angiography (MRA) are highly sensitive in confirming the diagnosis of dissection.[18] Another anatomical vascular abnormality that can cause a stroke is an aneurysmal dilation (called a "pseudoaneurysm"); it can become a source of emboli.

In a randomized trial of medical therapy of patients with a recent carotid or vertebral artery dissection, similar efficacy of antiplatelet and anticoagulant drugs was found.[19] From a practical standpoint, antiplatelets are easier to initiate and manage than anticoagulants. Thus, it is often the "go to" medication for patients with dissection (Case 12.2). Anticoagulants or IV heparin may be considered in cases with an intraluminal thrombus found on imaging.

Intracranial dissections carry a different risk profile because of the possibility of developing pseudoaneurysms, with a potential for rupture and subarachnoid hemorrhage. Intracranial dissections warrant a neurosurgical consultation.

3.5 Fibromuscular dysplasia

Fibromuscular dysplasia (FMD) is a nonatherosclerotic arterial pathology of an unknown cause, and it is considered a risk factor for ischemic stroke. The patient typically complains of "ringing" or "swooshing" sounds. Carotid bruit heard during auscultation of the neck is a common physical presentation of FMD. FMD can also be discovered on noninvasive imaging of carotid and vertebral arteries as an incidental finding (Case 12.3). Aspirin 81–325 mg daily is recommended for patients with both symptomatic and asymptomatic FMD.[20] Catheter-based interventions, including diagnostic angiography, are typically avoided in patients with FMD. Indications for EVT are failure of medical therapy, mostly in the setting of dissection or the presence of aneurysms with intracranial location and risk of subarachnoid hemorrhage.[20]

4 ANTICOAGULATION

Anticoagulation in ischemic stroke is reserved for specific conditions, of which atrial fibrillation (AF) is the most common one. Other disorders that benefit from anticoagulation typically include mechanical heart valves, intraluminal thrombi of the heart, and mobile thrombi of the aortic arch. Anticoagulation may also be beneficial in various hypercoagulable states.

4.1 Atrial fibrillation

In the past, warfarin was the only oral pharmacological agent used for stroke prevention in patients with newly diagnosed or known AF. The development and introduction of novel non-vitamin K oral anticoagulants (NOACs) to clinical practice has given clinicians and patients with sorely needed alternatives to warfarin. When compared to warfarin, NOACs offer a more rapid therapeutic effect and have more predictable pharmacokinetics, thus not requiring periodic dose adjustment and measurement of serum levels. Table 12.1 compares pharmacological characteristics of warfarin and NOAC agents. NOACs are currently approved for "nonvalvular" form of AF. "Nonvalvular" form is defined as AF in the absence of rheumatic mitral stenosis, a mechanical or bioprosthetic heart valve, or mitral valve repair. A clot forming within the atrial appendage is the most common mechanism of cerebral embolization.

CHADS$_2$ and its modified version, CHA$_2$DS$_2$-VASc are the two most widely used risk stratification scales designed to guide a clinician on whether chronic anticoagulation or an antiplatelet agent is indicated in patients with nonvalvular AF[21] (Box 12.1). Anticoagulation is recommended in patients with a cumulative score of or greater than 2.[21] The optimal timing of initiating oral anticoagulation therapy in patients with AF is a common clinical dilemma. This is because the benefit of preventing recurrent stroke from untreated AF is offset by an increased risk of ICH due to hemorrhagic transformation of the area of brain ischemia. The risk of hemorrhage often depends on the size and location of ischemic stroke, as well as the presence of additional risk factors, such as poorly controlled high BP and hyperglycemia. In a small-sized embolic stroke, anticoagulation may be safely initiated within the first few days of stroke onset. Patients with moderate or large embolic strokes

Table 12.1 PHARMACOLOGICAL PROPERTIES AND CLINICAL APPLICATION OF ORAL
ANTICOAGULANTS

Agent	Warfarin (Coumadin)	Dabigatran (Pradaxa)	Rivaroxaban (Xarelto)	Apixaban (Eliquis)	Edoxaban (Savaysa, Lixiana)
Target mechanism	vitamin K-dependent factors II, VII, IX, X	Direct thrombin inhibitor	Inhibits factor Xa	Inhibits factor Xa	Inhibits factor Xa
Monitoring	International normalized ratio (INR)	None required	None required	None required	None required
Regiment	Once daily, dosage adjustment based on INR	Once daily	Once daily	Twice a day	Once daily
Reversal of bleeding	Vitamin K, fresh frozen plasma (FFP), prothrombin complex concentrates (PCCs), recombinant-activated factor VII (Novoseven)	Idaruci-zumab (Praxbind)	Andexanet alfa (not US FDA approved)	Andexanet alfa (not US FDA approved)	Andexanet alfa (not US FDA approved)

from AF are typically treated with antiplatelet therapy first, and then transitioned to anticoagulation several weeks later (Case 12.4).

"Bridging" therapy—transitioning from IV heparin infusion or high-dose low molecular weight heparins to oral anticoagulants when initiating anticoagulation therapy for AF—is not indicated. Bridging increases the risk of serious or life-threatening bleeding and significantly offsets the benefit of preventing early stroke recurrence.[22]

4.2 Hypercoagulable states

Strokes due to hypercoagulable states are more common in younger patients. Venous thrombosis as a cause of stroke is discussed in a separate chapter. Arterial thrombosis in hypercoagulable states, especially from its inherited forms, often require long-term anticoagulation with warfarin. NOACs are currently not approved for this population of patients. From a practical standpoint, an extensive diagnostic laboratory workup is usually required to confirm an existing hypercoagulable state before initiating long-term anticoagulation. While the workup is often initiated in the hospital, it is typically completed as an outpatient. Box 12.2 lists the most frequently encountered conditions associated with hypercoagulable states.

Box 12.1

RISK STRATIFICATION SCORES FOR PATIENTS WITH NONVALVULAR ATRIAL FIBRILLATION

CHADS$_2$

- Risk factors and points assigned: congested heart failure—1, hypertension—1, age 75 or above—1, diabetes mellitus—1, stroke or TIA—2
- Maximus score of 6 corresponds to 18% adjusted stroke rate per year

CHA$_2$DS$_2$-VASc

- Risk factors and points assigned: congested heart failure—1, hypertension—1, age 75 or above—2, diabetes mellitus—1, stroke or TIA—2, vascular disease—1, age between 65 and 74—1, female sex—1
- Maximus score of 9 corresponds to 15% adjusted stroke rate per year

Oral anticoagulation is recommended for patients with score of 2 or greater

Adapted from 2014 AHA/ACC/HRS guideline for the management of AF.[21]

4.3 Restarting anticoagulation after intracerebral hemorrhage

When to restart anticoagulation in patients who developed intracerebral hemorrhage (ICH) while fully anticoagulated is a challenging clinical scenario. There are no randomized clinical trials to answer this question, and the decision is often made

Box 12.2

HYPERCOAGULABLE STATES ASSOCIATED WITH STROKE

- Protein C and S deficiency
- Antithrombin III deficiency
- Prothrombin G200210A mutation
- Activated protein C resistance and Factor V mutation
- Antiphospholipid syndrome
- Homocystinuria
- Sickle cell disease
- Pregnancy
- Cancer

after a multidisciplinary consultation, often taking into account the extent of the ICH and the risk of ischemic stroke without anticoagulation.

High scoring of CHADS$_2$ in patients with AF or other conditions, such as the presence of a mural thrombus, mechanical valves, or ventricular assist devices, would dictate a more aggressive medical regiment. For patients with AF, a wide range of the "optimal time" to resume anticoagulation is cited in the literature, ranging from 1 to 10 weeks after the hemorrhage.[23,24] It should be noted that most studies report their findings based on the safety data related to the use of warfarin, as large datasets on the use of NOACs after ICH are not yet available.

5 BLOOD GLUCOSE CONTROL

Hyperglycemia is commonly seen in patients with acute stroke, including patients without prior history of diabetes mellitus. Hyperglycemia is associated with poor outcomes in patients with ischemic stroke, including those treated with IV alteplase and EVT.[25,26] The recommended blood glucose level in patients with acute ischemic stroke is 140 to 180 mg/dL.[1] Over aggressive management of glucose levels may result in hypoglycemia, which can also have a damaging effect on brain function. Severe hypoglycemia can worsen or mimic acute neurologic deficits, and it should be treated if blood glucose value is below 60 mg/dL.[1] Both subcutaneous and IV insulin infusion protocols have been tested in clinical practice. Cochrane review of randomized trials of glycemic control in ischemic stroke showed no added benefit of IV insulin on functional outcome or mortality, but the number of hypoglycemic episodes significantly increased.[27]

6 DYSLIPIDEMIA

Comprehensive management of dyslipidemia, similar to controlling other modifiable stroke risk factors (such as hypertension, diabetes mellitus), requires a long-term relationship between a primary care physician and a patient. In an inpatient setting, acute management of dyslipidemia involves the use of statin agents with the long-term goal of lowering low-density lipoprotein <70 mg/dL. In addition to its lipid-lowering mechanisms, statins are believed to possess anti-inflammatory and antioxidant actions, potentially providing a neuroprotection function as well.

7 NEUROPROTECTION

To this date, despite promising preliminary data from multiple preclinical studies, no neuroprotective agents including hypothermia have shown a proven benefit in patients with acute ischemic stroke. The use of such agents remains experimental and is subject to several ongoing clinical trials, including patients treated with IV alteplase and EVT.[28] Less than 1% of patients with acute stroke are enrolled in clinical trials of neuroprotection within the "golden hour"—the first 60 minutes after onset of symptoms.[29] Active involvement of emergency medical services can improve early recruitment of patients into trials of neuroprotection, when such agents are believed to have the highest chance of clinical success.[30]

8 CLINICAL CASES

Case 12.1 Intracranial atherosclerosis

CASE DESCRIPTION
A patient with a history of hypertension, diabetes mellitus, and smoking was admitted with a fluctuating left arm and leg weakness lasting for several days. Systolic BP was 210 mm Hg on admission. Imaging revealed right hemispheric strokes and severe stenosis at the origin of the right middle cerebral artery (Figure 12.2).

PRACTICAL POINTS

- The presence of multiple vascular risk factors and imaging suggests that stenosis secondary to severe intracranial atheroscleorosis is the likely etiology of patient's strokes. The recommended medical management includes the use of dual antiplatelet therapy along with aggressive diabetes, BP control, and smoking cessation.
- In this case, caution is advised with lowering BP as patient's hypertension could be a compensatory mechanism to maintain cerebral perfusion. The hemodynamic rather than embolic nature of ischemic strokes is evident by "watershed" distribution of positive diffusion weighted imaging between the middle and anterior cerebral artery territories. Permissive hypertension in the first few days of admission is advised, along with aggressive hydration with IV fluids. Such patients may be quite sensitive to changes in position, where "lying flat" can result in temporary improvement of neurologic deficits, while sitting or standing up precipitates worsening of symptoms.
- While medical management of severe intracranial stenosis is recommended as a general rule, in patients with stereotypical symptoms with fluctuating severity, endovascular therapy with angioplasty or stenting may be considered.

Case 12.2 Vertebral artery dissection

CASE DESCRIPTION
A patient in his 30s with no significant past medical history presented to the ED with acute onset of headache, nausea, vomiting, and vertigo. The patient

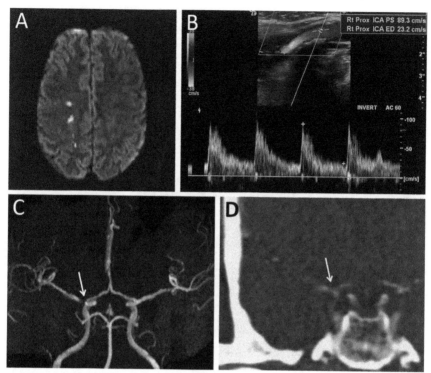

Figure 12.2 Right middle cerebral artery intracranial stenosis.

(A) Diffusion-weighted magnetic resonance (MR) images, axial view, demonstrate the hyperintense signal within the right hemisphere, at the borderline of the right anterior cerebral and middle cerebral arteries. Such pattern of the stroke is referred to as a "watershed" and signifies the hemodynamic mechanism of ischemia, often in a setting of critical stenosis and a transient episode of hypotension.

(B) A sonogram of the right common and internal carotid arteries shows normal systolic and diastolic velocities, with no evidence of hemodynamically significant stenosis.

(C) Time of flight (TOF) MR angiography shows complete occlusion of the right middle cerebral artery origin (arrow). This imaging technique allows visualization of flow within the vessel without the use of contrast, but can overcall the true degree of vessel narrowing.

(D) Computed tomography angiography demonstrated high-grade stenosis rather than occlusion of the arterial segment in question (arrow).

had a motor vehicle accident recently and has been complaining of neck pain. Magnetic resonance imaging (MRI) brain showed an acute infarct within the territory of the left posterior inferior cerebellar artery (PICA). MRA head and neck showed occluded left vertebral artery with an underlying dissection (Figure 12.3).

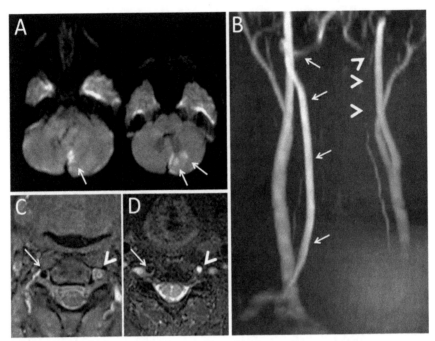

Figure 12.3 Stroke from vertebral artery dissection.
(A) Diffusion-weighted magnetic resonance (MR) images, axial view, demonstrate
the hyperintense signal within the left PICA distribution (arrows), suggestive of acute
ischemic stroke.
(B) MR angiography, 3D reconstruction, shows a patient right vertebral artery (arrows)
but lack of opacification of the left vertebral artery within its multiple segments
(arrowheads). More robust opacification of the very distal (V4) segment of the left
vertebral artery is seen. This alone is not diagnostic of a dissection, as severe vertebral
artery hypoplasia can present similarly.
(C) Axial T1- and (D) T2-weighted MR images obtained with fat saturation (often
referred to as "MRA dissection protocol") show a flow void surrounded by an intramural
hematoma (arrowhead). These imaging sequences are highly specific for diagnosing an
acute dissection. For comparison, note the appearance of a "normal" right vertebral artery
lumen (arrow). The appearance on the T1- and T2-weighted images depends on the
evolution of blood within the hematoma. This can help establish the approximate timing
of when dissection occurred.

Practical points

- Young age, absence of vascular risk factors and history of recent trauma,
  along with the location of ischemic changes on MRI (PICA territory
  infarct) raise the probability of arterial dissection as a cause of stroke.
- Modern noninvasive imaging, such as CTA or MRA are highly accurate
  in diagnosing carotid or vertebral artery dissection. Carotid ultrasound
  has limited value as a diagnostic tool, because carotid dissection often

involves middle to distal segments of the cervical segment, which are not well visualized with the Doppler. Besides, the ultrasound offers a limited window when assessing the vertebral arteries. Digital subtraction angiography can be considered if CTA or MRA are nondiagnostic, and the clinical suspicion of dissection remains high.

- As discussed earlier in this chapter, based on the results of the CADISS randomized trial, either an oral antiplatelet or an anticoagulation agent is equally effective in preventing future strokes.[19] In this clinical case, the size of the PICA distribution stroke is relatively small. Medium to large size cerebellar strokes carry an increased risk of hemorrhagic transformation. Repeat head CT may be considered when initiating antithrombotic or anticoagulation therapy in patients with large cerebellar strokes.
- PICA strokes of medium or large size also carry a risk of cerebellar (infratentorial) swelling with herniation.[31] Even if a patient with a cerebellar stroke "looks good" and has minimal neurologic deficits, as illustrated in this case, close observation in the intensive care unit for the first several days is advised. Frequent monitoring with neurologic exam for level of arousal and development of new deficits, including brainstem signs (e.g., pupillary anisocoria, pinpoint pupils) is needed. Repeat imaging to rule out further stroke expansion and hydrocephalus is indicated if worsening of neurological change in mental status.

Case 12.3 Fibromuscular dysplasia

CASE DESCRIPTION

A patient is admitted to the ED with complaints of a transient episode of left arm weakness lasting for 15 minutes. Past medical history is significant for hyperlipidemia. No acute stroke was seen on MRI brain. CT angiography of head and neck showed irregular appearance of the left internal carotid artery, interpreted by a neuroradiologist as FMD associated with a focal aneurysmal dilatation (Figure 12.4).

PRACTICAL POINTS

- FMD can often be diagnosed as an incidental finding, as illustrated in this case.
- Accurate diagnosis can be established with CT or MR angiography alone. Angiography may be required if intracranial aneurysms are suspected or alternative diagnosis such as vasculitis is sought.

Case 12.4 Atrial fibrillation

CASE DESCRIPTION

A male in his 80s with a prior history of hypertension and smoking presented with acute onset of word-finding difficulties (expressive aphasia). MRI brain

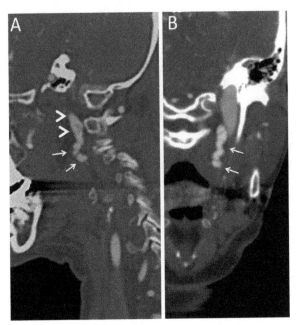

Figure 12.4 Fibromuscular dysplasia.
(A) Computed tomography angiography, sagittal and (B) axial views show multiple areas of alternating stenosis and dilatation, which is a classic finding in fibromuscular dysplasia (arrows). A pseudoaneurysm of the left cervical internal carotid artery is also present (arrowheads). This aneurysm has an extradural location. The likely cause of the aneurysm is from a dissection, which is suggested by the presence of a linear dissection flap, best visualized on the sagittal view.

confirmed the diagnosis of acute ischemic stroke with involvement of multiple vascular territories. Cardiac monitoring showed that that the patient was in AF (Figure 12.5).

PRACTICAL POINTS

- Given the involvement of multiple vascular territories on MRI imaging and documentation of AF, the suspected etiology of this stroke is cardioembolic.
- Based on age, history of hypertension, smoking, and stroke, the patient's $CHADS_2$ score is 4, which corresponds to 8.5% risk of stroke per year, and thus warrants long-term anticoagulation.
- Small size of embolic strokes indicates low risk of hemorrhagic transformation. Therefore, anticoagulation can be safely started relatively soon from stroke onset.
- Clinical scenarios that would alter the optimal timing of initiating anticoagulation therapy include the discovery of cardiac thrombus (in

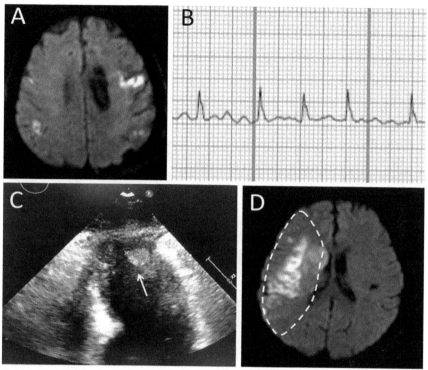

Figure 12.5 Stroke from atrial fibrillation.

(A) Diffusion-weighted magnetic resonance (MR) image, axial view, shows embolic-type strokes in bilateral middle cerebral artery territories, indicating the "central" source of the embolism.

(B) Electrocardiogram shows atrial fibrillation.

(C) Transthoracic 2D echocardiogram demonstrates an echodense structure in the left ventricular apex (arrow).

(D) Acute ischemic stroke involving half of the right middle cerebral artery (MRA) territory is shown on the diffusion-weighted MR image (the dotted line outlines a typical MCA territory distribution). Based on its large size, this area of ischemia is at high risk for bleeding if anticoagulation is started early.

which case earlier anticoagulation is needed; panel C of Figure 12.5) or large embolic stroke with high risk for hemorrhagic transformation (in such case, antithrombotic therapy is used for several weeks until it is safe to start anticoagulation; panel D of Figure 12.5). ASPECTS is a CT-based scoring system which can be also applied to MRI imaging. This score is described in the chapter on imaging of acute stroke. It can e applied to estimate the risk of hemorrhagic transformation.[32]

- Embolic stroke in a setting of cardiac thrombus represents one of rare examples where systemic anticoagulation with heparin infusion might be beneficial while transitioning to oral long-term anticoagulation with warfarin. The use of NOACs in this scenario is considered "off-label" by the Food and Drug Administration.

REFERENCES

1. Jauch EC, Saver JL, Adams HP, Jr., et al. Guidelines for the early management of patients with acute ischemic stroke: a guideline for healthcare professionals from the American Heart Association/American Stroke Association. *Stroke.* 2013;44(3):870–947.
2. Olavarria VV, Arima H, Anderson CS, et al. Head position and cerebral blood flow velocity in acute ischemic stroke: a systematic review and meta-analysis. *Cerebrovasc Dis.* 2014;37(6):401–408.
3. Munoz-Venturelli P, Arima H, Lavados P, et al. Head Position in Stroke Trial (HeadPoST)—sitting-up vs lying-flat positioning of patients with acute stroke: study protocol for a cluster randomised controlled trial. *Trials.* 2015;16:256.
4. Craig S Anderson HSC, Investigators and Coordinators. Head Position in Stroke Trial: An International Cluster Cross-over Randomized Trial. International Stroke Conference 2017; Houston.
5. Thompson HJ. Evidence-base for Fever interventions following stroke. *Stroke.* 2015;46(5):e98–e100.
6. Lyden P, Hemmen T, Grotta J, et al. Results of the ICTuS 2 Trial (Intravascular Cooling in the Treatment of Stroke 2). *Stroke.* 2016;47(12):2888–2895.
7. Kernan WN, Ovbiagele B, Black HR, et al. Guidelines for the prevention of stroke in patients with stroke and transient ischemic attack: a guideline for healthcare professionals from the American Heart Association/American Stroke Association. *Stroke.* 2014;45(7):2160–2236.
8. Wang Y, Wang Y, Zhao X, et al. Clopidogrel with aspirin in acute minor stroke or transient ischemic attack. *N Engl J Med.* 2013;369(1):11–19.
9. Zhang Q, Wang C, Zheng M, et al. Aspirin plus clopidogrel as secondary prevention after stroke or transient ischemic attack: a systematic review and meta-analysis. *Cerebrovasc Dis.* 2015;39(1):13–22.
10. Suri MF, Qiao Y, Ma X, et al. Prevalence of intracranial atherosclerotic stenosis using high-resolution magnetic resonance angiography in the general population: the atherosclerosis risk in communities study. *Stroke.* 2016;47(5):1187–1193.
11. De Silva DA, Woon FP, Lee MP, Chen CP, Chang HM, Wong MC. South Asian patients with ischemic stroke: intracranial large arteries are the predominant site of disease. *Stroke.* 2007;38(9):2592–2594.
12. Chimowitz MI, Lynn MJ, Howlett-Smith H, et al. Comparison of warfarin and aspirin for symptomatic intracranial arterial stenosis. *N Engl J Med.* 2005;352(13):1305–1316.
13. Chimowitz MI, Lynn MJ, Derdeyn CP, et al. Stenting versus aggressive medical therapy for intracranial arterial stenosis. *N Engl J Med.* 2011;365(11):993–1003.
14. Matsagas M, Jagroop IA, Geroulakos G, Mikhailidis DP. The effect of a loading dose (300 mg) of clopidogrel on platelet function in patients with peripheral arterial disease. *Clin Appl Thromb Hemost.* 2003;9(2):115–120.

15. Liu QZ, Hong T, Liu ZP, et al. [The effect of different loading doses of clopidogrel on platelet aggregation]. *Zhonghua Nei Ke Za Zhi.* 2007;46(2):107–110.
16. Lee DH, Arat A, Morsi H, Shaltoni H, Harris JR, Mawad ME. Dual antiplatelet therapy monitoring for neurointerventional procedures using a point-of-care platelet function test: a single-center experience. *Am J Neuroradiol.* 2008;29(7):1389–1394.
17. Hussein HM, Emiru T, Georgiadis AL, Qureshi AI. Assessment of platelet inhibition by point-of-care testing in neuroendovascular procedures. *Am J Neuroradiol.* 2013;34(4):700–706.
18. Rodallec MH, Marteau V, Gerber S, Desmottes L, Zins M. Craniocervical arterial dissection: spectrum of imaging findings and differential diagnosis. *Radiographics.* 2008;28(6):1711–1728.
19. investigators Ct, Markus HS, Hayter E, et al. Antiplatelet treatment compared with anticoagulation treatment for cervical artery dissection (CADISS): a randomised trial. *Lancet Neurol.* 2015;14(4):361–367.
20. Olin JW, Gornik HL, Bacharach JM, et al. Fibromuscular dysplasia: state of the science and critical unanswered questions: a scientific statement from the American Heart Association. *Circulation.* 2014;129(9):1048–1078.
21. January CT, Wann LS, Alpert JS, et al. 2014 AHA/ACC/HRS guideline for the management of patients with atrial fibrillation: executive summary: a report of the American College of Cardiology/American Heart Association Task Force on practice guidelines and the Heart Rhythm Society. *Circulation.* 2014;130(23):2071–2104.
22. Hallevi H, Albright KC, Martin-Schild S, et al. Anticoagulation after cardioembolic stroke: to bridge or not to bridge? *Arch Neurol.* 2008;65(9):1169–1173.
23. Pennlert J, Overholser R, Asplund K, et al. Optimal timing of anticoagulant treatment after intracerebral hemorrhage in patients with atrial fibrillation. *Stroke.* 2017;48(2):314–320.
24. Majeed A, Kim YK, Roberts RS, Holmstrom M, Schulman S. Optimal timing of resumption of warfarin after intracranial hemorrhage. *Stroke.* 2010;41(12):2860–2866.
25. Kim JT, Jahan R, Saver JL, Investigators S. Impact of glucose on outcomes in patients treated with mechanical thrombectomy: a post hoc analysis of the solitaire flow restoration with the intention for thrombectomy study. *Stroke.* 2016;47(1):120–127.
26. Masrur S, Cox M, Bhatt DL, et al. Association of acute and chronic hyperglycemia with acute ischemic stroke outcomes post-thrombolysis: findings from Get with the Guidelines-Stroke. *J Am Heart Assoc.* 2015;4(10):e002193.
27. Staszewski J, Brodacki B, Kotowicz J, Stepien A. Intravenous insulin therapy in the maintenance of strict glycemic control in nondiabetic acute stroke patients with mild hyperglycemia. *J Stroke Cerebrovasc Dis.* 2011;20(2):150–154.
28. Chamorro A, Dirnagl U, Urra X, Planas AM. Neuroprotection in acute stroke: targeting excitotoxicity, oxidative and nitrosative stress, and inflammation. *Lancet Neurol.* 2016;15(8):869–881.
29. Saver JL. The 2012 Feinberg Lecture: treatment swift and treatment sure. *Stroke.* 2013;44(1):270–277.

30. Sanossian N, Liebeskind DS, Eckstein M, et al. Routing ambulances to designated centers increases access to stroke center care and enrollment in prehospital research. *Stroke.* 2015;46(10):2886–2890.

31. Wijdicks EF, Sheth KN, Carter BS, et al. Recommendations for the management of cerebral and cerebellar infarction with swelling: a statement for healthcare professionals from the American Heart Association/American Stroke Association. *Stroke.* 2014;45(4):1222–1238.

32. Lin K, Zink WE, Tsiouris AJ, John M, Tekchandani L, Sanelli PC. Risk assessment of hemorrhagic transformation of acute middle cerebral artery stroke using multimodal CT. *J Neuroimaging.* 2012;22(2):160–166.

13

Medical Management of Hemorrhagic Stroke

SHASHANK SHEKHAR, SHREYAS GANGADHARA,
AND REBECCA SUGG ■

CONTENTS

1 INTRODUCTION

Hemorrhagic stroke accounts for about 10–20% of all strokes.[1] There are mainly five types of intracranial hemorrhages based on the location of the hematoma: intracerebral hemorrhage (ICH), subarachnoid hemorrhage (SAH), intraventricular hemorrhage (IVH), and subdural and epidural hematomas. When compared to ischemic stroke, hemorrhagic stroke has a worse prognosis with mortality rates of 35–52% at 30 days postdiagnosis.[2] Those who survive are often left with debilitating disabilities. Only about 20% attain functional independence at 6 months.[2] Early aggressive management in the acute stage impacts the long-term outcome of the patients. Therefore, hemorrhagic stroke is a true medical emergency.

The management of patients with IVH and subdural and epidural hematomas is discussed in Chapter 14. In this chapter, we will focus on the medical management of ICH in the acute setting (Figure 13.1). We will also review specific considerations related to the medical management of SAH.

Question 13.1: Can ischemic and hemorrhagic stroke be differentiated based on history and physical exam alone?

Answer: No, it is often very difficult to reliably differentiate ischemic from hemorrhagic stroke without neuroimaging.

2 CLINICAL PRESENTATION

Similar to ischemic stroke, hemorrhagic stroke usually presents with sudden onset of focal neurologic symptoms such as weakness, numbness, slurred speech, and visual deficits; however, altered mental state is also a common presentation. In comparison to ischemic stroke, patients with hemorrhagic stroke present more commonly with a headache, nausea, vomiting, seizures, altered mental status, and extremely elevated blood pressure (BP).

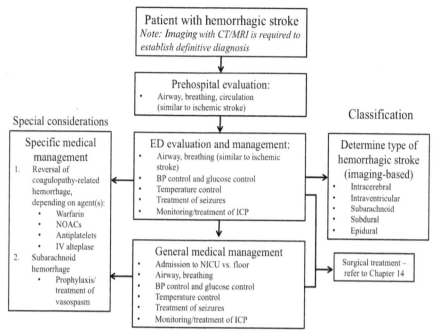

Figure 13.1 Basic algorithm of the medical management of hemorrhagic stroke.
ABBREVIATIONS: BP, blood pressure; CT, computed tomography; ED, emergency
department; ICP, intracranial pressure; IV, intravenous; MRI, magnetic resonance
imaging; NICU, neurointensive care unit; NOAC, non-vitamin K antagonists oral
anticoagulants.

3 PREHOSPITAL MANAGEMENT

The primary focus of management by the emergency medical services (EMS) should
include stabilizing the patient's respiratory and cardiovascular system (airway,
breathing, circulation; ABCs) and rapid transportation to the closest Emergency
Department (ED) equipped with facilities to care for stroke patients. A brief history (including time of onset or time of last known well if the time of onset is unknown), medical history, current medications, and illicit drug use history should also
be obtained (Box 13.1). Phone numbers for family members or witnesses should be
obtained to provide the treating physicians to help obtain any additional information
that may be needed.

Accurate differentiation between ischemic and hemorrhagic stroke requires neuroimaging, which is not available in the prehospital setting (except for mobile stroke
units and other portable imaging technologies designed specifically for ambulances,
which are considered experimental at this point). Thus, at this point, triage will depend on the patient's stability and severity of neurologic deficits.

Box 13.1

INITIAL ASSESSMENT IN THE EMERGENCY DEPARTMENT

- ABCs
  - Airway protection (intubation if GCS <8)
  - Maintain oxygenation saturation SaO_2 >94%
  - Hemodynamic resuscitation
- Focused history: time of onset or last known well, past medical history, medication history, history of coagulopathy
- Monitoring
  - Vital signs
  - Neurologic exam including GCS and NIHSS and signs of increased intracranial pressure
- Testing
  - Imaging (non-contrast head CT)
  - Labs: complete blood count, comprehensive metabolic panel, prothrombin time/partial thromboplastin time/INR, toxicology screen, cardiac enzymes
  - EKG

4 EMERGENCY DEPARTMENT EVALUATION

Initial management of the hemorrhagic stroke patient in the ED requires reassessment of the patient's ABCs, followed by rapid use of neuroimaging to establish the correct diagnosis (Box 13.2).

Comprehensive management of ICH requires tertiary care facility where appropriate specialties (neurology, neurosurgery, and neuroradiology) are available 24/7, either physically or via teleconsultation. Every ED should be prepared to treat ICH

Box 13.2

ADVANTAGES OF CT OVER MAGNETIC RESONANCE IMAGING

- Widespread availability in the ED
- Rapidity of the test
- Can be done in patients with contraindications to magnetic resonance imaging such as a pacemaker, defibrillator, or other implants
- Ease of obtaining images in patients who are intubated

or should have a plan for rapid transfer to higher level-of-care facilities. Assessment and classification of hemorrhagic strokes includes the following steps:

1. Note location of the hemorrhage: intracerebral, subarachnoid, subdural, or epidural. Also note whether there is an intraventricular extension of the hemorrhage.
2. If the hemorrhage is intraparenchymal, differentiation should be made concerning whether the hemorrhage is deep or cortical. A hemorrhage in deep structures such as basal ganglia, thalamus, brainstem, and cerebellum is usually secondary to hypertension whereas a cortical hemorrhage is often due to cerebral amyloid angiopathy.
3. The hematoma volume (such as using the ABC/2 formula described in Chapter 6), presence of "spot sign," and the ICH score (Box 13.3) should be calculated as it provides a rapid prognostic estimate.[3] For a SAH,

---

Box 13.3

SUMMARY OF THE INTRACEREBRAL HEMORRHAGE SCORE

The score is graded based on several components: GCS, hematoma volume and origin, presence of intraventricular hemorrhage, and age

- GCS score
  - GCS 3–4—2 points
  - GCS 5–12—1 point
  - GCS 13–15—0 point
- Hematoma volume, cm^3
  - 30 or above—1 point
  - <30—0 points
- Presence of Intraventricular hemorrhage
  - Yes—1 point
  - No—0 point
- Infratentorial origin of ICH
  - Yes—1 point
  - No—0 point
- Age, years
  - 80 or above—1 point
  - <80—0 point
- 30-day mortality is based on total ICH score: 0% with score of 0; 13% with score of 1; 26% with score of 2; 72% with score of 3; 97% with score of 4; 100% with score of 5 or 6.

Box 13.4

COMMONLY USED CLINICAL SUBARACHNOID HEMORRHAGE SCALES

Hunt and Hess grading scale

- Grade I—no/minimal headache, mild neck stiffness
- Grade II—moderate/severe headache, neck stiffness, cranial nerve palsy
- Grade III—drowsiness, confusion, minimal neurologic deficit
- Grade IV—stupor, moderate/severe hemiparesis
- Grade V—deep coma, decerebrate posture

World Federation of Neurological Surgeons grading scale

- Grade 1—GCS of 15, no focal deficits
- Grade 2—GCS 13–14, no focal deficits
- Grade 3—GCS 13–14 with focal deficits
- Grade 4—GCS 7–12
- Grade 5—GCS 0–6

its severity should be determined using the Hunt and Hess or World Federation of Neurologic Surgeons scores[4,5] (Box 13.4).
4. Special attention should be paid to a midline shift or any evidence of brain herniation.

Early neurologic deterioration is relatively common after hemorrhagic stroke. Often, this is due to expansion of the hematoma. About 30–40% of patients experience clinically significant hematoma expansion in the acute stage.[6] The hematoma expansion is believed to happen for up to first 6–8 hours, offering a therapeutic window for obtaining hemostasis (Case 13.1). Early hematoma expansion is one of the strongest predictors of 30-day mortality. The characteristics that help predict early neurologic deterioration are depicted in Box 13.5.

Box 13.5

FACTORS PREDICTIVE OF EARLY NEUROLOGIC DETERIORATION

- Large hematoma volume
- Antiplatelet and anticoagulant use
- Uncontrolled hypertension
- Low GCS score
- "Spot sign" on CT angiography

5 MEDICAL MANAGEMENT

5.1 Airway

Many patients with ICH will present obtunded or comatose or may require later intubation thus attention to airway and adequate oxygenation is required at all stages of management of these patients.

5.2 Blood pressure control

Uncontrolled hypertension is the most common cause of ICH and accounts for about 60–70% of all cases. The optimum BP goal after ICH remains unclear. Sustained elevation in BP is feared to cause expansion of hematoma, recurrent bleeding and perihematomal edema.[7-9] On the other hand, it was believed that rapid reduction in BP might cause perihematomal ischemia.[10]

Recently, the ATACH-2 and INTERACT-2 trials demonstrated that rapid and intensive BP lowering in patients with acute intracranial hemorrhage is safe, although it did not translate into decreased mortality or disability.[11,12] The 2015 American Heart Association (AHA) guidelines state that in patients presenting with a systolic BP of 150–220 mm Hg, acute lowering of SBP to 140 mm Hg is safe and improves outcome, whereas the BP goal in patients who present with initial SBP >220 is unclear.[13]

5.3 Coagulopathy related hemorrhage

Common causes for coagulopathy include anticoagulant medication use and acquired or congenital coagulation factor deficiency and platelet abnormalities. Most widely used oral anticoagulants currently approved by the Food and Drug Administration (FDA) in the United States are warfarin and novel oral anticoagulants (non-vitamin K antagonist oral anticoagulants). Patients with anticoagulant-related ICH have a poor outcome.[14] Uncorrected coagulopathy is one of the major factors for early hematoma expansion. Therefore, rapid identification and correction of the underlying coagulopathy is of utmost importance. In patients who require transfer to a higher level of care, this needs to be initiated before the transfer takes place.

5.3.1 WARFARIN

Although warfarin use is diminishing gradually with the introduction of non-vitamin K antagonist oral anticoagulants (NOACs, also commonly referred to as "novel oral anticoagulants"), it is still one of the most common anticoagulants currently in use. It works by antagonizing vitamin K dependent cofactors in the coagulation cascade: factors II, VI, IX, and X. Patients with warfarin-related ICH need rapid correction of international normalized ratio (INR).[15,16] The AHA recommends prompt withholding of warfarin, replacing the vitamin K-dependent coagulation factors and intravenous (IV) vitamin K administration.[13]

Two commonly available products for replacing coagulation factors include fresh-frozen plasma (FFP) and prothrombin complex concentrate (PCC), which contains factors II, VII, IX, and X. FFP has higher allergic and infusion reaction rates and requires longer processing time and a larger infusion volume. On the other hand, PCC corrects INR more rapidly than FFP. There has been a concern for prothrombotic complication with PCC based on the mechanism of action. However, trials have demonstrated the risk to be equal to FFP.[17,18] Therefore, PCC is preferred over FFP when available. Recombinant factor VII has been used for INR correction and even though it rapidly corrects the INR, it does not replace all the vitamin K-dependent factors and therefore is not recommended.

The recommended dose of vitamin K is 5 to 10 mg given slowly IV. Vitamin K is metabolized in the liver and has its onset of action at 2 hours, maximizing at 24 hours.[13,19] There is no consensus on target INR; however, various studies aim around <1.3 to <1.5.[20] Platelet transfusion has been widely used historically after ICH. However, the PATCH trial demonstrated higher mortality and adverse effects from platelet transfusion.[21] In light of this new evidence, authors do not recommend routine platelet transfusion.

5.3.2 NON-VITAMIN K ANTAGONISTS ORAL ANTICOAGULANTS

There are four FDA-approved NOACs currently available in the United States. They are dabigatran (Pradaxa), rivaroxaban (Xarelto), apixaban (Eliquis), and edoxaban (Sevaysa). Dabigatran is a direct thrombin inhibitor whereas rivaroxaban, apixaban, and edoxaban are factor Xa inhibitors. Currently, of all the NOACs, only dabigatran has the FDA-approved reversal agent idarucizumab.

Idarucizumab is a monoclonal antibody fragment that binds to dabigatran with an affinity that is about 350 times higher than that of thrombin. In the RE-VERSE AD trial, idarucizumab rapidly and completely reversed the anticoagulant effect of dabigatran in 88–98% of the patients who had elevated clotting times at baseline. There were no significant prothrombotic complications noted with idaracizumab. The recommended dose of idaracizumab is 5g IV once.[22]

For patients with ICH who are taking dabigatran, rivaroxaban, or apixaban, treatment with factor VIII inhibitor bypassing activity factor, other PCCs, or rFVIIa might be considered on an individual basis. Activated charcoal may be used if the most recent dose of dabigatran, apixaban, or rivaroxaban was taken within the first 2 hours. Hemodialysis may also be considered.[13]

Although, there are no currently available reversal agents for Factor Xa inhibitors, there are several drugs in the pipeline. Andexanet (andexanet alfa) is a recombinant modified human Factor Xa decoy protein that is catalytically inactive but binds to factor Xa inhibitors and restores the level of endogenous Factor Xa. It has shown promising results in preclinical and Phase 2 trials and is being investigated in two Phase 3 trials. If approved, it could be used for reversal of apixaban, rivaroxaban, and edoxaban.

Another promising drug in the pipeline is ciraparantag. It is a broad-spectrum anticoagulant reversal agent and is reported to antagonize all anticoagulants except warfarin and argatroban. It is currently being evaluated in Phase 2 trials and has shown promising results in preclinical trials.

Question 13.2: When is a safe time to restart antiplatelet therapy after ICH?

Answer: Currently, there is no good evidence-based answer. It should be considered on a case-by-case basis after evaluating the benefits and risks of resuming antiplatelet therapy.

5.3.3 ANTIPLATELET RELATED HEMORRHAGE

Although bleeding is a known complication of antiplatelet drug use, it is unclear if antiplatelet drugs worsen the outcome of hemorrhagic stroke. Antiplatelet drugs should be discontinued once ICH is diagnosed. According to the Neurocritical Care Society guidelines, platelet transfusion is not recommended in patients who will not undergo the neurosurgical procedure. However, in patients who will undergo neurosurgical interventions, such as placement of an external ventricular drain, platelet transfusion is recommended.[23]

5.3.4 THROMBOLYSIS-RELATED HEMORRHAGE

Symptomatic ICH occurred in 6.4% of patients treated with IV alteplase in the original National Institutes of Neurological Disorders and Stroke (NINDS) trial.[24] IV alteplase-related ICH is associated with high mortality and requires immediate attention. When a hemorrhage is suspected during IV alteplase administration, the thrombolytic agent should be discontinued immediately. An emergent non-contrast computed tomography (CT) should be obtained. Immediate reassessment of airway, breathing, and BP control is needed.

If the hemorrhage is symptomatic (i.e., when worsening of prior neurological deficits occurs), reversal of systemic thrombolytic is recommended. If the hemorrhagic transformation is asymptomatic and rather minor in size, conservative management may be considered on a case-by-case basis. Cryoprecipitate 10 units IV is recommended for all patients who experience a hemorrhagic complication from IV alteplase. If cryoprecipitate is contraindicated or unavailable, tranexamic acid 10–15 mg/kg IV over 20 min or e-aminocaproic acid 4–5 g IV as an alternative to cryoprecipitate should be considered. FFP may also be considered if none of the previously described options are available; however, larger volume of FFP is needed due to the low concentration of fibrinogen. Fibrinogen should be checked after administration of the reversal agent, and if its level is greater than 150 mg/dl, an additional dose of the reversal agent should be considered.[23]

5.4 Blood glucose control

Hyperglycemia at presentation has been associated with increased risk of mortality in both non-diabetic and diabetic patients.[25] In animal experiments, hyperglycemia results in brain edema, hematoma enlargement, and perihematomal cell death.[26,27] Both hyperglycemia and hypoglycemia could worsen outcome and should be avoided.

5.5 Temperature control

Hyperthermia also impairs outcome in ICH patients, presumably due to elevation in intracranial pressure.[28] On the other hand, hypothermia has not proved to improve outcomes. Therefore, the goal should be normothermia.

5.6 Seizures

Seizures frequently occurs after ICH, especially if hemorrhage is located cortically.[29-31] The reported frequency of clinical seizures is as high as 16% within one week after the occurrence of ICH.[29,30] The frequency of subclinical seizures may be even higher. In 1 study, 1 in 3 patients showed electrographic seizures.[31,32]

Despite this high incidence of seizure, prophylactic use of antiepileptic drugs is not recommended. Prophylactic use of phenytoin after ICH has shown higher morbidity and mortality rates.[33,34] A meta-analysis studying the use of phenytoin (Dilantin) versus levetiracetam (Keppra) also suggested similar outcomes.[35] However, once the patient has been diagnosed with clinical or electrographic seizures, there is a clear benefit from antiepileptic therapy.[13] In patients with altered mental status that is believed to be out of proportion to the hemorrhage, continuous electroencephalography (EEG) monitoring should be considered.

> **Question 13.3:** Can steroids be used to decrease elevated intracranial pressure (ICP) in ICH?
>
> **Answer:** No, steroids do not decrease ICP in ICH. In fact, they are known to worsen outcome.

5.7 Management of intracranial pressure

ICP is associated with worse prognosis. The increase in ICP results in lower the cerebral perfusion pressure, which in turn causes tissue hypoxia. Cerebral perfusion pressure less than 70–80 mm Hg is associated with poor outcome. Basic principles of ICP management include elevating head of bed to 30°, positioning head in midline,

---

Box 13.6

BASIC PRINCIPLES OF INTRACRANIAL PRESSURE MANAGEMENT

- Head elevation at 30°
- Head in a midline position
- Mild sedation
- Avoiding tight cervical collar
- Hyperventilation, mannitol, or hypertonic saline in impending herniation

---

mild sedation, and avoiding tight cervical collar or endotracheal ties (Box 13.6). In an acute setting with impending herniation, hyperventilation with the goal of pCO_2 <35 mm Hg rapidly reduces ICP; however, the effect is short lasting. Osmotic therapy, despite little evidence for its efficacy, is widely used in patients with increased ICP. Mannitol and hypertonic saline are the two commonly used hyperosmolar agents. Mannitol is commonly used as a 20% solution and is given at a dose of 0.5–1 g/kg IV every 4–6 hours. A serum osmolality goal of 320 mOsm/kg is recommended. Hypertonic saline is available in various strengths. Commonly used strengths are 3%, 7%, and 23% solutions. Hypertonic saline can be used either as a continuous infusion or a bolus administration every 4–6 hours. Bolus administration is thought to be more effective; however, the data is limited. Commonly used bolus doses include 250 ml of 3% solution or 75 ml of 7% solution or 30 ml of 23% solution. A central venous line is preferred for hypertonic saline administration. Serum sodium should be monitored every 6 hours with a target level of 155–160 mmol/L. Alternatively, serum osmolality with target 320 mOsm/kg may also be considered.[36]

6 DISPOSITION FROM THE EMERGENCY DEPARTMENT

Close monitoring and an intensive care unit (ICU) level of care is recommended at least for the first 24 hours. Studies have shown the benefit of early admission to neuroscience ICU (NSICU) or stroke unit rather than a prolonged stay in the ED.[37] Delay in admission is associated with higher morbidity and mortality. A study comparing medical ICU and NSICU showed better outcome in patients cared for at NSICU.[38]

> **Question 13.4:** When can heparin or enoxaparin be started for deep venous thrombosis (DVT) prophylaxis after ICH?
>
> **Answer:** Chemical prophylaxis for DVT can be started in 1–4 days after documenting cessation of hematoma expansion. Sequential compression devices can be used immediately.

7 DEEP VENOUS THROMBOSIS PROPHYLAXIS

Patients with hemorrhagic stroke are at high risk of venous thrombosis.[39] The incidence of DVT after ICH is about 0.5–13% and pulmonary embolism is 0.7–55%.[40] The CLOTS 3 trial demonstrated that the use of intermittent pneumatic compression started on the day of admission reduces the occurrence of proximal DVT.[41] Low dose subcutaneous low-molecular-weight heparin or unfractionated heparin should be considered for early DVT prophylaxis. For the treatment of DVT or pulmonary embolism, systemic anticoagulation with heparin or enoxaparin, or inferior vena cava filter (IVC) filter placement, may be considered. An IVC filter is preferred in patients who are at risk for hematoma expansion or rebleeding.

8 SPECIAL CONSIDERATIONS IN SUBARACHNOID HEMORRHAGE

There are some specific considerations related to SAH management:

1. Unlike in ICH, there are no clinical trials evaluating optimum BP goal in SAH. The AHA guideline recommends goal SBP <160.
2. Oral nimodipine should be administered to all patients within 96 hours from the onset of SAH. The recommended dose is 60 mg oral every 4 hours. It should be continued until day 21. Nimodipine has been shown to improve neurological outcomes but does not prevent cerebral vasospasm. The utility of other calcium antagonists is uncertain.
3. The prophylactic use of "triple H" therapy (hypervolemia, hypertension, and hemodilution) before the development of vasospasm is not beneficial and can be potentially harmful and, therefore, is not recommended. Rather, maintenance of euvolemia is advised.
4. Monitoring for cerebral vasospasm using daily transcranial Doppler is recommended.[42]

9 CLINICAL CASES

Case 13.1 Intracranial hemorrhage with hematoma expansion

CASE DESCRIPTION

A 67-year-old right-handed woman with a history of hypertension develops sudden onset left face, arm, and leg weakness. Initial vital signs at the scene include BP 218/110 mmHg, heart rate 84, pulse oxygen saturation 96%, and temperature 98.0 F. On neurological examination, the patient is alert and fully oriented. The National Institutes of Health Stroke Scale (NIHSS) score is 10, and Glasgow Coma Scale (GCS) is 15. Non-contrast head CT shows the right basal ganglia hemorrhage as shown in Figure 13.2A. Shortly after the CT is completed, the patient becomes unresponsive and her GCS worsens to 5.

PRACTICAL POINTS

- The differential diagnosis for early neurologic deterioration after ICH includes expansion of the hematoma and non-convulsive seizures. Failure to provide rapid BP control is one of potential mechanisms for early hematoma expansion in this case.
- After stabilizing the ABCs, a repeat head CT should be obtained to rule out hematoma expansion (Figure 13.2B). If the hematoma is stable, a non-convulsive seizure should be suspected, in which case a bed-side EEG is required. Commonly used drugs in the ED include fosphenytoin 10–20 mg/kg or levetiracetam 1 gram IV load, followed by maintenance therapy.

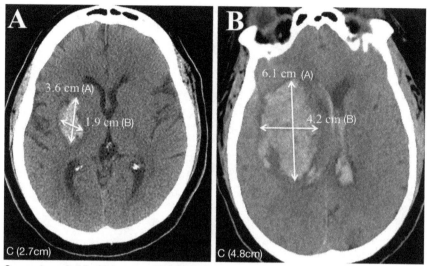

C= number of slide thickness x thickness of each slice (cm)

Figure 13.2 Anticoagulation related intracranial hemorrhage.
(A) Non-contrast computed tomography (CT), axial view, showing a left occipital intraparenchymal hematoma with a fluid level (arrowheads). A midline shift (7 mm) is also present A and B are perpendicular width of the hematoma and C is the number of slide thickness × thickness of each slice (cm) thus ABC/2 hematoma volume is 3.6 × 1.9 × 2.7/2 = 9.2 cm³.
(B) Repeat CT study with evidence of significantly enlarged right parenchymal hematoma, now also with an intraventricular bleeding component. The new ABC/2 hematoma volume is 6.1 × 4.2 × 4.8/2 = 61.5 cm³.

Case 13.2 Anticoagulation related intracranial hemorrhage

CASE DESCRIPTION

A 78-year-old female with past medical history significant for atrial fibrillation and hypertension presents with sudden onset headache and loss of consciousness. The patient takes warfarin at home. On EMS arrival, the patient's GCS is 4, and she is immediately intubated and transported to the ED. Her vitals sign show BP 140/90 mm Hg, oxygen saturation of 98% on arrival to the ED. Non-contrast head CT is shown in Figure 13.3. Laboratory studies are significant for INR 4.0.

PRACTICAL POINTS

- CT shows a large left occipital intraparenchymal hematoma with a fluid level that suggests ongoing active bleeding and is commonly seen in anticoagulant-related hemorrhages. The hypodense part of the hemorrhage represents the unclotted blood.
- The INR is supratherapeutic, which is the likely etiology for the hemorrhage. In accordance with AHA guidelines, 10mg IV vitamin K, and dose-appropriate PCC should be administered immediately. Also, given the large size of hemorrhage, emergent neurosurgery consultation should be obtained.

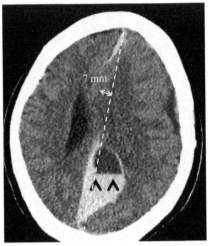

Figure 13.3 Intracranial hemorrhage with hematoma expansion.
Non-contrast computed tomography, axial view, showing a left occipital intraparenchymal hematoma with a fluid level (arrowheads). A midline shift (7 mm) is also present.

Case 13.3 Thrombolysis-related intraventricular hemorrhage

CASE DESCRIPTION

56-year-old woman presents with right hemiparesis and slurred speech. Her NIHSS score is 9, and non-contrast head CT is unremarkable. She receives IV alteplase. Shortly after initiating the drip of alteplase, she develops a severe headache along

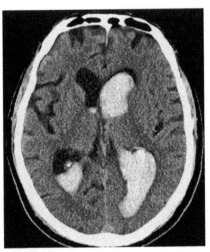

Figure 13.4 Thrombolysis-related intraventricular hemorrhage.
Non-contrast computed tomography, axial view, showing a large intraventricular hemorrhage.

with projectile vomiting and becomes unresponsive. Vital signs show bradycardia, elevated BP, and irregular breathing. The drip is discontinued immediately, the patient gets intubated, and a repeat CT is obtained (Figure 13.4).

Practical points

- The patient demonstrates clinical signs of increased intracranial pressure, which include bradycardia, hypertension, and irregular breathing. Hyperventilation, administration of mannitol or hypertonic saline, and a stat neurosurgical consultation for a placement of an external ventricular drain is needed.
- Simultaneously, alteplase reversal protocol should be initiated immediately.

Case 13.4 Aneurysmal subarachnoid hemorrhage

Case description
A 21-year-old female with no significant past medical history arrives to the ED with a sudden onset of severe headache. Neurological exam is significant for lethargy and neck rigidity. BP is 170/100 mm Hg, pulse is 106/minute, respiratory rate is 22/minute, and temperature was 98.8°F. Non-contrast head CT is performed in the ED (Figure 13.5A).

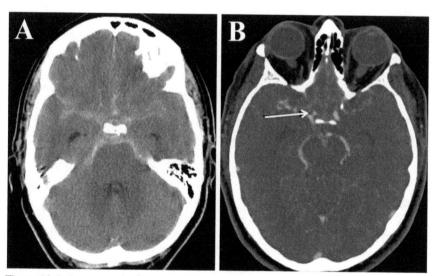

Figure 13.5 Aneurysmal subarachnoid hemorrhage.
(A) Non-contrast computed tomography (CT), axial view, showing a diffuse subarachnoid hemorrhage.
(B) CT angiography, axial view, showing a small right internal carotid artery (terminus segment) aneurysm (arrow). This is the source of the patient's hemorrhage.

PRACTICAL POINTS

- The non-contrast head CT shows SAH. CT or MR angiography should be performed next to rule out an intracranial aneurysm.
- In this case, CT angiography showed a small ruptured aneurysm of the right internal carotid artery (Figure 13.5B). An immediate neurosurgical consultation is needed.
- CT angiography (CTA) has 98% sensitivity for aneurysms greater than 3 mm but is less sensitive for very small aneurysms.[43] Catheter digital subtraction angiogram is considered the gold standard test for aneurysm evaluation and should be pursued if CTA study is "negative" for an aneurysm.

REFERENCES

1. Feigin VL, Lawes CM, Bennett DA, Barker-Collo SL, Parag V. Worldwide stroke incidence and early case fatality reported in 56 population-based studies: a systematic review. *Lancet Neurol.* 2009;8(4):355–369.
2. Caceres JA, Goldstein JN. Intracranial hemorrhage. *Emerg Med Clin North Am.* 2012;30(3):771–794.
3. Hemphill JC, 3rd, Bonovich DC, Besmertis L, Manley GT, Johnston SC. The ICH score: a simple, reliable grading scale for intracerebral hemorrhage. *Stroke.* 2001;32(4):891–897.
4. Hunt WE, Hess RM. Surgical risk as related to time of intervention in the repair of intracranial aneurysms. *J Neurosurg.* 1968;28(1):14–20.
5. Report of World Federation of Neurological Surgeons Committee on a Universal Subarachnoid Hemorrhage Grading Scale. *J Neurosurg.* 1988;68(6):985–986.
6. Specogna AV, Turin TC, Patten SB, Hill MD. Factors associated with early deterioration after spontaneous intracerebral hemorrhage: a systematic review and meta-analysis. *PLoS ONE.* 2014;9(5):e96743.
7. Zhang Y, Reilly KH, Tong W, et al. Blood pressure and clinical outcome among patients with acute stroke in Inner Mongolia, China. *J Hypertens.* 2008;26(7):1446–1452.
8. Rodriguez-Luna D, Pineiro S, Rubiera M, et al. Impact of blood pressure changes and course on hematoma growth in acute intracerebral hemorrhage. *Eur J Neurol.* 2013;20(9):1277–1283.
9. Sakamoto Y, Koga M, Yamagami H, et al. Systolic blood pressure after intravenous antihypertensive treatment and clinical outcomes in hyperacute intracerebral hemorrhage: the stroke acute management with urgent risk-factor assessment and improvement-intracerebral hemorrhage study. *Stroke.* 2013;44(7):1846–1851.
10. Naval NS, Nyquist PA, Carhuapoma JR. Management of spontaneous intracerebral hemorrhage. *Neurol Clin.* 2008;26(2):373–384, vii.
11. Anderson CS, Heeley E, Huang Y, et al. Rapid blood-pressure lowering in patients with acute intracerebral hemorrhage. *N Engl J Med.* 2013;368(25):2355–2365.

12. Qureshi AI, Palesch YY, Barsan WG, et al. Intensive blood-pressure lowering in patients with acute cerebral hemorrhage. *N Engl J Med.* 2016;375(11):1033–1043.

13. Hemphill JC, 3rd, Greenberg SM, Anderson CS, et al. Guidelines for the management of spontaneous intracerebral hemorrhage: a guideline for healthcare professionals from the American Heart Association/American Stroke Association. *Stroke.* 2015;46(7):2032–2060.

14. Steiner T, Al-Shahi Salman R, Beer R, et al. European Stroke Organisation (ESO) guidelines for the management of spontaneous intracerebral hemorrhage. *Int J Stroke.* 2014;9(7):840–855.

15. Holbrook A, Schulman S, Witt DM, et al. Evidence-based management of anticoagulant therapy: Antithrombotic Therapy and Prevention of Thrombosis, 9th ed: American College of Chest Physicians Evidence-Based Clinical Practice Guidelines. *Chest.* 2012;141(2 Suppl):e152S–e184S.

16. Hanley JP. Warfarin reversal. *J Clin Pathol.* 2004;57(11):1132–1139.

17. Leissinger CA, Blatt PM, Hoots WK, Ewenstein B. Role of prothrombin complex concentrates in reversing warfarin anticoagulation: a review of the literature. *Am J Hematol.* 2008;83(2):137–143.

18. Sarode R, Milling TJ, Jr., Refaai MA, et al. Efficacy and safety of a 4-factor prothrombin complex concentrate in patients on vitamin K antagonists presenting with major bleeding: a randomized, plasma-controlled, phase IIIb study. *Circulation.* 2013;128(11):1234–1243.

19. Dentali F, Ageno W, Crowther M. Treatment of coumarin-associated coagulopathy: a systematic review and proposed treatment algorithms. *J Thromb Haemost.* 2006;4(9):1853–1863.

20. Steiner T, Rosand J, Diringer M. Intracerebral hemorrhage associated with oral anticoagulant therapy: current practices and unresolved questions. *Stroke.* 2006;37(1):256–262.

21. Baharoglu MI, Cordonnier C, Al-Shahi Salman R, et al. Platelet transfusion versus standard care after acute stroke due to spontaneous cerebral haemorrhage associated with antiplatelet therapy (PATCH): a randomised, open-label, phase 3 trial. *Lancet.* 2016;387(10038):2605–2613.

22. Pollack CV, Jr., Reilly PA, Eikelboom J, et al. Idarucizumab for dabigatran reversal. *N Engl J Med.* 2015;373(6):511–520.

23. Frontera JA, Lewin JJ, 3rd, Rabinstein AA, et al. Guideline for reversal of antithrombotics in intracranial hemorrhage: a statement for healthcare professionals from the Neurocritical Care Society and Society of Critical Care Medicine. *Neurocrit Care.* 2016;24(1):6–46.

24. Intracerebral hemorrhage after intravenous t-PA therapy for ischemic stroke. The NINDS t-PA Stroke Study Group. *Stroke.* 1997;28(11):2109–2118.

25. Fogelholm R, Murros K, Rissanen A, Avikainen S. Admission blood glucose and short term survival in primary intracerebral haemorrhage: a population based study. *J Neurol Neurosurg Psychiatry.* 2005;76(3):349–353.

26. Song EC, Chu K, Jeong SW, et al. Hyperglycemia exacerbates brain edema and perihematomal cell death after intracerebral hemorrhage. *Stroke.* 2003;34(9):2215–2220.

27. Liu J, Gao BB, Clermont AC, et al. Hyperglycemia-induced cerebral hematoma expansion is mediated by plasma kallikrein. *Nat Med*. 2011;17(2):206–210.

28. Rossi S, Zanier ER, Mauri I, Columbo A, Stocchetti N. Brain temperature, body core temperature, and intracranial pressure in acute cerebral damage. *J Neurol Neurosurg Psychiatry*. 2001;71(4):448–454.

29. De Herdt V, Dumont F, Henon H, et al. Early seizures in intracerebral hemorrhage: incidence, associated factors, and outcome. *Neurology*. 2011;77(20):1794–1800.

30. Beghi E, D'Alessandro R, Beretta S, et al. Incidence and predictors of acute symptomatic seizures after stroke. *Neurology*. 2011;77(20):1785–1793.

31. Bladin CF, Alexandrov AV, Bellavance A, et al. Seizures after stroke: a prospective multicenter study. *Arch Neurol*. 2000;57(11):1617–1622.

32. Szaflarski JP, Rackley AY, Kleindorfer DO, et al. Incidence of seizures in the acute phase of stroke: a population-based study. *Epilepsia*. 2008;49(6):974–981.

33. Naidech AM, Garg RK, Liebling S, et al. Anticonvulsant use and outcomes after intracerebral hemorrhage. *Stroke*. 2009;40(12):3810–3815.

34. Messe SR, Sansing LH, Cucchiara BL, et al. Prophylactic antiepileptic drug use is associated with poor outcome following ICH. *Neurocrit Care*. 2009;11(1):38–44.

35. Zafar SN, Khan AA, Ghauri AA, Shamim MS. Phenytoin versus Leviteracetam for seizure prophylaxis after brain injury—a meta analysis. *BMC Neurol*. 2012;12:30.

36. Ropper AH. Hyperosmolar therapy for raised intracranial pressure. *N Engl J Med*. 2012;367(8):746–752.

37. Terent A, Asplund K, Farahmand B, et al. Stroke unit care revisited: who benefits the most? A cohort study of 105,043 patients in Riks-Stroke, the Swedish Stroke Register. *J Neurol Neurosurg Psychiatry*. 2009;80(8):881–887.

38. Diringer MN, Edwards DF. Admission to a neurologic/neurosurgical intensive care unit is associated with reduced mortality rate after intracerebral hemorrhage. *Crit Care Med*. 2001;29(3):635–640.

39. Gregory PC, Kuhlemeier KV. Prevalence of venous thromboembolism in acute hemorrhagic and thromboembolic stroke. *Am J Phys Med Rehab*. 2003;82(5):364–369.

40. Chan S, Hemphill JC, 3rd. Critical care management of intracerebral hemorrhage. *Critical care clinics*. 2014;30(4):699–717.

41. Collaboration CT, Dennis M, Sandercock P, et al. Effectiveness of intermittent pneumatic compression in reduction of risk of deep vein thrombosis in patients who have had a stroke (CLOTS 3): a multicentre randomised controlled trial. *Lancet*. 2013;382(9891):516–524.

42. Connolly ES, Jr., Rabinstein AA, Carhuapoma JR, et al. Guidelines for the management of aneurysmal subarachnoid hemorrhage: a guideline for healthcare professionals from the American Heart Association/american Stroke Association. *Stroke*. 2012;43(6):1711–1737.

43. Agid R, Lee SK, Willinsky RA, Farb RI, terBrugge KG. Acute subarachnoid hemorrhage: using 64-slice multidetector CT angiography to "triage" patients' treatment. *Neuroradiology*. 2006;48(11):787–794.

14

Surgical Treatment of Hemorrhagic Stroke

VLADIMIR LJUBIMOV, TRAVIS DAILEY, AND SIVIERO AGAZZI ∎

CONTENTS

1 INTRODUCTION

Although hemorrhagic strokes account for only 10–15% of all the strokes, they are the most fatal with a 30-day mortality of up to 40%.[1] Only one-third of survivors will recover to functional independence. Hemorrhagic stroke can often be managed with medical therapy alone. Great controversy currently exists on the role of surgery in its overall management strategy. Past trials dealing with the surgical evacuation of the blood clot have failed to show much benefit, yet more recent trials, including minimally invasive surgical approaches and new emerging technologies, hold promise for treatment. Here, we discuss the decision-making process for surgical treatment of intracerebral and intraventricular hemorrhages (IVHs), epidural and subdural hematomas (SDHs), and subarachnoid hemorrhage (SAH) (Figure 14.1).

Question 14.1: What is considered the "normal" intracranial pressure (ICP)?

Answer: The normal range of ICP depends on patient's age. In adults, ICP below 10–15 mm Hg is considered normal.

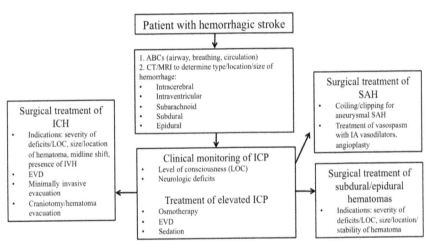

Figure 14.1 Surgical management of hemorrhagic stroke.
ABBREVIATIONS: CT, computed tomography; EVD, external ventricular drain; IA, intra-arterial; ICH, Intracerebral hemorrhage, ICP, intracranial pressure; IVH, Intraventricular hemorrhage; LOC, level of consciousness; MRI, magnetic resonance imaging; SAH, subarachnoid hemorrhage.

2 BASIC PRINCIPLES OF INTRACRANIAL PATHOPHYSIOLOGY

Published commentary on the effects of elevated ICP goes back to at least the description provided in 1783 by Monroe.[2] Kellie further expanded on it in 1824.[3] Over time, their collective work became known as the Monroe–Kellie doctrine. It describes the intracranial compartment as the set of three physiologic components: the brain, the cerebrospinal fluid (CSF), and the blood.

Because the skull is a closed and rigid structure, additional intracranial elements will cause displacement of the existing physiologic components and/or an increase in the ICP. Displacement can produce radiographic findings such as compression of the basilar cisterns, compression of the ventricles, midline shift, effacement of the sulci, and displacement of the brain parenchyma.

Elevation of the ICP, in additional to radiographic characteristics, may produce a combination of clinical findings including headaches, confusion, nausea, emesis, decrease in mental status, pupillary abnormalities, coma, loss of brainstem reflexes, and, finally, brain death. In the Emergency Department (ED), the diagnosis of an intracranial hemorrhage relies on radiographic findings (non-contrast computed tomography [CT] scan and magnetic resonance imaging [MRI]). The evidence of rising ICP is heavily factored in the decision-making process for medical versus surgical treatment (Figure 14.1).

As demonstrated in Figure 14.2, the rise in intracranial volume will initially cause only a very minor rise in ICP. This compensation mechanism is mostly mediated by a shift of CSF away from the brain into the lumbar spinal cistern. A critical aspect of this pressure volume curve is the "genu" of the curve or "critical volume." Once the critical volume has been reached, further fluid shifts are not possible, and the brain is now devoid of any compensating mechanism. From this point forward, even a small increase in the intracranial volume will cause a dramatic increase in the ICP.

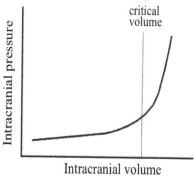

Figure 14.2 The Monroe Kelley doctrine and the intracranial pressure–volume curve.

3 INITIAL CLINICAL EVALUATION IN THE EMERGENCY DEPARTMENT

The initial clinical assessment of a patient with hemorrhagic stroke should be aimed at determining the presence of increased ICP and immediately taking action to treat and prevent further elevation.

3.1 Awake patient

A patient arriving to the ED with an intracranial hemorrhage who is fully conscious has a normal cerebral perfusion pressure. However, he or she could still be in danger of deteriorating if the intracranial volume is approaching the knee of the pressure/volume curve and should therefore be closely monitored with frequent assessment of their neurological status. Increasing headaches, nausea and vomiting, and progressive somnolence should be considered alarming signs of impending neurological deterioration.

3.2 Somnolent or comatose patient

A patient with an intracranial hemorrhage arriving at the ED with an altered mental status should be considered as having an elevated ICP. The longer the period of elevated ICP is, the higher the risk of permanent damage to the brain is. Therefore, in these patients, steps should be taken quickly to measure and treat the ICP, and neurosurgical consultation should be immediately obtained. Administration of osmotic agents (mannitol and hypertonic saline), insertion of an external ventricular drain (EVD), or emergent evacuation of the hematoma should be considered depending on the overall condition and prognosis of the patient (Case 14.1). The American Heart Association (AHA) guidelines on the surgical management of increased ICP are summarized in Box 14.1.

Box 14.1

SURGICAL MONITORING AND TREATMENT OF INTRACRANIAL PRESSURE

- Consider ICP monitoring and treatment in patients with a GCS score of ≤8, those with clinical evidence of transtentorial herniation, or those with significant IVH or hydrocephalus.
- Do not use corticosteroids for treatment of elevated ICP in ICH.
- Extraventricular drainage is reasonable as treatment for hydrocephalus, especially in patients with decreased level of consciousness.

Adapted from the 2015 AHA guidelines for the management of spontaneous ICH.[20]

Box 14.2

SURGICAL MONITORING AND TREATMENT OF INTRACEREBRAL HEMORRHAGE

- In patients with supratentorial ICH, the benefit of surgery is not well established.
- The effectiveness of minimally invasive clot evacuation with stereotactic or endoscopic aspiration is uncertain.
- Decompressive craniectomy with/without hematoma evacuation might reduce mortality for patients with supratentorial ICH who are in a coma, have large hematomas with midline shift, or have elevated ICP refractory to medical management.
- Emergent surgical removal of the hemorrhage in patients with cerebellar hemorrhage who are deteriorating neurologically or who have brainstem compression and/or hydrocephalus from ventricular obstruction.

Adapted from the 2015 AHA guidelines for the management of spontaneous ICH.[20]

3.3 Posterior fossa hemorrhage

The posterior fossa is a small space and contains some of the most critical cerebral structures such as the brainstem. Elevated pressure, compression of the brainstem, and herniation can occur there much more rapidly as compared to other locations that may require a larger volume of displacement.

Clinical evidence of neurological deterioration and radiographic effacement of the posterior fossa cisterns and fourth ventricle are considered to be an indication for evacuation of a posterior fossa hematoma (Box 14.2). Herniation of the cerebellar tonsils can result in brainstem compression and irreversible coma. In the setting of a posterior fossa hematoma, insertion of an external ventricular drain should be considered with great care as it could precipitate brainstem compression by upward transtentorial herniation.

Question 14.2: What are the indications for surgical treatment of intracerebral hemorrhage (ICH)?

Answer: Severity of neurological deficits, the size and location of the hematoma, and the presence of midline shift.

4 SURGICAL MANAGEMENT OF INTRACEREBRAL HEMORRHAGE

The current AHA guidelines on the surgical treatment of ICH are summarized in Box 14.2. The landmark trials on surgical evacuation of ICH are reviewed in the following discussion.

4.1 The STICH trial series

Among the first trials to evaluate surgical intervention for hemorrhagic stroke was the Surgical Treatment for IntraCerebral Hemorrhage (STICH) trial in 2005.[4] The trial evaluated early surgical intervention versus non-operative management in patients with spontaneous supratentorial intracerebral hematomas. The study randomized 1033 patients to early surgery (within 96 hours) or conservative measures. The study showed no difference in mortality or functional outcome between the two groups. However, during subgroup analysis, it was found that lobar ICHs within 1 cm from the surface had an 8% absolute increase in good outcomes following surgery. Patients with deeper ICH randomized to early surgery tended to do poorly compared to the conservatively managed group. The trial ultimately concluded that there was no surgical benefit overall, and in patients with low Glasgow Coma Scale (GCS) scores, surgery was likely harmful.

The original STICH trial was criticized on a few points. First, 26% of patients in the medical management arm crossed over to the surgical arm. Generally, these patients were in grave condition. They had lower GCS scores and worse prognosis, and if they were not to have surgery, their presence in the medical group would have increased the group's morbidity and mortality. Second, there were concerns as to the lack of standardization of surgical timing and the operation performed. The so-called early group had surgery on average within 30 hours postbleed, which could have contributed to poor outcomes.

In 2013 the STICH II trial was published.[5] Like its predecessor, it examined early surgery versus initial conservative management of intracerebral hematomas. This trial aimed to address the weaknesses of the original STICH study. This study randomized 607 patients with spontaneous ICH, and early craniotomy was performed within 12 hours in the surgical arm. Inclusion criteria were depth of the hematoma <1 cm from the cortical surface; ICH volume of 10–100 ml, no IVH, and GCS >6. The overall outcome did not show any benefit with surgery. Within the subgroup analysis, the strongest benefit came in patients with poor predicted prognosis. This trial also faced criticism due to its high crossover rate of 21% and variability in the medical management of the nonsurgical arm.

4.2 Minimally invasive surgery

New technologies are evolving for ways of minimally invasive clot removal. Traditionally, large craniotomies were done for clot evacuation, and it was postulated that the poor outcome demonstrated by the early studies could be explained by surgical damage to surrounding brain tissue, in particular during access to deep-seated hematomas.

With advances in technology, including the widespread availability of intra-operative navigation, an attempt was made at evacuation of the blood clot with minimal damage to surrounding brain. Stereotactic needle aspiration and other less invasive methods are becoming more widespread (Case 14.1).

Stereotactic needle aspiration works by using imaging as a virtual intraoperative GPS, allowing the surgeon to know the precise location of the needle by looking at a rendered image on the screen, showing the tip of the navigation probe relative to the head. This allows precise insertion of a needle into the clot, with a desired trajectory bypassing critical structures and fiber tracts of the brain.

One of the first trials to assess minimally invasive surgery was the safety and efficacy of Minimally Invasive Surgery plus Tissue Plasminogen Activator (alteplase) in Intracerebral Hemorrhage Evacuation (MISTIE) pilot trial in 2005. The trial evaluated minimally invasive surgery for ICH evacuation plus alteplase administration and concluded in 2016.[6] The trial evaluated 30-day mortality, 7-day procedure related mortality, 72-hour symptomatic bleeding, and 30-day CNS infections. There were no differences observed in primary outcomes assessed. It was found that hematoma evacuation was associated with lower perihematomal edema, considered by some to inflict cytotoxicity of surrounding tissue. Currently, the MISTIE III trial is ongoing with expected completion in 2019, with plans to enroll 500 patients in multiple countries.

Another surgical technique is image-guided endoscopic surgery. The Intraoperative Stereotactic Computer Tomography-Guided Endoscopic Surgery (ICES) trial enrolled 20 patients to test the safety for suction and transendoscopic irrigation of hematomas without alteplase. Based on its results, it was concluded that image-guided endoscopic surgery was safe and effective.[7] The ongoing Evaluation of Minimally Invasive Subcortical Parafascicular Access for Clot Evacuation (MISPACE) trial focuses on assessing surgical performance while secondarily assessing complications and outcomes at 30- and 90-day intervals.[8]

Brain Path® is a new minimally invasive technology that aims to reduce subcortical injury by attempting to part cortical fibers without tearing them.[9] Prior to surgery, advanced MRI diffusion tensor imaging allows for the identification of the major white matter fiber tracts. Then surgical trajectory is planned from the brain surface to the hematoma by using access routes parallel to those tracts, thereby displacing rather than transecting them. This new technology was tested at Cleveland Clinic in a single center trial on 18 patients. In this small trial, there were no hemorrhagic recurrences during the hospital stay, and median GCS improved from 10 before surgery to 14 afterwards.[10]

5 INTRAVENTRICULAR HEMORRHAGE

IVH occurs in nearly half of patients with ICH.[11] The main danger in these situations is the formation of obstructive hydrocephalus. As blood fills the ventricles, it will clot and may interrupt CSF flow. This, in turn, may lead to dangerous increases in ICP. Patients with IVH who have a GCS score less than 8 or are at high risk for transtentorial herniation should undergo placement of an EVD. Unfortunately, even with a drainage system in place, depending on the clot burden, obstruction of the EVD may occur.

The CLEAR III trial evaluated how intraventricular clot lysis affects outcomes. The investigators used alteplase to help lyse the clot, with the rationale that this will resolve the IVH faster, reduce ICP, and decrease CSF diversion.[12] The trial showed that the use of low-dose alteplase had an acceptable safety profile and reduced time of clot elimination from the ventricular system. In a subgroup analysis, it was found that the best results were in patients with larger clots and with more than 20 mL of clot degradation. As far as the outcomes, clot lysis via EVD did not increase good functional recovery. There was no significant difference in Rankin score outcomes in the two groups. However, the use of alteplase resulted in a 10% reduction in mortality without an increase in poor functional outcome.

6 EPIDURAL HEMATOMA

Epidural hematomas are most frequently seen after trauma. Although uncommon, they are especially dangerous due to the arterial source of hemorrhage in 85% of the cases. One of the more common vascular structures damaged is the middle meningeal artery. Other rare nontraumatic causes exist such as iatrogenic postoperative complications, infection, coagulopathies, vascular malformations, tumors, and lupus among others.

Due to the arterial nature of the bleed, these hematomas can expand at a very rapid rate, which does not give the brain time to adapt to pressure changes and can lead to acute deterioration and death within hours of the original insult. Epidural hematomas are, therefore, surgical emergencies. The ICP increase can be very rapid, and surgical evacuation is the preferred treatment.

Epidural hematomas of smaller volume may electively be monitored. These patients will need vigilant neurological examinations and serial non-contrast CT images of the head, usually with the first 6 hours after the initial scan. If depression or lethargy is noted during an examination, a repeat CT scan is warranted immediately. If the hematoma expands on imaging, the patient should be taken to the operating room for evacuation without delay, to prevent further neurological decline or death.

All patients presenting with epidural hematomas should have anticoagulation stopped, coagulation factors assessed, and anticoagulants reversed. Generally, the risk of reversal of anticoagulation in patients in the context of epidural hematomas is less than the benefit incurred from stopping the hematoma spread.

7 SUBDURAL HEMATOMA

Similar to epidural hematomas, SDHs are often the result of trauma to the head, whether it is blunt force injury or rapid deceleration. SDHs are most often venous bleeds caused by rupture of bridging veins. The vulnerable populations for these are on opposite ends of the age spectrum: the infants and the elderly. SDHs can also form from low ICP, such as after a CSF leak or overdrainage in shunt patients.

SDH can range from acute to chronic. Acute SDHs can present very similarly to acute epidural hematomas. About half of acute SDH patients are comatose after their original injury. Chronic SDHs take a more insidious course. Because of the generally slower nature of the bleed, they may have a longer delay after the original trauma (up to weeks) before becoming symptomatic. These patients can present with headaches, confusion, light-headedness, apathy, or seizures. Chronic SDH found in neurologically intact patients might be observed with serial imaging and clinical exam.

In general, acute SDH with symptoms of elevated ICP should be managed similar to epidural hematomas. Symptoms may be associated with increased ICP and should be treated appropriately with head-of-bed elevation, hyperventilation, mannitol or hypertonic saline, and reversal of any anticoagulation, and the patient should be taken to the operating room for evacuation.

8 SUBARACHNOID HEMORRHAGE

SAH is bleeding within the subarachnoid space between the arachnoid and the pia. These areas are normally filled with CSF. The most frequent cause of SAH is trauma. In the non-trauma population, the majority of SAH are from intracranial aneurysmal rupture.

8.1 Presentation

The most common presentation of SAH is the classic "thunderclap" headache, which patients frequently describe as the worst headache of their lives, which occurs acutely with an almost ictal onset. This can be associated with loss of consciousness, seizures, nausea, and meningeal signs.

8.2 Surgical and endovascular treatment

The current treatment for ruptured aneurysms is endovascular coiling or surgical clipping. The approach depends on aneurysm location, patient's age, and comorbidities (Case 14.2). According to the *Cochraine Database Review*, in aneurysms suitable for both endovascular and surgical treatment, coiling is associated with a better clinical outcome.[13] For aneurysms with challenging surgical approach, especially in the posterior circulation, endovascular coiling is preferred.

In more easily surgically accessed aneurysms, such as the middle cerebral artery trifurcation/bifurcation or ones that have a wide neck, craniotomy and surgical clipping may be preferred. Clipping is the more definitive treatment but carries higher risk due to being a more invasive procedure, whereas coiling has better outcomes but has higher chances of aneurysm recurrence.[14,15]

Question 14.3: What is the most common time of onset of vasospasm in SAH?

Answer: It typically occurs on day 6–10. However, in some cases, the onset can be as early as day 2–3 and as late as 3–4 weeks after the occurrence of SAH.

8.3 Treatment of complications

Complications of SAH include rebleeding, delayed cerebral ischemia from vasospasm, hydrocephalus, and increased ICP increase among others.[16]Patients with SAH should be admitted to an intensive care unit for close neurological and hemodynamic monitoring with appropriate neurocritical care management. In patients with decreased level of consciousness, it is advised to place an EVD that can treat hydrocephalus, a common complication of SAH, as well as to monitor ICP.

Vasospasm occurs in SAH, which can cause devastating cerebral ischemia. Nimodipine is believed to be protective against delayed cerebral ischemia from vasospasm, however, the exact mechanism is still debated. It does improve outcomes in SAH, and thus every SAH patient should be placed on nimodipine.[17] In cases of severe vasospasm, patients can be taken to the angiography suite for intraarterial vasodilator infusions or balloon angioplasty.[18,19]

9 CLINICAL CASES

Case 14.1 Intracerebral hemorrhage

CASE PRESENTATION

A 65-year-old male with a history of hypertension was brought to the ED after he was found at home unresponsive. Upon arrival, the patient was obtunded and had a complete right-sided hemiplegia. His GCS was 7. Non-contrast CT of the head revealed a left hemispheric hematoma measuring about 7 × 4 cm with mass effect and a 6 mm of shift on the midline structures (Figures 14.3A and 14.3B). A small amount of IVH was also present.

PRACTICAL POINTS

- Although a hypertension-induced ICH was suspected, CT angiography was performed to rule out other causes of hemorrhage such as a middle cerebral artery aneurysm or an arteriovenous malformation/fistula. The study was unremarkable.
- Intravenous mannitol was administered first, and the patient then underwent immediate surgical evacuation of the clot due given severe neurological deficit, evidence of midline shift, and high risk for herniation (Figure 14.3C).

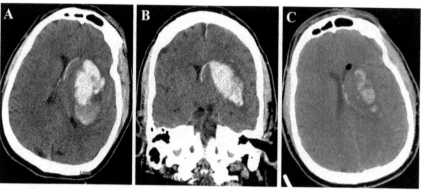

Figure 14.3 Intracerebral hemorrhage.
(A) Non-contrast computed tomography, axial and (B) coronal views showing an intracerebral hematoma associated with significant midline shift. The hematoma is measuring 7 × 4 cm (approximately 40 ml of blood).
(C) Repeat non-contrast computed tomography after minimally invasive endoscopic evacuation of the hematoma. A small amount of residual blood is present.

- Access to the hematoma was gained using a minimally invasive technique with tubular retractors. The patient's mentation improved after the evacuation of the hematoma, and after a short stay in the neurosurgical intensive care unit, he was transferred out to the floor and then to inpatient rehabilitation. The patient never recovered a functional right hemibody but was able to be discharged home with his family and home health support.

Case 14.2 Subarachnoid hemorrhage

CASE PRESENTATION
A 42-year-old female with no prior medical history was admitted to the ED after sudden onset of "thunderclap" headache, followed by loss of consciousness. Her GCS was 6. Non-contrast CT head showed a diffuse SAH (Figure 14.4A).

PRACTICAL POINTS

- This presentation fits a classic description of SAH. The first step is treatment of increased ICP and hydrocephalus with an external ventricular drain.
- Once the patient is stabilized, an emergent CT or MR angiography is needed to rule out an intracranial aneurysm. In this case, a 7 mm right internal carotid artery saccular aneurysm was identified. The aneurysm was treated with endovascular coiling (Figures 14.4B and 14.4C). The patient had a prolonged hospitalization course complicated by severe delayed vasospasm requiring intra-arterial verapamil infusion and intracranial balloon angioplasty.

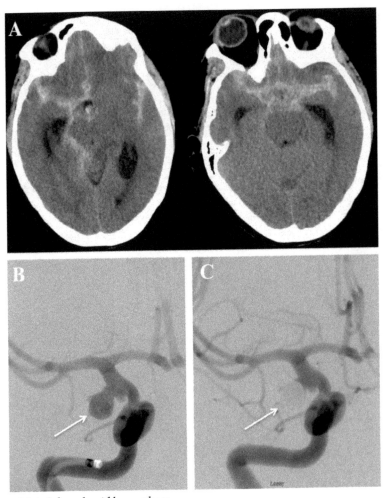

Figure 14.4 Subarachnoid hemorrhage.
(A) Non-contrast computed tomography showing a diffuse subarachnoid hemorrhage. Hydrocephalus is present in this case.
(B) Digital subtraction angiography, right internal carotid artery injection showing a 7 mm posterior communicating artery region aneurysm (arrow). The aneurysm has irregular shape and is the suspected source of the hemorrhage.
(C) The aneurysm was treated successfully with endovascular coiling (arrow).

REFERENCES

1. Lichtman JH, Jones SB, Leifheit-Limson EC, Wang Y, Goldstein LB. 30-day mortality and readmission after hemorrhagic stroke among Medicare beneficiaries in Joint Commission primary stroke center-certified and noncertified hospitals. *Stroke.* 2011;42(12):3387–3391.

2. Monro, A. *Observations on the structure and function of the nervous system.* Edinburgh, UK: Creech & Johnson, 1783.

3. Kelly, G. Appearances observed in the dissection of two individuals; death from cold and congestion of the brain. *Trans Med Chir Sci Edinb.* 1824;1:84–169.

4. Mendelow AD, Gregson BA, Fernandes HM, et al. Early surgery versus initial conservative treatment in patients with spontaneous supratentorial intracerebral haematomas in the International Surgical Trial in Intracerebral Haemorrhage (STICH): a randomised trial. *Lancet.* 2005;365(9457):387–397.

5. Mendelow AD, Gregson BA, Rowan EN, et al. Early surgery versus initial conservative treatment in patients with spontaneous supratentorial lobar intracerebral haematomas (STICH II): a randomised trial. *Lancet.* 2013;382(9890):397–408.

6. Hanley DF, Thompson RE, Muschelli J, et al. Safety and efficacy of minimally invasive surgery plus alteplase in intracerebral haemorrhage evacuation (MISTIE): a randomised, controlled, open-label, phase 2 trial. *Lancet Neurol.* 2016;15(12): 1228–1237.

7. Vespa P, Hanley D, Betz J, et al. ICES (Intraoperative Stereotactic Computed Tomography-Guided Endoscopic Surgery) for brain hemorrhage: a multicenter randomized controlled trial. *Stroke.* 2016;47(11):2749–2755.

8. Ritsma B, Kassam A, Dowlatshahi D, Nguyen T, Stotts G. Minimally Invasive Subcortical Parafascicular Transsulcal Access for Clot Evacuation (Mi SPACE) for intracerebral hemorrhage. *Case Rep Neurol Med.* 2014;2014:102307.

9. Labib MA, Shah M, Kassam AB, et al. The safety and feasibility of image-guided brainpath-mediated transsulcul hematoma evacuation: a multicenter study. *Neurosurgery.* 2017;80(4):515–524.

10. Andrew M. Bauer PAR, Mark D. Bain. Initial single-center technical experience with the brainpath system for acute intracerebral hemorrhage evacuation. *Oper Neurosurg.* 2017;13(1):69–76.

11. Hinson HE, Hanley DF, Ziai WC. Management of intraventricular hemorrhage. *Curr Neurol Neurosci Rep.* 2010;10(2):73–82.

12. Ziai WC, Tuhrim S, Lane K, et al. A multicenter, randomized, double-blinded, placebo-controlled phase III study of Clot Lysis Evaluation of Accelerated Resolution of Intraventricular Hemorrhage (CLEAR III). *Int J Stroke.* 2014;9(4):536–542.

13. van der Schaaf I, Algra A, Wermer M, et al. Endovascular coiling versus neurosurgical clipping for patients with aneurysmal subarachnoid haemorrhage. *Cochrane Db Syst Rev.* 2005(4):CD003085.

14. Molyneux AJ, Kerr RS, Yu LM, et al. International Subarachnoid Aneurysm Trial (ISAT) of neurosurgical clipping versus endovascular coiling in 2143 patients with ruptured intracranial aneurysms: a randomised comparison of effects on survival, dependency, seizures, rebleeding, subgroups, and aneurysm occlusion. *Lancet.* 2005;366(9488):809–817.

15. Molyneux AJ, Birks J, Clarke A, Sneade M, Kerr RS. The durability of endovascular coiling versus neurosurgical clipping of ruptured cerebral aneurysms: 18 year follow-up of the UK cohort of the International Subarachnoid Aneurysm Trial (ISAT). *Lancet.* 2015;385(9969):691–697.

16. Solenski NJ, Haley EC, Jr., Kassell NF, et al. Medical complications of aneurysmal subarachnoid hemorrhage: a report of the multicenter, cooperative aneurysm

study. participants of the multicenter cooperative aneurysm study. *Crit Care Med.* 1995;23(6):1007–1017.

17. Pickard JD, Murray GD, Illingworth R, et al. Effect of oral nimodipine on cerebral infarction and outcome after subarachnoid haemorrhage: British aneurysm nimodipine trial. *BMJ.* 1989;298(6674):636–642.

18. Aburto-Murrieta Y, Marquez-Romero JM, Bonifacio-Delgadillo D, Lopez I, Hernandez-Curiel B. Endovascular treatment: balloon angioplasty versus nimodipine intra-arterial for medically refractory cerebral vasospasm following aneurysmal subarachnoid hemorrhage. *Vasc Endovascular Surg.* 2012;46(6):460–465.

19. Jun P, Ko NU, English JD, et al. Endovascular treatment of medically refractory cerebral vasospasm following aneurysmal subarachnoid hemorrhage. *Am J Neuroradiol.* 2010;31(10):1911–1916.

20. Hemphill JC, 3rd, Greenberg SM, Anderson CS, et al. Guidelines for the management of spontaneous intracerebral hemorrhage: a guideline for healthcare professionals from the American Heart Association/American Stroke Association. *Stroke.* 2015;46(7):2032–2060.

15

Cerebral Venous Thrombosis

JUAN RAMOS-CANSECO AND MAXIM MOKIN ■

CONTENTS

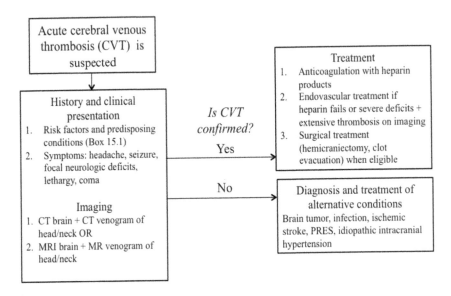

Figure 15.1 Algorithm for the diagnosis and management of cerebral venous thrombosis. ABBREVIATIONS: CT, computed tomography; CVT, cerebral venous thrombosis; MRI, magnetic resonance imaging; PRES, posterior reversible encephalopathy syndrome.

1 INTRODUCTION

Establishing the diagnosis of cerebral venous thrombosis (CVT) can often be challenging to physicians. This condition is quite rare, accounting for less than 1% of all strokes.[1] A good clinical history, exam, and radiologic imaging will help the physician establish the correct diagnosis for prompt treatment. In 2011, the American Heart Association (AHA) released evidence-based recommendations on the diagnosis and treatment of CVT, which are cited and reviewed throughout this chapter.[2] An algorithm for the diagnosis and management of CVT is shown in Figure 15.1.

The first medical description of a patient with thrombosis of major cerebral sinuses dates back to 1825 by Ribes.[3] Before the wide spread use of brain imaging, the diagnosis was largely made at the time of autopsy. Death from CVT remained significant, as high as 40% until trials in early 1990s showed the benefit of anticoagulation therapy in reducing mortality from CVT.

2 CLINICAL PRESENTATION

CVT affects women more commonly than men. Box 15.1 lists the most common conditions that can cause CVT. The fact that CVT presents with variable symptoms and typically affects a younger patient population are likely factors underlying why the diagnosis is often missed, resulting in delay in treatment.[4] Sometimes physical

Box 15.1

RISK FACTORS AND PREDISPOSING CONDITIONS FOR CVT

- Prothrombotic states:
  - Antithrombin III deficiency, protein C and S deficiency, antiphospholipid and anticardiolipin antibodies, activated protein C resistance and Factor V mutation, prothrombin G200210A mutation, hyperhomocysteinemia
- Pregnancy and postpartum
- Medications
  - Oral contraceptives, hormone replacement therapy
- Malignancy
- Infection
  - Mastoiditis, sinusitis, face and neck infection
- Trauma
- Internal jugular vein catheters
- Hematologic disorders
  - Polycythemia, sickle cell disease, thrombotic thrombocytopenic purpura, paroxysmal nocturnal hemoglobinuria
- Systemic diseases
  - Systemic lupus erythematosus, Behcet's disease, inflammatory bowel disease, sarcoidosis, thyroid disease, liver cirrhosis, dehydration

Adapted from the 2011 AHA guidelines[2] and Lee et al.[34]

manifestations are not commonly seen on exam, further making diagnosis difficult to establish, especially when patients present to facilities with limited resources and access to subspecialty care.[5] (Case 15.1)

The International Study on Cerebral Vein and Dural Sinus Thrombosis (ISCVT) was a large prospective multicenter study that included hundreds of patients with CVT.[6] In this study, the average delay from onset of symptoms to admission was 4 days and from onset of symptoms to diagnosis, 7 days.

2.1 Headache

About 90% of patients with CVT present with a headache.[6] The headache is believed to be caused by increased intracranial hypertension via thrombosis of the major sinuses and/or draining veins. The headache can be sudden in onset or gradual in evolution. With headache being a common presentation in the Emergency Department,[7-9] and with its variable etiology, it explains why patients with CVT are often misdiagnosed as having a migraine headache, idiopathic intracranial hypertension, or brain tumor.

2.2 Seizure

Nearly 40% of patients with CVT have seizures at presentation, including focal and generalized seizures.[6,10] Intracerebral hemorrhage and cortical vein thrombosis are predictors of early seizures in patients with CVT.[11] Seizures are more commonly seen as a presenting symptom in younger patients. Status epilepticus is associated with a threefold increase in mortality.[10]

2.3 Focal neurologic deficits

Focal deficits can include cranial nerve deficits, weakness, aphasia, and ataxia. Patients can also experience psychiatric symptoms and visual deficits. Analysis of ISCVT outcomes showed that the correct diagnosis of CVT was established earlier in patients who showed more severe clinical presentations, including decreased level of consciousness, seizure, and motor deficits than in patients with more benign presentation.[12]

In some cases, decreased level of consciousness without any focal deficits may be the only clinical finding of CVT. Such diagnostically challenging presentation may occur as a result of unilateral or bilateral thalamic involvement from the thrombosis of the deep cerebral venous system.[13]

Question 15.1: What is the best imaging test to diagnose acute CVT?

Answer: There is no single "best" test. In the emergency setting, a combination of magnetic resonance imaging (MRI) and magnetic resonance venography (MRV) or computed tomography (CT) and CT venography (CTV) is highly accurate.

3 IMAGING

Unlike many other types of neurologic disorders in which the diagnosis can often be correctly established solely on history and clinical findings alone, brain imaging is a critical component when evaluating a patient with suspected CVT. Different imaging modalities are currently available in the repertoire of the treating physician, with variable sensitivity/specificity in diagnosing CVT and carrying different risk profiles.

3.1 Computed tomography

In the emergency setting, a non-contrast CT scan is often the first radiographic test a patient is subjected to when evaluated for any intracranial cause of change in symptoms or appearance upon examination. CT offers excellent accuracy in detecting intracranial hemorrhage, which is present in up 40% of cases of CVT.[6] The ability of CT to detect the regions of ischemic stroke is variable; hyperacute stroke can be missed until the area of ischemia evolves into an area of clearer hypodensity. The mechanism underlying ischemic stroke in CVT is venous congestion (an outflow obstruction) and thus spares the arterial territories. Seeing this helps the physician to differentiate between typical imaging patterns of ischemic versus venous strokes.

A hyperattenuating ("bright") appearance of the affected sinus from a fresh thrombus is one of the classic imaging features of acute CVT on non-contrast CT of the brain. (Case 15.2) Unfortunately, this imaging finding has rather low sensitivity. This radiographic sign can also be falsely "positive" in patients with elevated hemoglobin and hematocrit levels secondary to dehydration or diseases such as polycythemia.[14,15] Another pathologic finding that is frequently cited in the literature is the "empty delta sign" on contrast-enhanced CT of the brain. This finding describes a filling defect within the sinus. Cortical edema can also be seen surrounding the thrombosed veins.

3.2 Magnetic resonance imaging

MRI of the brain can also provide useful information for diagnosing CVT. Depending on the acuteness of CVT, the appearance of the thrombus on MRI (hypo-, iso-, or hyperintense) varies on T1- and T2-weighted sequences.

Contrasted imaging with gadolinium can show contrast enhancement of the sinus secondary to organized thrombus,[16] or parenchymal enhancement showing disruption of the blood brain barrier. The pattern of diffusion-weighted imaging/apparent diffusion coefficient (ADC) can also be quite variable due to the presence of both cytotoxic and vasogenic edema, distinguishing CVT from acute ischemic stroke, where the ADC sequence almost always appears "dark." Overall, in comparison to CT, MRI is more sensitive and specific in establishing the diagnosis of CVT, especially if contrast-enhanced 3D gradient echo sequences T1-weighted MRI imaging sequence is used.[17,18]

> **Question 15.2:** My patient is diagnosed with acute CVT. Should I order catheter angiography to confirm the diagnosis?
>
> **Answer:** Diagnostic catheter angiography is not required unless noninvasive imaging and clinical presentation are inconclusive.

3.3 CT and MR venography

Advances in CTV and MRV have largely replaced catheter angiography. Both tests can be rapidly performed in the emergency setting, and the choice between CT and MR depends on the individual patient's characteristics such as age (pediatric vs. adult patients), pregnancy, and renal function.

Time-of-flight (TOF) MRV is commonly used to evaluate the patency of cerebral venous sinuses because it does not require intravenous contrast administration. However, TOF MRV can erroneously overcall venous thrombosis. Therefore, contrast-enhanced MRV is superior to TOF MRV in establishing the correct diagnosis.[19,20]

3.4 Digital subtraction angiography

Digital subtraction angiography (DSA) is the gold standard for diagnosis of venous sinus thrombosis. Benefits of DSA over other imaging modalities include a better view of all intracranial vessels, the ability to rule out other causes of intracranial bleeding, and its use as treatment when patients fail to respond to medical therapy.

The use of DSA for diagnosing CVT has declined in recent years. This is due to the invasive nature, price, and complexity of arranging for a DSA in the face of continuous improvements in accuracy of noninvasive tests such as CT and MR angiography for diagnosis of venous sinus thrombosis. DSA should still be considered in cases where the diagnosis is not clear such as when thrombosis of deep cortical veins is suspected. DSA is also critically important in ruling out other causes of intracranial bleeding, for example, when a dural arteriovenous fistula is suspected, given that this condition can resemble the radiographic appearance of CVT including thrombosis of major cortical sinuses.

3.5 Normal anatomical variants

The most common anatomical "abnormality" encountered in imaging is hypoplasia and atresia of the transverse sinuses. These variant anatomical anomalies appear in up to 50% of all patients imaged. (Case 15.3) Arachnoid granulations are a second structural anomaly seen in the transverse sinuses that mimic thrombosis, presenting as a filling defect in imaging.

Rather than relying on a single "best" imaging modality, clinicians should carefully analyze the information combined from several imaging tests such as MRI and MRV or CT and CTV when such anatomical variants are encountered. Other frequently encountered anomalies such as flow gaps in venography, variation in signal intensity of the sinuses, and other anatomical variants (i.e., hypoplasia or atresia of the anterior portion of the superior sagittal sinus) must be expected when considering CVT as cause of patient's symptoms in correlation to imaging abnormalities.

Question 15.3: Can novel oral antiocoagulants (NOACs) be used for the treatment of CVT?

Answer: NOACs are currently not approved for this indication. Studies evaluating safety and efficacy of this class of anticoagulants for CVT are underway.

4 TREATMENT

The current AHA guidelines recommend initial evaluation and assessment by a stroke neurologist with admission to a stroke unit.[2] Specialized care has been shown to reduce morbidity and mortality.[21,22]

4.1 Anticoagulation

The initial treatment, after diagnosis of CVT is established, requires anticoagulation with unfractioned heparin or low molecular weight heparin, which is typically transitioned to oral anticoagulation with warfarin. Anticoagulation is indicated even if there is evidence of hemorrhage on brain imaging. The goal of acute treatment is to facilitate recanalization of the occluded sinuses and veins and prevent further thrombus propagation. Long-term anticoagulation is needed to prevent recurrent thrombosis. The duration of treatment depends on the cause of CVT and whether there is recurrence.[23]

4.2 Endovascular treatment

There are no well-established guidelines on when it is appropriate to initiate endovascular recanalization in acute CVT. Unlike the treatment of acute ischemic stroke, which has been studied in multiple randomized trials, the experience with endovascular therapy of CVT is limited to case series with significant variability in individual institution protocols and approaches to recanalization.[24] The AHA guidelines recommend endovascular interventions when neurological deterioration occurs despite intensive anticoagulation treatment. Some centers consider a more aggressive approach to endovascular procedures for patients when radiographic evidence of brain edema or hemorrhage and poor neurological status is present on admission without waiting for medical therapy to "fail" first.[25,26] (Case 15.1) A variety of endovascular approaches are available; local pharmacological thrombolysis delivered via a microcatheter, stent retriever thrombectomy, direct aspiration of the thrombus with a large bore catheter, and angioplasty/stenting.

4.3 Surgical treatment

Decompressive surgery with craniectomy or hematoma evacuation is typically reserved for CVT patients with large parenchymal lesions causing herniation.[27] Such treatment can result in good functional outcome even in the most severe cases of CVT.[27,28]

5 CLINICAL CASES

Case 15.1 Extensive CVT

CASE DESCRIPTION

A woman with a past medical history of hypertension is brought to the hospital after being found down, unresponsive. During transport to the hospital, the patient had a seizure with clonic movements lasting approximately 4 minutes. The daughter notes that the patient had been complaining of headache and blurry vision for a week and was seen in an outside facility where she got a CT scan, which was noted to be unremarkable, and the patient was discharged home. Repeat imaging showed extensive thrombosis of the superior sagittal sinus (Figure 15.2).

PRACTICAL POINTS

- Patient's symptoms of blurry vision were likely due to increased intracranial pressure even though papilledema was not seen.[29] Papilledema is not often found acutely and takes 1–2 weeks to develop.
- Endovascular treatment of CVT was pursued in this case within 24 hours of patient's admission to the hospital. The decision to escalate therapy was based on (a) significant amount of thrombus, (b) poor neurological function on admission, and (c) lack of early response to systemic heparin infusion.
- In a patient with CVT presenting with a seizure, early initiation of antiepileptic drugs for is recommended.

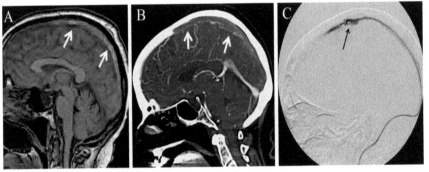

Figure 15.2 Extensive cerebral venous thrombosis.
(A) Sagittal view, magnetic resonance imaging brain without contrast showing hyperintense signal within the superior sagittal sinus (SSS).
(B) Computed tomography venography confirms the presence of a filling defect within the middle and posterior portions of the SSS indicating significant clot burden.
(C) Endovascular treatment with direct clot aspiration via a large bore distal aspiration catheter (the arrow points to the tip of the aspiration catheter).

Case 15.2 CVT in trauma

CASE DESCRIPTION
An elderly patient presents to the emergency room after a fall. Patient notes he had a brief loss of consciousness. Imaging is performed in the ED, showing thrombosis of the left transverse sinus, as well as a subdural hematoma of the left hemisphere (Figure 15.3).

PRACTICAL POINTS

- This patient is an example of CVT resultant from trauma. It is important to consider further imaging studies whenever an intracranial fracture is observed that is adjacent to the major venous structures in the brain.[30,31]
- A small subdural hematoma introduces additional complexity in this case; the main treatment of CVT is anticoagulation. However, anticoagulation might cause worsening of this patient's acute subdural hematoma.

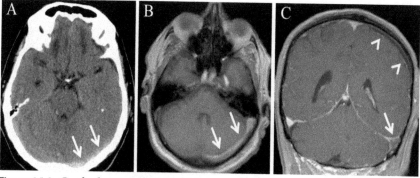

Figure 15.3 Cerebral venous thrombosis in trauma.
(A) Non-contrast head computed tomography (CT) shows hyperdensity within the left transverse sinus (arrows). This finding is not necessarily specific for cerebral venous thrombosis and can be seen in other conditions such as dehydration or polycythemia.
(B) Axial view, magnetic resonance imaging (MRI) brain, T1 sequence without contrast showing an area of increased signal intensity (arrow) at the same location. This finding is more specific for a thrombus than non-contrast CT.
(C) Coronal view, MRI brain T1 sequence with contrast showing a subdural convexity fluid collection (arrowhead) and lack of contrast enhancement of the left transverse sinus secondary to a thrombus (arrow).

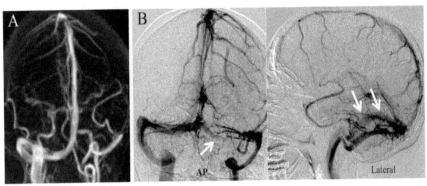

Figure 15.4 Hypoplasia of the left transverse sinus.
(A) Contrast-enhanced magnetic resonance venography with absence flow within the left transverse sinus, raising concern for acute left transverse sinus thrombosis.
(B) Digital subtraction angiography showing hypoplastic appearance of the left transverse sinus representing a normal anatomical variant (arrows). This is best appreciated on the lateral view.

Case 15.3 Hypoplastic sinus

CASE DESCRIPTION

A woman with a history of migraines presents to the ED with complaints of new severe headache with gradual onset, with photophobia (sensitivity to light), phonophobia (sensitivity to sound), and nausea. Her neurologic exam is unremarkable. MRV is performed in the Emergency Department. The study is interpreted as possible transverse sinus thrombosis (Figure 15.4A).

PRACTICAL POINTS

- Additional imaging such as a non-contrast CT or MRI should be carefully reviewed to look for additional signs of acute thrombosis of the suspected transverse sinus (i.e., hyperattenuation of the affected sinus)
- In addition, catheter angiography can be performed, which can reveal a hypoplastic sinus confused for a thrombosed vessel (Figure 15.4B). Studies show that asymmetry and hypoplasia or even absence of a sinus represent anatomic variants which can be mistaken for CVT.[32,33]

REFERENCES

1. Bousser MG, Ferro JM. Cerebral venous thrombosis: an update. *Lancet Neurol.* 2007;6(2):162–170.
2. Saposnik G, Barinagarrementeria F, Brown RD, Jr., et al. Diagnosis and management of cerebral venous thrombosis: a statement for healthcare professionals from the American Heart Association/American Stroke Association. *Stroke.* 2011;42(4): 1158–1192.

3. MF R. Des recherches faites sur la phlebite. *Revue Médicale Française Etrangère Journal de Clinique de l'Hôtel-Dieu et de la Charité de Paris.* 1825;3:5–41.

4. Newman-Toker DE, Moy E, Valente E, Coffey R, Hines AL. Missed diagnosis of stroke in the Emergency Department: a cross-sectional analysis of a large population-based sample. *Diagnosis.* 2014;1(2):155–166.

5. Rim HT, Jun HS, Ahn JH, et al. Clinical Aspects of Cerebral Venous Thrombosis: Experiences in Two Institutions. *J Cerebrovasc Endovasc Neurosur.* 2016;18(3):185–193.

6. Ferro JM, Canhao P, Stam J, Bousser MG, Barinagarrementeria F. Prognosis of cerebral vein and dural sinus thrombosis: results of the International Study on Cerebral Vein and Dural Sinus Thrombosis (ISCVT). *Stroke.* 2004;35(3):664–670.

7. Torelli P, Campana V, Cervellin G, Manzoni GC. Management of primary headaches in adult Emergency Departments: a literature review, the Parma ED experience and a therapy flow chart proposal. *Neurol Sci.* 2010;31(5):545–553.

8. Ramirez-Lassepas M, Espinosa CE, Cicero JJ, Johnston KL, Cipolle RJ, Barber DL. Predictors of intracranial pathologic findings in patients who seek emergency care because of headache. *Arch Neurol.* 1997;54(12):1506–1509.

9. Dermitzakis EV, Georgiadis G, Rudolf J, et al. Headache patients in the Emergency Department of a Greek tertiary care hospital. *J Headache Pain.* 2010;11(2):123–128.

10. Masuhr F, Busch M, Amberger N, et al. Risk and predictors of early epileptic seizures in acute cerebral venous and sinus thrombosis. *Eur J Neurol.* 2006;13(8):852–856.

11. Ferro JM, Canhao P, Bousser MG, Stam J, Barinagarrementeria F, ISCVT Investigators. Early seizures in cerebral vein and dural sinus thrombosis: risk factors and role of antiepileptics. *Stroke.* 2008;39(4):1152–1158.

12. Ferro JM, Canhao P, Stam J, et al. Delay in the diagnosis of cerebral vein and dural sinus thrombosis: influence on outcome. *Stroke.* 2009;40(9):3133–3138.

13. Wieshmann NH, Amin S, Hodgson R. A case of unilateral thalamic hemorrhagic infarction as a result of the vein of Galen and straight sinus thrombosis. *J Stroke Cerebrovasc Dis.* 2009;18(1):28–31.

14. Black DF, Rad AE, Gray LA, Campeau NG, Kallmes DF. Cerebral venous sinus density on noncontrast CT correlates with hematocrit. *Am J Neuroradiol.* 2011;32(7):1354–1357.

15. Al-Ryalat NT, AlRyalat SA, Malkawi LW, Al-Zeena EF, Najar MS, Hadidy AM. Factors affecting attenuation of dural sinuses on noncontrasted computed tomography scan. *J Stroke Cerebrovasc Dis.* 2016;25(10):2559–2565.

16. Sadigh G, Mullins ME, Saindane AM. Diagnostic performance of MRI sequences for evaluation of dural venous sinus thrombosis. *Am J Roentgenol.* 2016;206(6):1298–1306.

17. Patel D, Machnowska M, Symons S, et al. Diagnostic performance of routine brain MRI sequences for dural venous sinus thrombosis. *Am J Neuroradiol.* 2016;37(11):2026–2032.

18. Sari S, Verim S, Hamcan S, et al. MRI diagnosis of dural sinus—cortical venous thrombosis: immediate post-contrast 3D GRE T1-weighted imaging versus unenhanced MR venography and conventional MR sequences. *Clin Neurol Neurosurg.* 2015;134:44–54.

19. Fu JH, Lai PH, Hsiao CC, et al. Comparison of real-time three-dimensional gadolinium-enhanced elliptic centric-ordered MR venography and two-dimensional

time-of-flight MR venography of the intracranial venous system. *J Chin Med Assoc.* 2010;73(3):131–138.

20. Klingebiel R, Bauknecht HC, Bohner G, Kirsch R, Berger J, Masuhr F. Comparative evaluation of 2D time-of-flight and 3D elliptic centric contrast-enhanced MR venography in patients with presumptive cerebral venous and sinus thrombosis. *Eur J Neurol.* 2007;14(2):139–143.

21. Stroke Unit Trialists' Collaboration. Organised inpatient (stroke unit) care for stroke. *Cochrane Db Syst Rev.* 2013(9):CD000197.

22. Saposnik G, Fang J, O'Donnell M, Hachinski V, Kapral MK, Hill MD. Escalating levels of access to in-hospital care and stroke mortality. *Stroke.* 2008;39(9):2522–2530.

23. Einhaupl K, Stam J, Bousser MG, et al. EFNS guideline on the treatment of cerebral venous and sinus thrombosis in adult patients. *Eur J Neurol.* 2010;17(10):1229–1235.;9(11);1086–1092.

25. Nyberg EM, Case D, Nagae LM, et al. The addition of endovascular intervention for dural venous sinus thrombosis: single-center experience and review of literature. *J Stroke Cerebrovasc Dis.* 2017;26(10):2240–2247.

26. Tsai FY, Kostanian V, Rivera M, Lee KW, Chen CC, Nguyen TH. Cerebral venous congestion as indication for thrombolytic treatment. *Cardiovasc Intervent Radiol.* 2007;30(4):675–687.

27. Ferro JM, Crassard I, Coutinho JM, et al. Decompressive surgery in cerebrovenous thrombosis: a multicenter registry and a systematic review of individual patient data. *Stroke.* 2011;42(10):2825–2831.

28. Zuurbier SM, Coutinho JM, Majoie CB, Coert BA, van den Munckhof P, Stam J. Decompressive hemicraniectomy in severe cerebral venous thrombosis: a prospective case series. *J Neurol.* 2012;259(6):1099–1105.

29. Steffen H, Eifert B, Aschoff A, Kolling GH, Volcker HE. The diagnostic value of optic disc evaluation in acute elevated intracranial pressure. *Ophthalmology.* 1996;103(8):1229–1232.

30. Matsushige T, Nakaoka M, Kiya K, Takeda T, Kurisu K. Cerebral sinovenous thrombosis after closed head injury. *J Traum.* 2009;66(6):1599–1604.

31. Delgado Almandoz JE, Kelly HR, Schaefer PW, Lev MH, Gonzalez RG, Romero JM. Prevalence of traumatic dural venous sinus thrombosis in high-risk acute blunt head trauma patients evaluated with multidetector CT venography. *Radiology.* 2010;255(2):570–577.

32. Surendrababu NR, Subathira, Livingstone RS. Variations in the cerebral venous anatomy and pitfalls in the diagnosis of cerebral venous sinus thrombosis: low field MR experience. *Indian J Med Sci.* 2006;60(4):135–142.

33. Ayanzen RH, Bird CR, Keller PJ, McCully FJ, Theobald MR, Heiserman JE. Cerebral MR venography: normal anatomy and potential diagnostic pitfalls. *Am J Neuroradiol.* 2000;21(1):74–78.

34. Lee SK, Kim BS, Terbrugge KG. Clinical presentation, imaging and treatment of cerebral venous thrombosis (CVT). *Interv Neuroradiol.* 2002;8(1):5–14.

Note: Page numbers followed by *b, f, and t* indicate a box, figure, and table.